Allogeneic Immunotherapy for Malignant Diseases

BASIC AND CLINICAL ONCOLOGY

Editor

Bruce D. Cheson, M.D.

National Cancer Institute
National Institutes of Health
Bethesda, Maryland

1. Chronic Lymphocytic Leukemia: Scientific Advances and Clinical Developments, *edited by Bruce D. Cheson*
2. Therapeutic Applications of Interleukin-2, *edited by Michael B. Atkins and James W. Mier*
3. Cancer of the Prostate, *edited by Sakti Das and E. David Crawford*
4. Retinoids in Oncology, *edited by Waun Ki Hong and Reuben Lotan*
5. Filgrastim (r-metHuG-CSF) in Clinical Practice, *edited by George Morstyn and T. Michael Dexter*
6. Cancer Prevention and Control, *edited by Peter Greenwald, Barnett S. Kramer, and Douglas L. Weed*
7. Handbook of Supportive Care in Cancer, *edited by Jean Klastersky, Stephen C. Schimpff, and Hans-Jörg Senn*
8. Paclitaxel in Cancer Treatment, *edited by William P. McGuire and Eric K. Rowinsky*
9. Principles of Antineoplastic Drug Development and Pharmacology, *edited by Richard L. Schilsky, Gérard A. Milano, and Mark J. Ratain*
10. Gene Therapy in Cancer, *edited by Malcolm K. Brenner and Robert C. Moen*
11. Expert Consultations in Gynecological Cancers, *edited by Maurie Markman and Jerome L. Belinson*
12. Nucleoside Analogs in Cancer Therapy, *edited by Bruce D. Cheson, Michael J. Keating, and William Plunkett*
13. Drug Resistance in Oncology, *edited by Samuel D. Bernal*
14. Medical Management of Hematological Malignant Diseases, *edited by Emil J Freireich and Hagop M. Kantarjian*
15. Monoclonal Antibody-Based Therapy of Cancer, *edited by Michael L. Grossbard*
16. Medical Management of Chronic Myelogenous Leukemia, *edited by Moshe Talpaz and Hagop M. Kantarjian*
17. Expert Consultations in Breast Cancer: Critical Pathways and Clinical Decision Making, *edited by William N. Hait, David A. August, and Bruce G. Haffty*
18. Cancer Screening: Theory and Practice, *edited by Barnett S. Kramer, John K. Gohagan, and Philip C. Prorok*

19. Supportive Care in Cancer: A Handbook for Oncologists: Second Edition, Revised and Expanded, *edited by Jean Klastersky, Stephen C. Schimpff, and Hans-Jörg Senn*
20. Integrated Cancer Management: Surgery, Medical Oncology, and Radiation Oncology, *edited by Michael H. Torosian*
21. AIDS-Related Cancers and Their Treatment, *edited by Ellen G. Feigal, Alexandra M. Levine, and Robert J. Biggar*
22. Allogeneic Immunotherapy for Malignant Diseases, *edited by John Barrett and Yin-Zheng Jiang*
23. Cancer in the Elderly, *edited by Carrie P. Hunter, Karen A. Johnson, and Hyman B. Muss*

ADDITIONAL VOLUMES IN PREPARATION

Tumor Angiogenesis and Microcirculation, *edited by Emile E. Voest and Patricia A. D'Amore*

Allogeneic Immunotherapy for Malignant Diseases

edited by

John Barrett

National Institutes of Health
Bethesda, Maryland

Yin-Zheng Jiang

Yale New Haven Health
Bridgeport, Connecticut

MARCEL DEKKER, INC.   NEW YORK • BASEL

ISBN: 0-8247-6781-0

This book is printed on acid-free paper.

Headquarters
Marcel Dekker, Inc.
270 Madison Avenue, New York, NY 10016
tel: 212-696-9000; fax: 212-685-4540

Eastern Hemisphere Distribution
Marcel Dekker AG
Hutgasse 4, Postfach 812, CH-4001 Basel, Switzerland
tel: 41-61-261-8482; fax: 41-61-261-8896

World Wide Web
http://www.dekker.com

The publisher offers discounts on this book when ordered in bulk quantities. For more information, write to Special Sales/Professional Marketing at the headquarters address above.

Current printing (last digit):
10 9 8 7 6 5 4 3 2 1

PRINTED IN THE UNITED STATES OF AMERICA

To all our patients,
whose bravery in adversity is an inspiration for us
to improve our understanding of disease processes
and devise better ways to treat and cure.

Series Introduction

The current volume, *Allogeneic Immunotherapy for Malignant Diseases,* is the twenty-second in the Basic and Clinical Oncology series. Many of the advances in oncology have resulted from close interaction between the basic scientist and the clinical researcher. The current volume illustrates the success of this relationship as demonstrated by new insights into clinical drug resistance and means of circumventing this potential obstacle to effective cancer treatment.

As editor of the series, my goal is to recruit volume editors who not only have established reputations based on their outstanding contributions to oncology, but who also have an appreciation for the dynamic interface between the laboratory and the clinic. To date, the series has consisted of monographs on topics that are of a high level of current interest. *Allogeneic Immunotherapy for Malignant Diseases* certainly fits into this category and is a most important addition to the series.

Volumes in progress focus on tumor angiogenesis and microcirculation, and cancer in the elderly. I anticipate that these books will provide a valuable contribution to the oncology literature.

Bruce D. Cheson

Preface

Allogeneic stem-cell transplantation is becoming an essential component of clinical hematology and oncology practice. The curative effect of allogeneic stem cell transplantation is attributed at least partially to an allogeneic immune response: the graft-versus-leukemia (GVL) or graft-versus-tumor (GVT) effect. For the last decade or so, our perception of the GVL phenomenon has changed dramatically. We observed in the mid-'80s that depletion of T cells from the graft dramatically increased the rate of leukemia relapse; subsequently it became evident that remissions could be reinduced by donor lymphocyte transfusions to patients with leukemia relapsing after bone marrow transplantation. Although variable in its expression, the allogeneic GVT effect appears to extend to a variety of acute and chronic myeloid and lymphoid malignancies and possibly solid tumors. With new insights into the cellular and molecular biology of GVL, we have advanced from the stage of trying to prove the existence of a GVL effect to understanding it better and applying it more effectively.

Anyone reading current publications on bone marrow transplantation will have noticed a growing number of original papers and review articles on GVL which signal an increased awareness and demand for information on the topic. Alongside the applied research in GVL, there are continuing advances in cellular immunology and tumor immunology that improve our understanding of the alloresponse to malignancies. Looking forward to the next decade, the use of allogeneic cells promises important therapeutic benefits for our patients. In this book, authors who are leaders in their respective fields provide a comprehensive review of the GVL/GVT effect, from descriptions of the alloimmune responses to the clinical applications of GVL. We hope this book will bring to its readership state-of-the-art knowledge on the subject and also indicate directions for future research and therapeutic applications in GVL.

John Barrett
Yin-Zheng Jiang

ACKNOWLEDGMENT

To my parents for their diligent work to support me through my education; to my wife, Junhua, for her sacrifice to free me to pursue my career.

Y-Z J

Contents

Contributors

John Barrett, M.D., F.R.C.P., F.R.C.Path. Chief, Bone Marrow Transplant Unit, Hematology Branch, National Heart, Lung and Blood Institute, National Institutes of Health, Bethesda, Maryland

Rami Ben-Yosef, M.D. Department of Bone Marrow Transplantation, Cancer Immunotherapy and Immunobiology Research Center, Hadassah University Hospital, Jerusalem, Israel

Bruce R. Blazar, M.D. Professor, Division of Bone Marrow Transplantation, Department of Pediatrics, University of Minnesota, Minneapolis, Minnesota

Hal E. Broxmeyer, Ph.D. Chairman, Department of Microbiology and Immunology, Indiana University School of Medicine, and Professor and Scientific Director, Walther Cancer Institute, Indianapolis, Indiana

Richard E. Champlin, M.D. Chief, Section of Blood and Marrow Transplantation, University of Texas, M. D. Anderson Cancer Center, Houston, Texas

Richard W. Childs, M.D. Senior Clinical Investigator, Bone Marrow Transplant Unit, Hematology Branch, National Heart, Lung and Blood Institute, National Institutes of Health, Bethesda, Maryland

J. H. Frederick Falkenburg, M.D., Ph.D. Professor, Laboratory of Experimental Hematology, Department of Hematology, Leiden University Medical Center, Leiden, The Netherlands

Jay Gaddy, Ph.D. Department of Microbiology and Immunology, Indiana University School of Medicine, and Walther Cancer Institute, Indianapolis, Indiana

Carlo Gambacorti-Passerini, M.D. Senior Investigator, Department of Experimental Oncology, National Cancer Institute, Milan, Italy

Sergio A. Giralt, M.D. Associate Professor, Section of Blood and Bone Marrow Transplantation, University of Texas, M. D. Anderson Cancer Center, Houston, Texas

Els Goulmy, Ph.D. Professor, Department of Immunohematology and Blood Bank, Leiden University Medical Center, Leiden, The Netherlands

John G. Gribben, M.D., Ph.D., F.R.C.P., F.R.C.Path. Associate Professor, Department of Adult Oncology and Medicine, Harvard Medical School, Dana-Farber Cancer Institute, and Brigham Women's Hospital, Boston, Massachusetts

Helen E. Heslop, M.D., F.R.A.C.P., F.R.C.P.A. Professor, Center for Cell and Gene Therapy, Baylor College of Medicine, Houston, Texas

Yin-Zheng Jiang, M.D., Ph.D. Department of Internal Medicine, Bridgeport Hospital, Yale New Haven Health, Bridgeport, Connecticut

Bryon D. Johnson, Ph.D. Assistant Professor, Department of Pediatrics, Medical College of Wisconsin, Milwaukee, Wisconsin

Hans-Jochem Kolb, M.D., Ph.D. Professor, Department of Medicine, Klinikum Grosshadern, Ludwig Maximilian's University, Munich, Germany

Robert Korngold, Ph.D. Professor, Kimmel Cancer Institute, Jefferson Medical College, Philadelphia, Pennsylvania

Robert I. Lechler, Ph.D., F.R.C.Path., F.R.C.P. Professor, Department of Immunology, Imperial College School of Medicine, Hammersmith Hospital, London, United Kingdom

Onno C. Leeksma, M.D., Ph.D. Department of Immunohematology and Blood Bank, Leiden University Medical Center, Leiden, The Netherlands

Graham M. Lord, M.A., M.R.C.P. Research Fellow, Department of Immunology, Imperial College School of Medicine, Hammersmith Hospital, London, United Kingdom

Dimitrios Mavroudis, M.D., Ph.D. Department of Medical Oncology, University General Hospital, Heraklion, Crete, Greece

Jayesh Mehta, M.D. Professor and Clinical Director, Myeloma and Lymphoma Program, Division of Transplantation Medicine, Richland Memorial Hospital and South Carolina Cancer Center, Columbia, South Carolina

Cornelis J. M. Melief, M.D., Ph.D. Professor of Immunology, Department of Immunohematology and Blood Bank, Leiden University Medical Center, Leiden, The Netherlands

Jeffrey J. Molldrem, M.D. Chief, Section of Transplantation Immunology, Department of Blood and Marrow Transplantation, University of Texas, M. D. Anderson Cancer Center, Houston, Texas

Shoshana Morecki, Ph.D. Department of Bone Marrow Transplantation, Cancer Immunotherapy and Immunobiology Research Center, Hadassah University Hospital, Jerusalem, Israel

Koichi Moriwaki, M.D. Postdoctoral Associate, Center for Cell and Gene Therapy, Baylor College of Medicine, Houston, Texas

Tuna Mutis, M.D., Ph.D. Department of Immunohematology and Blood Bank, Leiden University Medical Center, Leiden, The Netherlands

Arnon Nagler, M.D., M.S.C. Department of Bone Marrow Transplantation, Cancer Immunotherapy and Immunobiology Research Center, Hadassah University Hospital, Jerusalem, Israel

Elizabeth Naparstek, M.D. Department of Bone Marrow Transplantation, Cancer Immunotherapy and Immunobiology Research Center, Hadassah University Hospital, Jerusalem, Israel

Reuven Or, M.D. Department of Bone Marrow Transplantation, Cancer Immunotherapy and Immunobiology Research Center, Hadassah University Hospital, Jerusalem, Israel

Pierluigi Porcu, M.D.* Division of Hematology/Oncology, Department of Medicine, Indiana University School of Medicine, and Walther Cancer Institute, Indianapolis, Indiana

Joachim L. Schultze, M.D. Department of Adult Oncology, Harvard Medical School, Dana-Farber Cancer Institute, Boston, Massachusetts

Shimon Slavin, M.D. Chief, Department of Bone Marrow Transplantation, Cancer Immunotherapy and Immunobiology Research Center, Hadassah University Hospital, Jerusalem, Israel

Paul M. Sondel, M.D., Ph.D. Professor, Departments of Pediatrics, Human Oncology, and Genetics, University of Wisconsin, Madison, Wisconsin

George J. A. ten Bosch, M.D., Ph.D. Department of Immunohematology and Bloodbank, Leiden University Medical Center, Leiden, The Netherlands

Robert Townsend, Ph.D. Kimmel Cancer Institute, Jefferson Medical College, Philadelphia, Pennsylvania

Robert L. Truitt, Ph.D. Professor, Departments of Pediatrics and Microbiology and Molecular Genetics, Medical College of Wisconsin, Milwaukee, Wisconsin

Frits van Rhee, M.D., Ph.D., M.R.C.P., M.R.C.Path. Associate Professor and Director of Cellular Immunotherapy, Division of Transplantation Medicine, University of South Carolina, Columbia, South Carolina

Gabor Varadi, M.D. Department of Bone Marrow Transplantation, Cancer Immunotherapy and Immunobiology Research Center, Hadassah University Hospital, Jerusalem, Israel

Roelof Willemze, M.D., Ph.D. Professor, Department of Hematology, Leiden University Medical Center, Leiden, The Netherlands

* *Current affiliation*: Assistant Professor, Division of Hematology, Department of Internal Medicine, The Ohio State University School of Medicine, Columbus, Ohio

1

Introduction

The Graft-Versus-Leukemia Effect

Paul M. Sondel
University of Wisconsin
Madison, Wisconsin

I. INTRODUCTION AND HISTORY

The clinical phenomenon of the graft versus-leukemia (GVL) effect is linked to predictions made a century ago that immune reactivity could be used beneficially as an antitumor mechanism. Distinct perspectives led Ehrlich to propose a "magic bullet," Metchnikoff to pursue the potent phagocyte, and Coley to pursue bacterial toxins as antitumor activators [1]. With over one hundred years of data and progress, these three philosophies are now best visualized in the mechanisms of (1) T cell–and antibody-mediated tumor recognition, as magic bullets of sorts; (2) macrophages, natural killer cells, granulocytes, and the diverse functions associated with the "innate" immune system [2]; and (3) therapeutic utilization of recombinant cytokines or cytokine activators.

Preclinical testing, in vitro and in murine models, focused on manipulations that may induce immune destruction of cancers growing within autologous or syngeneic animals. This includes pioneering work by the teams of Prehn, Gross, and Fefer in murine solid tumors and virally induced leukemias, respectively [4–6]. Leukemia-bearing animals undergoing hematopoietic ablation and reconstitution with syngeneic marrow could, under certain experimental conditions, be cured of leukemia [7]. However, the paucity of human leukemia patients with syngeneic (identical twin) donors [8] forced the pursuit of allogeneic bone marrow transplantation (BMT).

The severe graft-versus-host disease (GVHD) associated with histoincompatible donations could be circumvented in part by picking HLA-identical sibling donors, utilizing HLA serological testing pioneered by VanRood and Dausset, and mixed lymphocyte culture matching developed by Bach [9]. The clinical era of successful allogeneic bone marrow transplantation began in 1968 [10,11]. Efficacy of BMT as treatment for leukemia was demonstrated first by Thomas and colleagues, who documented far better survival for leukemia patients transplanted with allogeneic marrow while in remission [12].

As teams around the world began performing allogenic transplants for leukemia patients, occasional patients were noted to have an unusual GVL response. One well-documented case [13] involved a patient whose leukemia was recurring following allogeneic transplant and who then developed GVHD and, coincidentally, achieved hematologic remission. Weiden et al. summarized the clinical experience of the Seattle transplant team in 1979 [14]. These data indicated that patients developing GVHD had a decreased chance for leukemic relapse following allogeneic BMT from an HLA-identical sibling. Murine models provided further support for this concept [7].

One decade later, the International Bone Marrow Transplant Registry evaluated data [15] from 2254 patients receiving BMT as treatment for early-stage leukemia [acute lymphoblastic leukemia (ALL) or acute nonlymphoblastic leukemia (ANLL) in first remission and chronic myelocytic leukemia (CML) in chronic phase]. The large patient numbers analyzed in this report helped provide the statistical power to make three distinct conclusions relevant to the GVL phenomenon:

1. Patients experiencing GVHD had a decreased incidence of leukemic relapse following BMT than patients who did not develop GVHD.
2. Among patients who did not develop any GVHD, the recipients of identical-twin donor marrow had a greater chance of leukemic relapse (approximately 46%) than the recipients of HLA-identical sibling marrow (approximately 25% chance of relapse).
3. Among patients who did not develop GVHD, the recipients of T cell–depleted HLA-identical sibling marrow had a greater chance of leukemic relapse (41%), than those receiving ''nondepleted'' HLA-identical sibling marrow (25%).

This critical analysis [15] clearly documented the association of GVHD with an antileukemic effect; but, more importantly, it documented the importance of allorecognition in the antileukemic reaction and showed that T cells were at least partly responsible for this reaction.

Although the original clinical intent of allogeneic BMT for leukemia was to provide ''allogeneic stem-cell rescue'' following ablation of host hematopoietic tissue and leukemia, these GVL data argue that a separate mechanism, the antileukemic effect of the allogeneic marrow itself, may be just as important. The high relapse rate of nearly 50% for recipients of marrow from an identical twin suggests that nearly half of early leukemia patients would relapse after transplant if not given allogeneic T cells. In contrast, only 16% (7–25%, depending on the severity of GVHD) of early leukemia patients relapse if they receive marrow (that is not depleted of T cells) from an HLA-identical sibling. These relapse data indicate that nearly one-third of leukemia patients who are alive today following allogeneic HLA-identical sibling BMTs are in fact alive because of an effective GVL reaction that was being mediated by their sibling's immune cells. Current estimates from the international BMT registry suggest that more than 10,000 leukemia patients are now alive following allogeneic BMT [16]; one-third of these are estimated to be survivors *because of the GVL effect*. It seems likely that this group of more than 3000 "GVL survivors" far exceeds the number of cancer patients worldwide who are alive as a result of *all other forms* of effective immunotherapy used to treat preexistent cancer.

More importantly, these preclinical and clinical GVL findings demand further research in this area in order to identify the mechanisms responsible for this antileukemic effect, to clarify how to prospectively control the antitumor immune mechanisms involved, to determine how to more safely and controllably direct these immune reactions against hematopoietic malignancies, and to determine what other malignant conditions may be amenable to allogeneic-mediated "graft versus tumor" reactions. These important and timely issues are all addressed later in this volume.

II. TARGETS FOR GVL

As thousands of patients appear to have been protected from recurrent leukemia by the GVL effect without succumbing to lethal GVH, there has been much focus and speculation on the potential separability of the GVH and GVL mechanisms. For murine models of virally induced leukemias, the identification of leukemia-specific cytotoxic T cells and helper T cells, each recognizing distinct MHC restricted virally controlled peptides, proves that in certain settings truly "leukemia-specific" immune recognition can occur [17]. However, the majority of human leukemias do not seem to be caused by or associated with expression of exogenous viral proteins. Thus, the recognition structures seen on allogeneic human leukemias might not be analogous to the viral peptides on murine leukemic cells recognized by syngeneic T cells. Thus it is important to evaluate both qualitatively and quantitatively distinct pathways that might allow immune cells to preferentially (if not specifically) destroy HLA-identical allogeneic leukemic cells while sparing nonleukemic somatic tissues. These issues are the primary focus of Part 1 of this text, including seven chapters devoted to the biological basis of the GVL effect. If leukemia cells are eradicated in vivo, without irreversible destruction of normal tissues, this implies that the leukemia cells are either preferentially recognized or preferentially destroyed by some component of an immune response that is mediated by the allogeneic cells from the donor.

Even though immune reactions are initiated by specific molecular recognition events, one need not assume that the GVL effect involves selective or preferential recognition of leukemic cells following allogeneic BMT. The diverse alloantigens (major, minor, and tissue-restricted) might be expressed comparably on leukemic cells and certain other nonleukemic normal tissues. If so, the clinically observed GVL effect without lethal GVH would imply that either (a) the leukemia cells may be more susceptible to the mechanisms of cell destruction mediated by the immune effector cells than the normal host tissues, which are recognized similarly in the allograft reaction but are not destroyed to the degree that the leukemia cells are, or (b) the leukemia and certain nonleukemia cells are recognized equally and destroyed similarly; however, precursors of the normal tissue (for example, undifferentiated stem cells) might not be completely destroyed while the leukemic cells and their transformed precursors may well be completely eradicated by the immune reaction.

In addition, several distinct mechanisms might allow preferential recognition of the leukemia cells by the cells of the allogeneic donor's immune system. These include the following:

1. Leukemia-''specific'' molecules controlled by exogenous viruses [such as Epstein-Barr virus (EBV) and human T-cell leukemia virus (HTLV)], which are exogenous to the host, might serve as truly ''foreign'' antigenic determinants [18,19].
2. Minor histocompatibility antigens might be better recognized if they were expressed in greater quantity on the leukemia cells than nonleukemic cells [20–22].
3. Minor histocompatibility antigens expressed similarly on a variety of leukemic and nonleukemic tissues might be presented better on the leukemic cells due to better expression of antigen-presenting MHC molecules or costimulatory molecules [20–23].
4. Tissue-''specific'' antigens might be preferentially expressed by the leukemia cells and certain ''nonessential'' host tissues. The best example of these might be differentiation antigens expressed selectively by the host's hematopoietic tissues. Recognition and destruction of cells bearing these molecules would result in complete eradication of the leukemia as well as the host's hematopoietic system [24]. The latter would be of no clinical consequence, as the hematopoietic system is being ''rescued'' by reconstitution with the donor's allogeneic marrow.
5. The malignant process itself can generate point mutations and chromosomal rearrangements that are selectively and specifically linked to the neoplastic process and expressed by the malignant cells themselves.

These include the BCR-ABL and RAR-α fusion proteins associated with CML and APML respectively [25,26].

6. Although T cells do play a role in the GVL effect, their role may be the recognition of host alloantigens and induction of a ''generalized'' alloantigenic recognition, with subsequent release of immunologically active cytokines. The selective antileukemic effect that is observed might be mediated by cells of the ''innate'' immune system [including natural killer (NK) cells] that are activated by these cytokines [2], such as IL-2. If so, leukemia cells (at least from certain patients) might preferentially express activation molecules recognized mainly by NK cells [27].

Detailed in vitro analyses and in vivo murine model systems provide some support for each of the above potential mechanisms [18–27]. Even so, it may be that different mechanisms are at work in the GVL reaction occurring in distinct patients. Moreover, many of these GVL mechanisms might be at work simultaneously within any given patient. The current clinical challenge is to determine how best to apply this interesting yet still incomplete mechanistic information to provide benefits for patients currently diagnosed with malignancies and being considered as candidates for allogeneic stem-cell transplants. Future studies will need to better control the reactions involved in each of the antileukemic mechanisms in order to prospectively induce and enhance a more specific antileukemic reaction in vivo.

III. GVL AND CLINICAL PRACTICE

Historical data documenting the GVL effect came largely from analyses of BMT from HLA-identical siblings [14,15]. Somewhat distinct patterns were observed for the strength of the GVL effect in the settings of ALL, ANLL, and CML [15], with differential roles observed for acute and chronic GVHD in the process. More recently, graft-versus-tumor (GVT) effects appear to be observed for treatment of other hematopoietic malignancies, including myeloma and lymphoma. In contrast, it has been more difficult to document any allogeneic GVT effect against nonhematopoetic malignancies, such as neuroblastoma [28] or breast cancer. The inability to detect GVT for nonhematopoietic malignancies might indicate differences in the immunobiology of hematopoietic and nonhematopoietic malignancies. However, relatively small patient numbers and other clinical factors influencing the choice of treatment [28], may have influenced the ability of these clinical studies to detect a potential GVT effect.

Over the past decade, the practice of allogeneic hematopoietic stem-cell transplantation has been modified by the use of alternative sources, other than bone marrow, for stem cells, particularly umbilical cord blood and peripheral blood stem cells. The number, potency, and immunologic reactivity of contaminating T cells within cord blood and peripheral blood stem-cell populations is expected to be different than that for conventionally aspirated harvests of allogeneic marrow. Therefore the GVL observations obtained with infusions of HLA-identical sibling marrow might not be exactly reproduced with infusions of HLA-identical siblings' cord blood or peripheral blood stem cells. Furthermore, the variables associated with the use of alternative donor stem cells [HLA-matched or partially matched, unrelated or related, marrow or blood (peripheral or cord) stem cells, with or without T cell–depletion procedures] could also influence the multiple variables involved in the balance between the GVH and GVL phenomena [29].

These issues are discussed in detail in the six chapters in Part 2 of this text. Furthermore, additional infusions of donor lymphocytes, distinct from those provided with the stem cells themselves, have been pioneered by Slavin et al. [30], and subsequently by Kolb et al. [31], and several others [32] as a mechanism for inducing a lymphocyte mediated antileukemic effect for some patients that have relapsed after BMT. This has been designated donor lymphocyte infusion (DLI). For high-risk patients likely to relapse, the prospective use of this DLI approach following BMT may potentially prove to have some benefit in preventing leukemic relapse. Furthermore, the ability of donor lymphocytes to eradicate host hematopoietic tissue provides an alternative strategy for destruction of host-derived leukemic cells and normal hematopoietic cells. Recent studies by Slavin et al. show that this approach may provide for the hematopoietic ablation of the host without requiring the previously standard supralethal doses of chemotherapy and radiation therapy [33].

IV. MODULATION AND APPLICATION OF THE GVL EFFECT

Many distinct types of donor-derived cell types may be mediating the GVL reactivity through recognition of a variety of distinct membrane structures expressed on the leukemia cell surfaces and through activation of multiple distinct effector pathways able to destroy the leukemia cells [34]. If one could preferentially deplete the donor-derived immune cells that are not required for the antileukemic effect or, alternatively, increase the numbers or activation state of the donor cells most involved in the anti leukemic effect, it might be possible to functionally "separate" quantitatively the GVL effect from the GVHD effect. A number of clinical strategies are now under way testing potential strategies based on this hypothesis. Some clinical trials are providing infusions of stem cells and lymphocytes that have been depleted of subpopulations potentially more important in alloreactivity and less important in the antileukemic mechanisms. However, the specific cell subtypes that are essential for GVL have not been clarified in a uniform way for clinical application. Therefore distinct strategies are being tested by different clinical research teams. Some involve depletions of CD8 lymphocytes [35] while others involve the depletion of all T lymphocytes [36] in order to focus on the activity of NK cells [37]. Some of these are based on a presumed major antileukemic role for the NK population, while others are anticipating a greater antileukemic effect to be mediated by CD4+ cells.

Particularly in those clinical settings where known molecular targets on the neoplastic cells are potentially recognized by antitumor effector cells, mechanisms are being tested to preferentially activate and expand immune cells with selective antitumor specificity. Current clinical studies are testing in vitro or in vivo activation of donor immune reactivity against the recipient's malignant cells. The antigenic targets on the malignant cells include immunoglobulin idiotype determinants expressed on B-cell lymphomas [38], EBV-controlled peptides [18] associated with posttransplant lymphoproliferative disorders or Hodgkin's disease [39], and oncogenic fusion proteins exclusively expressed within the neoplastic cells, such as BCR-ABL [25].

Clinical trials testing virtually all of these possibilities are now under way and reflect attempts to preferentially control and manipulate the GVL reaction in a prospective clinical way. These approaches are summarized in the six chapters comprised by Part 3 of this book.

V. FUTURE PERSPECTIVES

In the 1970s it was demonstrated that ablative chemoradiotherapy followed by syngeneic or HLA-identical sibling stem-cell reinfusion could be curative for a major fraction of patients undergoing such treatment for hematologic malignancy [8,12]. Such treatment has since proven lifesaving for thousands of leukemia patients worldwide. Over 3000 of these are thought to be survivors because of the mechanisms involved in a ''subclinical'' GVL effect that eradicated residual leukemia in the absence of clinically significant GVHD. For certain nonneoplastic diseases currently being treated with BMT [including diseases caused by single gene defects, such as severe combined immunodeficiency (SCID), sickle cell disease, thalassemia, and other stem-cell defects], the future may herald effective therapies that involve ''genetic repair'' through insertion of nonmutated genes into autologous hematopoietic stem cells. For neoplastic diseases, a myriad of preclinical and clinical paradigms are being pursued in order to activate a patient's autologous immune system to preferentially destroy endogenous neoplastic cells. If effective, such an approach may, in the future, supersede the need for allogeneic stem-cell transplantation. Whether and when the hope of inducing autologous tumor specific immunity will be realized remains speculative [40]. This elusive goal of effective autologous antitumor immunity must be contrasted with the thousands of patients who have already benefited from the allogeneic GVL effect.

The survival benefits of allogeneic BMT initially seemed applicable only to those with an HLA-identical sibling. Recently, the use of alternative donors and alternative sources of stem cells is extending the technology of stem-cell transplantation to the vast majority of patients with ''transplantable'' hematopoietic malignancies. The clinical results of these alternative donor transplants do not yet match those obtained for recipients of HLA-identical sibling's stem cells [41–43]. Quantitative or qualitative mechanisms in the GVL/GVH paradigm are likely the source of these differences in clinical results for leukemic recipients of alternative donor stem-cell transplants. For the present and near future, expanding our ability to provide alternative donor transplants and selectively enhance the GVL reactions should prove beneficial. The components of successful allogeneic BMT for leukemia involve (1) cytoreduction of residual leukemia; (2) host hematopoietic ''ablation''; (3) donor stem-cell reconstitution; (4) GVH ''prophylaxis''; (5) antileukemic effects provided by donor-derived lymphocytes; and (6) infection control and supportive care. These components are all somewhat separable. Future protocols may best provide innovative approaches toward each of these therapeutic targets independently. For example, treatment of leukemia by stem-cell transplantation in the near future might include combinations of the following approaches. First, innovative approaches toward ablating host hematopoietic cells (either with donor-derived alloreactive lymphocytes [33] or with radiolabeled monoclonal antibodies [44] directed against hematopoietic elements). Such innovations might preferentially eradicate host leukemic cells and host hematopoietic cells without the level of nonspecific somatic cell toxicity observed with current supralethal radiotherapy and chemotherapy ''ablation'' regimens. Second, if adequate immunosuppressive ''conditioning'' is provided to the host during the peritransplant period, purified donor-derived stem-cell populations, virtually devoid of mature immune elements, would be expected to engraft even across histocompatibility barriers. Third, once engraftment has been initiated and the tissue destruction associated with the peritransplant period has been adequately repaired by restoration of normal cellular metabolism and myeloid function, the differentiating donor-derived immune elements should recognize host tissues as ''self'' and become ''tolerant.'' At that time, infusion of graded numbers [30] of donor-derived immune cells (possibly selected for subtype) might best provide antileukemic mechanisms without inducing GVHD. Finally, in vitro and in vivo manipulations to increase the antileukemic specificity of the infused lymphocytes may well enhance their in vivo antitumor potential.

VI. SUMMARY

The GVL reaction following allogeneic BMT is very real and thousands of patients are alive because of it. This text celebrates and clarifies our current understanding regarding the mechanisms responsible for this clinically important effect and identifies ongoing approaches in order to better utilize the mechanisms involved so as to provide more selective GVL benefits for an even greater number of leukemia patients. This is clearly an example of tumor immunotherapy that is already working and is most certainly going to become even more effective.

ACKNOWLEDGMENTS

The author thanks Roxanne Albertson for the preparation of this manuscript. Supported by grants CA32685, CA57746, CA68334, CA61498, CA14520.

REFERENCES

1. Coley WB. Late results of the treatment of inoperable sarcoma by the mixed toxins of erysipelas and Bacillus prodigiosus. Am J Med Sci 1906; 131:373.
2. Frederick M, Grimm E, Krohn E, Smid C, Yu TK. Cytokine-induced cytotoxic function expressed by lymphocytes of the innate immune system: distinguishing characteristics of NK and LAK based on functional and molecular markers. J Interferon Cytokine Res 1997; 17:435–447.
3. Sondel PM, Rakhmilevich, DeJong JLO, Hank JA. Cellular immunity and cytokines. In: Mendelsohn J, ed. The Molecular Basis of Cancer. W.B. Saunders Co. Philadelphia, PA. In press, 1999.
4. Prehn RT, Main JM. Immunity to methyl cholanthrene induced sarcomas. J Natl Cancer Inst 1957; 18:769.
5. Gross L. Intradermal immunization of C3H mice against a sarcoma that originated in an animal of the same line. Cancer Res 1943; 3:326–333.
6. Berenson JR, Einstein AB Jr, Fefer A. Syngeneic adoptive immunotherapy and chemoimmunotherapy of a Friend leukemia: requirement for T cells. J Immunol 1975; 115:234–238.
7. Bortin MM, Truitt RL, Rimm AA, Bach FH. Graft vs leukemia reactivity induced by alloimmunization without augmentation of graft vs host reactivity. Nature 1979; 281:490–491.
8. Fefer A, Einstein AB, Thomas ED, Buckner CD, Clift RA, Glucksberg H, Neiman PE, Storb R. Bone marrow transplantation for hematologic neoplasia in 16 patients with identical twins. N Engl J Med 1974; 290:1389–1393.
9. Bach FH, Van Rood JJ. The major histocompatibility complex—genetics and biology (first of three parts). N Engl J Med 1976; 295:806–813.
10. Gatti RA, Meuwissen HJ, Allen HD, Hong R, Good RA. Immunological reconstitu-

tion of sex-linked lymphopenic immunological deficiency. Lancet 1968; 2:1366–1369.

11. Bach FH, Albertini RJ, Joo P, Anderson JL, Bortin MM. Bone marrow transplantation in a patient with the Wiskott-Aldrich syndrome. Lancet 1968; 2:1364–1366.
12. Thomas ED, Storb R, Clift RA, Fefer A, Johnson L, Neiman PE, Lerner KG, Glucksberg H, Buckner CD. Bone marrow transplantation (second of two parts). N Engl J Med 1975; 292:832–843 and 895–902.
13. Odom LF, August CS, Githens JH, Humbert JR, Morse H, Peakman D, Sharma B, Rusnak SL, Johnson FB. Remission of relapsed leukemia during a graft-versus-host reaction: a ''graft-versus-leukemia reactions'' in man? Lancet 1978; 2:537–540.
14. Weiden PL, Fluornoy N, Thomas ED, Prentice R, Fefer A, Buckner CD, Storb R. Antileukemic effects of graft versus host disease in human recipients of allogeneic marrow grafts. N Engl J Med 1979; 300:1068.
15. Horowitz MM, Gale RP, Sondel PM, Goldman JM, Kersey J, Kolb HJ, Rimm AA, Ringden O, Rozman C, Speck B, Truitt RL, Zwaan FE, Bortin MM. Graft-versus-leukemia reactions after bone marrow transplantation. Blood 1990; 75:555–562.
16. Batturini A, Gale RP. Allogeneic bone marrow transplantation for leukemia. Curr Opin Hematol 1994; 1:402–405.
17. Greenberg PD. Adoptive T cell therapy of tumors: mechanisms operative in the recognition and elimination of tumor cells. Adv Immunol 1991; 49:281–291.
18. Rooney CM, Smith CA, Ng CY, Loftin SK, Sixhey JW, Gan Y, Srivastava DK, Bowman LC, Krance RA, Brenner MK, Heslop HE. The use of gene modified virus specific T lymphocytes to control Epstein-Barr virus related lymphoproliferation. Lancet 1995; 345:9.
19. Mitsuya H, Matis LA, Megson M, Bunn PA, Murray C, Mann DL, Gallo RC, Broder S. Generation of an HLA-restricted cytotoxic T cell line reactive against cultured tumor cells from a patient infected with human T cell leukemia/lymphoma virus. J Exp Med 1983; 158:994–999.
20. Sondel PM, Hank JA, Wendel T, Flynn B, Bozdech MJ. HLA identical leukemia cells and T cell growth factor activate cytotoxic T cell recognition of minor locus histocompatibility antigens in vitro. J Clin Invest 1983; 71:1779–1786.
21. Dolstra H, Fredrix H, Preijers F, Goulmy E, Figdor CG, deWitte TM, van de Wiel-van Kemenade E. Recognition of a B-cell leukemia associated minor histocompatibility antigen by CTL. J Immunol 1997; 152:560–565.
22. Mutis T, Schrama E, van Lyxemburg-Heijs SA, Falkenburg JH, Melief CJ, Goulmy E. HLA class II restricted T-cell reactivity to a developmentally regulated antigen shared by leukemic cells and CD34+ early progenitor cells. Blood 1997; 90:1083–1090.
23. Dermine S, Mavroudis D, Jiang YZ, Hensel N, Molldrem J, Barrett AJ. Immune escape from a graft versus leukemia effect may play a role in the relapse of myeloid leukemias following allogeneic bone marrow transplantation. Bone Marrow Transplant 1997; 19:989–999.
24. Sprent J, Surh CD, Agus D, Hurd M, Sutton S, Heath WR. Profound atrophy of the bone marrow reflecting major histocompatibility complex class II restricted destruction of stem cells by CD4+ cells. J Exp Med 1994; 180:307–317.

25. Bocchia M, Korontsvit T, Xu Q, Mackinnon S, Yang SY, Sette A, Scheinberg DA. Specific human cellular immunity to bcr-abl oncogene-derived peptides. Blood 1996; 87:3587–3592.
26. Gambacorti-Passerini C, Grignani F, Arienti F, Pandolfi PP, Pelicci PG, Parmiani G. Human CD4 lymphocytes specifically recognize a peptide representing the fusion region of the hybrid protein pml/RARα present in acute promyelocytic leukemia cells. Blood 1993; 81:1369–1375.
27. O'Reilly RJ. Minimal residual disease is more common in patients who have mixed T-cell chimerism after bone marrow transplantation for chronic myelogenous leukemia. Blood 1994; 83:3409–3416.
28. Matthay KK, Seeger RC, Reynolds CP, Stram DO, O'Leary MC, Harris RE, Selch M, Atkinson JB, Haase GM, Ramsay NK. Allogeneic versus autologous purged bone marrow transplantation for neuroblastoma: a report from the Childrens Cancer Group. J Clin Oncol 1994; 12:2382–2389.
29. Keever-Taylor CA, Passweg J, Kawanishi I, Flomenberg N, Baxter-Lowe LA. Association of donor-derived host-reactive cytolytic and helper T cells with outcome following alternative donor T cell–depleted bone marrow transplantation. Bone Marrow Transplant 1997; 19:1001–1009.
30. Slavin S, Naparstek E, Nagler A, Ackerstein A, Samuel S, Kapelushnik J, Brautbar C, Or R. Allogeneic cell therapy with donor peripheral blood cells and recombinant human interluekin-2 to treat leukemia relapse after allogeneic bone marrow transplantation. Blood 1996; 87:2195–2204.
31. van Rhee F, Kolb HJ. Donor leukocyte transfusions for leukemic relapse. Curr Opin Hematol 1995; 2:423–430.
32. Collins RH Jr, Shpilberg O, Drobyski WR, Porter DL, Giralt S, Champlin R, Goodman SA, Wolff SN, Hu W, Verfaillie C, List A, Dalton W, Ognoskie N, Chetrit A, Antin JH, Nemunaitis J. Donor leukocyte infusions in 140 patients with relapsed malignancy after allogeneic bone marrow transplantation. J Clin Oncol 1997; 15: 433–441.
33. Slavin S, Nagler A, Naparstek E, Kapelushnik Y, Aker M, Cividalli G, Varadi G, Kirschbaum M, Ackerstein A, Samuel S, Amar A, Brautbar C, Ben-Tal O, Eldor A, Or R. Nonmyeloablative stem cell transplantation and cell therapy as an alternative to conventional bone marrow transplantation with lethal cytoreduction for the treatment of malignant and nonmalignant hematologic diseases. Blood 1998; 91: 756–763.
34. Sosman JA, Sondel PM. The graft-vs.-leukemia effect. Implications for post-marrow transplant antileukemia treatment. Am J Pediatr Hematol Oncol 1993; 15:185–195.
35. Champlin R, Giralt S, Gajewski J. T cells, graft-versus-host disease and graft-versus-leukemia: innovative approaches for blood and marrow transplantation. Acta Haematol 1996; 95:157–163.
36. Papadopoulos EB, Carabasi MH, Castro-Malaspina H, Childs BH, Mackinnon S, Boulad F, Gillio AP, Kernan NA, Small TN, Szabolcs P, Taylor J, Yahalom J, Collins NH, Bleau SA, Black PM, Heller G, O'Reilly RJ, Young JW. T-cell-depleted allogeneic bone marrow transplantation as postremission therapy for acute myelogenous leukemia: freedom from relapse in the absence of graft-versus-host disease. Blood 1998; 91:1083–1090.

37. Robertson MJ, Ritz J. Biology and clinical relevance of human natural killer cells. Blood 1990; 76:2421.
38. Kwak LW, Taub DD, Duffey PL, Bensiger WI. Bryant EM, Reynolds CW. Longo DL. Transfer of myeloma idiotype-specific immunity from an actively immunized marrow donor. Lancet 1995; 345:1016.
39. Sing AP, Ambinder RF, Hong DJ, Jensen M, Batten W, Petersdorf E, Greenberg PD. Isolation of Epstein-Barr virus (EBV)-specific cytotoxic T lymphocytes that lyse Reed-Sternberg cells: implications for immune-mediated therapy of EBV+ Hodgkin's disease. Blood 1997; 89:1978–1986.
40. Wagner JE, Kurzberg J. Cord blood stem cells. Curr Opin Hematol 1997; 4:413–418.
41. Gajewski J, Champlin R. Bone marrow transplantation from unrelated donors. Curr Opin Oncol 1996; 8:84–88.
42. Korbling M, Champlin R. Peripheral blood progenitor cell transplantation: a replacement for marrow auto- or allografts. Stem Cells 1996; 14:185–195.
43. Press OW, Eary JF, Appelbaum FR, Bernstein ID. Myeloablative radio labeled antibody therapy with autologous bone marrow transplantation for relapsed B cell lymphomas. Cancer Treat Res 1995; 76:281–297.

2

The Immune Response to Alloantigens

Graham M. Lord and Robert I. Lechler
Hammersmith Hospital
London, United Kingdom

I. INTRODUCTION

Tissues that are mismatched for major histocompatibility complex (MHC) molecules can induce uniquely strong primary immune responses *in vitro*, as reflected by the mixed lymphocyte reaction (MLR), and provoke allograft rejection, graft-versus-host disease (GVHD), and the graft-versus-leukemia effect (GVL) *in vivo*. In fact, the investigation of the targets of the immune responses to allografts led to the discovery of MHC molecules, which were initially called transplantation antigens.

Responses to alloantigens are strong, reflecting to some extent the high precursor frequency of alloreactive T cells within the normal repertoire. The precursor frequency of T cells reactive to conventional antigens is approximately 1:150,000–1:350,000 [1], whereas alloreactive T-cell precursor frequencies may be as high as 1:1000 [2]. This finding is surprising given the phenomenon of self-MHC restriction, whereby a T cell is positively selected in the thymus on the basis of recognizing peptide antigen in association with syngeneic MHC molecules [3–5].

The cellular and molecular basis for the recognition of alloantigens has only recently become clear, as information regarding MHC and T-cell receptor (TCR) structure and function has become available. The mechanisms that contribute to the development of an alloresponse and the responses to minor histocompatibility complex (mHC) molecules are the subjects of this chapter. In addition, strategies to subvert the mechanisms of self-tolerance in order to induce tolerance to transplanted tissues will be discussed.

II. THE MOLECULAR BASIS OF ALLORECOGNITION

The first challenge in accounting for the strength of anti-MHC alloresponses is to explain the uniquely high frequencies of alloreactive precursor T cells. As mentioned above, T cells recognize peptide antigen when it is presented in association with self (syngeneic) MHC molecules owing to the nature of T-cell selection that occurs during T-cell development in the thymus [3]. The vigor of the T-cell response to allogeneic MHC molecules would seem to contradict the basic tenet of self-MHC restriction. There are two theories as to how this may occur, and these are not mutually exclusive. The first is that the TCRs may recognize allogeneic MHC molecules directly, irrespective of the specific peptide antigen bound in the groove of the MHC molecule. This is referred to as the *high ligand density model* [6], discussed below. The second hypothesis is that the TCRs of allospecific T cells are specific for complexes of allogeneic MHC molecules and individual naturally processed peptides. Owing to polymorphism in the peptide-binding groove, allogeneic MHC molecules are usually occupied by a different repertoire of peptides to which the recipient T cells have not been previously exposed. Thus, a single MHC incompatibility can stimulate a very large number of alloreactive T-cell clones. This is known as the *multiple binary complex model* [7].

A. High Ligand Density

As MHC molecules display marked polymorphism, it is possible that alloreactive T cells recognize polymorphic residues directly on the allogeneic MHC molecule. In this case, the nature of the bound peptide is of secondary importance. This concept is more readily understood in the context of the structure of MHC molecules. Figure 1 shows a space-fill and a ribbon diagram of a human class II MHC molecule. The molecule is a transmembrane heterodimer composed of an invariant DRα chain and a polymorphic DRβ chain, which are noncovalently associated. Each chain has two domains (α1, α2, β1, β2), and the peptide-binding groove is formed by the α1 and β1 helical domains with a β pleated sheet structure in the floor of the groove. Class I MHC molecules have a similar structure but are made up of a heavy chain with three α-helical domains noncovalently associated with β2-microglobulin. The peptide-binding groove of class I molecules is made up from the α1 and α2 domains of the heavy chain, forming a groove that is closed at either end, in contrast to the class II molecule, which has open ends to the groove, allowing longer peptides to be bound. The TCR recognizes a trimolecular complex of two MHC chains and bound peptide. Evi-

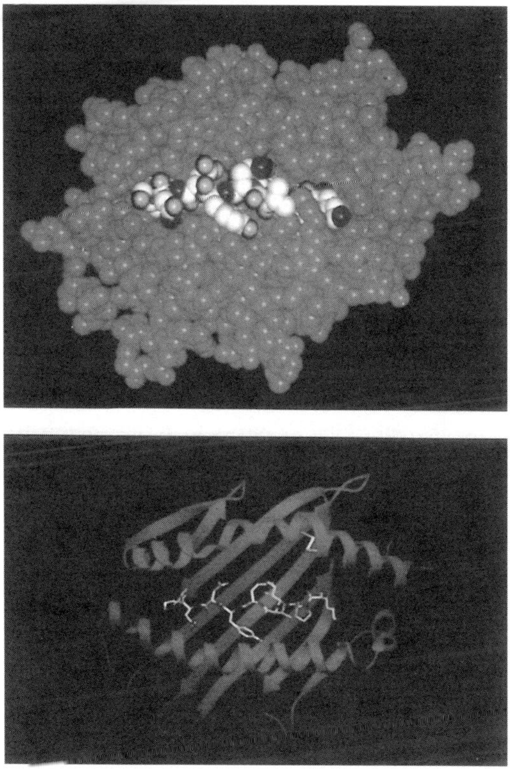

Figure 1 Upper panel: Space-fill diagram of a human class II MHC molecule complexed with a viral peptide, viewed from above. Lower panel: Ribbon diagram of the same class II molecule complexed with peptide, demonstrating the peptide groove and β-pleated sheet at the floor of the groove, viewed from above.

dence that, in the alloresponse, the TCR directly recognizes foreign MHC molecules is provided by studies of cell lines expressing mutated MHC genes [8–10]. Mutation of residues pointing up from the α helix, which influence TCR contact but not peptide binding, can abrogate many alloresponses. In one particular study, the peptides recognized in the alloresponse were associated with both syngeneic and allogeneic molecules [11], showing that a self-peptide can be immunogenic when presented by allogeneic MHC.

Further evidence comes from experiments which demonstrate that synthetic peptides corresponding to the sequence of the TCR-contacting regions of the allo-MHC molecule can block specific alloresponses [12,13], presumably by blocking the TCR-MHC contact required for T-cell activation. This has been demonstrated both in human and murine systems for allorecognition of class I and class II molecules [14].

There is also evidence that some allospecific T cells may not require endogenous peptide for allorecognition. In a cell-free system, class I MHC molecules were reconstituted from light and heavy chains in the absence of peptide. These molecules were then able to stimulate proliferation of allospecific T cells [15]. Analogously, some T-cell clones are able to recognize class I on the surface of antigen-processing defective mutants such as T2 or RMA-S [16,17].

Thus, in some circumstances, alloreactive T cells may interact directly with exposed regions of an allo-MHC molecule, bound peptide being of secondary importance. In these cases, all the MHC molecules of a given type on the surface of an allogeneic cell could act as ligands for the alloreactive T cell (approximately 10^5 class II molecules of a given isotype are expressed on the surface of a B cell). This represents at least a 100-fold higher determinant density than is available for an antigen-specific, self MHC–restricted T cell. In this latter case, it is unlikely that more than 1% of the MHC molecules of a particular type become occupied with any one individual peptide derived from a processed protein antigen. Thus, T cells, with a lower specific affinity for their ligand than would be required for an antigen-specific response, can be recruited into an alloresponse. This would be reflected in a higher precursor frequency of T cells to alloantigens. Figure 2 shows a schematic illustration of this concept.

B. Multiple Binary Complexes

The multiple binary complex model [7] (Figure 2) proposes that anti-MHC alloresponses are analogous to antigen responses in that they are mediated by T cells specific for peptide-MHC complexes. In this case the peptide is a naturally processed peptide derived from a serum or cellular protein and the MHC molecule is allogeneic. This would account for the high frequencies of anti-MHC alloreactive T cells, because of the wide diversity of different naturally processed peptides displayed by cell-surface MHC molecules. It has been estimated that 2000 different species of peptides may be bound to a single type of MHC molecule at any one time [18]. Thus a single MHC alloantigen could stimulate a large number of different T-cell clones, each specific for a different peptide/MHC complex.

There is experimental evidence for this model of alloreactivity. Incubation of cells expressing MHC class II with exogenous peptide capable of binding class II inhibits allorecognition by alloreactive T cells [19,20]. The interpretation of these data is that the exogenous peptide can displace or compete with the peptide of self origin for presentation to the allospecific T cell. Alloreactive human T-cell clones have been reported that are specific for either class I [21,22] or class II [23] MHC molecules that require the expression of a second MHC molecule

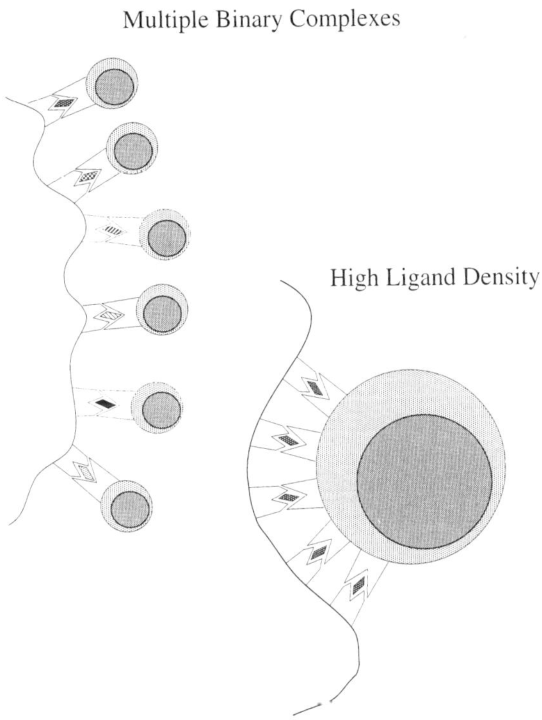

Figure 2 Schematic representation of the two hypotheses that have been proposed to explain the high precursor frequency of anti-MHC alloreactive T cells.

for allorecognition. In this case, it is probably necessary for a peptide derived from the second MHC molecule to be presented by the first MHC molecule.

Additionally, there are many descriptions of alloreactive T-cell clones that discriminate between MHC molecules differing at residues that lie within the peptide-binding groove [24–27]. These would therefore produce no alteration in the three-dimensional structure of the MHC molecule that directly contacted the TCR unless a conformational change was induced at a site distant from the mutation. The only difference would therefore be in the peptides bound in the MHC groove.

The nature of the antigen presenting cell (APC) can also influence alloreactivity. There have been reports of alloreactive T cells that distinguish between the same MHC molecules displayed on either murine or human APCs, even though these different cells can present peptide with equal efficiency to antigen-specific T cells [28–31]. This could be explained by the fact that a species-specific peptide is required for an alloresponse to be generated. In one experimental system, allorecognition of a murine class I molecule on a human APC could only be restored by the addition of murine-derived peptides [32]. Cell type–specific allorecognition has also been observed whereby alloreactive T cells distinguish between the same MHC molecule expressed on different cell lines, probably owing to the requirement for a peptide from a particular lineage of cell [29].

Further evidence to support the peptide dependence of some alloresponses comes from studies on the antigen-processing mutant cell line T2. When T2 cells were transfected with a cDNA clone encoding a murine class I molecule, there appeared to be a very limited diversity of peptides present in its groove when expressed at the surface of the cell. These class I molecules were not recognized by allospecific T-cell clones until the transfected T2 cells were exposed to mouse cell–derived peptides. Additionally, each clone recognized a different specific peptide [16]. In a similar set of experiments, MHC class II–transfected T2 cells were used in limiting dilution assays to determine the frequencies of allogeneic CD4+ T cells capable of responding to these cells or similarly transfected wild-type cells. T2 cells transfected with a class II MHC molecule expressed only sodium dodecyl sulfate (SDS)–unstable (i.e., empty or invariant chain peptide–associated) class II molecules and were poor stimulators of primary and secondary alloreactive CD4+ T-cell responses. Incubation of these transfectants with a class II–binding peptide derived from another class II molecule generated SDS-stable cell surface class II expression and enabled these cells to stimulate alloreactive CD4+ T cells that had been primed by the same peptide-MHC complex [33].

III. ALLOGENEIC IMMUNE RESPONSES AND THYMIC SELECTION

There is thus experimental evidence supporting both the high-ligand-density and the multiple-binary-complex models of alloreactivity. The models are not mutually exclusive, and there may be situations *in vivo* where the alloresponse is focused on the foreign MHC molecule or is more peptide-specific. However, neither model addresses the fundamental question of why the mature T-cell repertoire, which has been selected in the thymus for self-MHC restriction, contain such a high frequency of alloreactive precursors.

Consideration of structural aspects of MHC molecules may provide a mechanistic explanation of allorecognition that can be accommodated within the framework of positive selection of the T-cell repertoire in the thymus for self-MHC restriction. We have considered this issue in the context of the allorecognition of the human class II molecule, HLA-DR, and proposed that two distinct models may be required to resolve the issue [34].

The first is illustrated by considering the alloresponse between a DR1 responder and certain DR4 subtypes. The amino-terminal domains of these molecules are illustrated schematically in Figure 3. As shown, the amino acid sequences that make up the α-helical portions of these two molecules are highly conserved. Since it is these regions that contact the TCR and impose the constraints of self-MHC restriction, it seems reasonable to assume that the developing thymocytes from a DR1 responder will recognize the surface of DRB1*0401 as being very similar to self and utilize it as a restriction element. If this is the case, it begs the question of why DR1-restricted T cells recognize DRB1*0401 as an alloantigen. The explanation may be that there are multiple sequence differences in the floor of the β1 domains between these two molecules, leading to the display of a different set of naturally processed peptides. Therefore, in this type of responder-stimulator combination, the specificity of the alloresponse is likely to be for peptides bound and displayed by DR4 but not by DR1. The T-cell repertoire from a DR1 individual would therefore not be tolerant to the DR4-bound peptides and, owing to the conserved TCR-contacting regions of

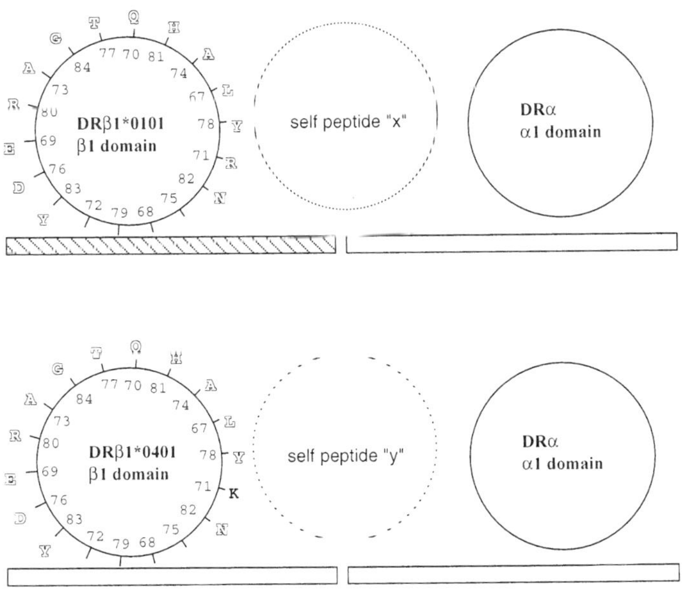

Figure 3 Schematic representation of a cross-section through the α helices (solid circles) and the antiparallel strands (rectangles) forming the floor of the peptide-binding groove that constitute HLA-DR1 (above) and HLA-DR4 (below). The orientation of individual amino acid residues of the β1 domain α helix from positions 67 to 84 is shown.

these two molecules, these peptides could be recognized by T cells selected for DR1 restriction in a manner that mimics self-MHC restriction. This model is applicable to a large number of responder:stimulator combinations, since DRβ chain sequences fall into groups that have conserved sequences in the α-helical regions of their β1 domains. This model is analogous to the multiple-binary-complex hypothesis of allorecognition described above.

However, this cannot account for all situations, since strong alloresponses are still generated when responders and stimulators have multiple sequence differences in the TCR contact regions of their MHC molecules. This situation is illustrated by considering the responder-stimulator combination of DRw17 and DRw11 (Figure 4). It is impossible to invoke any mimicking of self-MHC restriction in such a responder-stimulator combination, since the TCR-contacting residues are so different. We have proposed that the specificity of allorecognition in such combinations is due to recognition of the exposed MHC polymorphisms. Thymic positive selection for self-MHC restriction is thought to select thymocytes whose receptors have an intermediate affinity for thymically expressed MHC molecules. If a maturing thymocyte has a high affinity for self MHC, it is deleted in order to avoid autoreactivity (negative selection). Thymocytes whose receptors display low affinity for MHC molecules die from neglect, since they receive no signals for further differentiation and would serve no purpose in the mature T-cell repertoire [35]. In this context it is reasonable to predict that a small percentage of T cells selected on the basis of having intermediate affinity for self-MHC may cross-react with higher affinity to allogeneic MHC molecules. This would occur as a chance event and would need to apply to only 1:1000 T cells to account for the observed alloreactive precursor frequencies observed.

Support for this model comes from the finding that alloreactive T cells in a responder-stimulator combination, differing extensively at the TCR-contacting

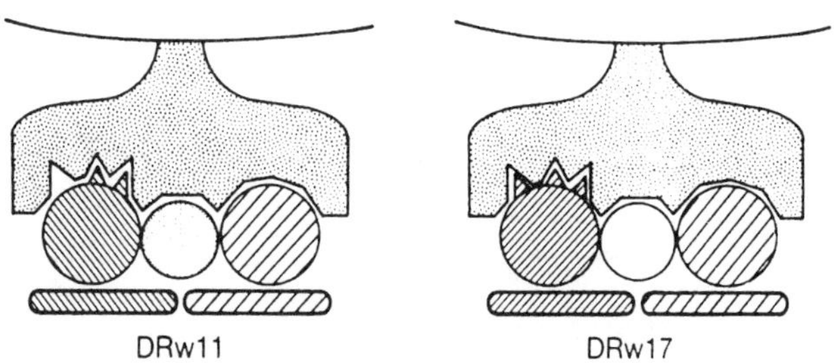

Figure 4 Allorecognition between responder:stimulator combinations with disparate MHC TCR contact surfaces may result from a chance high-affinity cross reaction. The complex of MHC class II molecule and bound peptide (middle small circle) involved in DR11-restricted anti-DR17 allospecific recognition by the same T-cell clone is shown. The basis of this cross-reaction is explained in the text.

surfaces, show biased Vβ gene usage [36]. The CDR1 and CDR2 regions of the TCR contact the third variable region of the MHC α and β chains and are encoded by germ-line V gene sequences, thus indicating that the TCRs of alloreactive cells in combinations of this type are focused on polymorphic MHC residues. Conversely, alloreactive T cells from responder-stimulator combinations with very similar TCR-contacting surfaces, for which it would be predicted that bound peptide contributes significantly to allorecognition, show no such bias.

Many responder-stimulator combinations will fall between these two extremes, and in these cases allorecognition will depend upon a combination of specificities for MHC polymorphisms and for differentially bound peptides. Based on these considerations, it is possible to accommodate allorecognition of foreign MHC molecules within a self-restricted TCR repertoire.

These considerations may be important in the future design of strategies to specifically inhibit allorecognition. Where the alloresponse seems to be focused on bound peptide, the administration of MHC-binding peptides that will compete for occupancy of the allogeneic MHC molecules may be advantageous; whereas in the situation where MHC polymorphisms contribute to T-cell activation, monoclonal antibodies or peptides that block TCR-MHC interaction may be more effective.

IV. PATHWAYS OF ALLORECOGNITION

All of the above discussion has been focused on "direct" allorecognition, whereby T cells recognize the MHC-peptide alloantigen in an intact form on the surface of an allogeneic cell. Recent experimental data have shown that there is another pathway for alloantigen-mediated T-cell activation, known as "indirect" allorecognition [37]. Based on results obtained in a rodent transplantation model, we proposed over 15 years ago that this pathway may play an important role in late, more chronic forms of allograft rejection.

Direct alloimmunization may be the prerogative of allogeneic cells with specialized APC function, such as dendritic cells and macrophages. This is supported by experimental models of kidney [38] and thyroid [39,40] transplantation in which depletion of donor-derived ("passenger") APCs from the transplanted tissue led to greatly extended or indefinite graft survival. Indirect allorecognition occurs when allogeneic MHC molecules are taken up and processed by recipient APCs and presented to recipient T cells in association with syngeneic MHCs (Figure 5). Thus, indirect allorecognition occurs through the same pathway as does recognition of other foreign antigens, such as viral peptides. It has been argued that this pathway plays an important role in mediating allograft rejection, although it has been difficult until recently to demonstrate its importance separately from the direct pathway. It has been shown that immunization of graft recipients with peptides of allogeneic MHC antigens (which could only stimulate

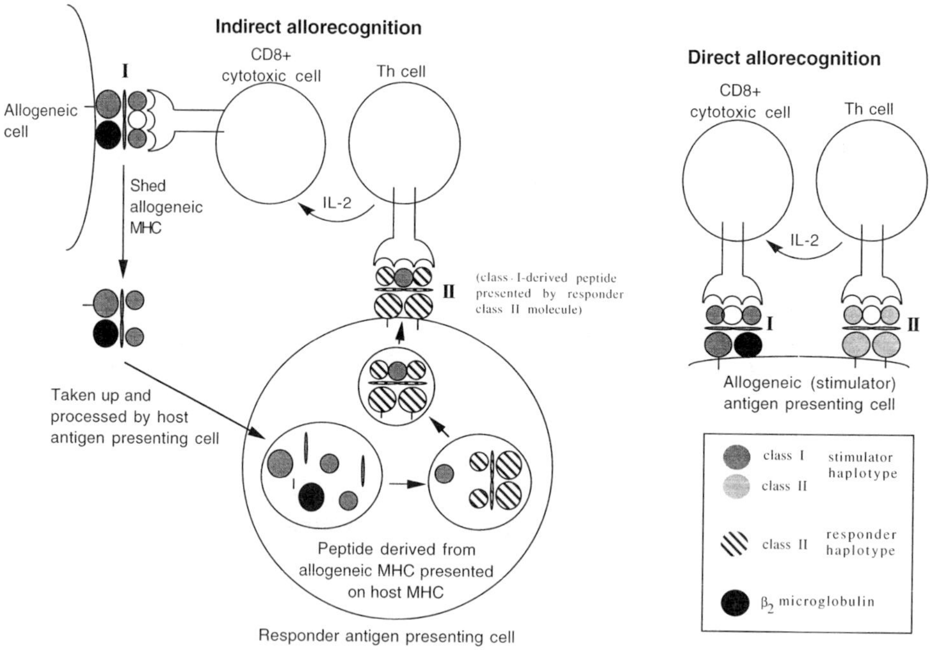

Figure 5 Indirect versus direct allorecognition. Direct allorecognition entails responder T cells recognizing foreign MHC molecules directly on the surface of allogeneic APCs. Indirect allorecognition entails recognition of alloantigens that are shed from the allogeneic cell and taken up and processed by APCs of recipient origin in association with host MHC molecules.

an indirect response) led to accelerated graft rejection [41]. Additionally, allografts from MHC class II knockout mice are rejected swiftly in a CD4+ T cell–dependent manner [42], demonstrating the importance of this pathway, since these grafts are unable to stimulate a direct alloresponse from CD4+ T cells. Furthermore, downregulation of T-cell responses by thymic administration of peptides from allogeneic MHC antigens can lead to prolonged survival of subsequent allografts [43].

V. MINOR HISTOCOMPATIBILITY ANTIGENS AND ALLORESPONSES

Minor histocompatibility antigens (H) were originally defined by allograft rejection responses in mice that were matched for MHC loci. It was possible, by backcrossing experiments, to observe the segregation of individual mHC loci and to develop congenic strains that differed only at a single mHC locus [44]. It became apparent that while antigens encoded by single loci elicited delayed rejection times, differences at multiple minor loci could stimulate rejection almost as rapid as that seen with MHC mismatches. In humans, the significance of minor H antigens is illustrated by the potential to develop severe GVHD in recipients of bone marrow transplants from HLA-identical siblings [45,46]. Additionally, patients receiving a kidney from an HLA-identical sibling still require immunosuppression because of minor H antigen mismatch, although graft survival is much longer than for MHC-mismatched grafts.

In vitro, primary mixed lymphocyte reactions (MLRs) occur against allogeneic MHC antigens, characterized by proliferation of CD4+ T cells and the development of CD8+ cytotoxic T cells specific for MHC class I disparities. MLRs against minor H antigens can be obtained only with responder T cells from individuals previously immunized *in vivo* by skin grafting or with spleen cells expressing the relevant antigen [47,48]. In contrast with the immune response to MHC molecules, no antibodies are made to minor H molecules. However, both CD4+ and CD8+ T-cell clones specific for components of mHC antigens can be isolated from secondary mixed lymphocyte cultures, and the minor H antigen specificities defined by these T-cell clones cosegregate with the loci encoding minor H antigens defined by *in vivo* skin grafting [49]. It has been shown that separate epitopes need to be recognized by CD4+ and CD8+ T cells in order to stimulate graft rejection [50,51]. Minor H antigen–specific cells are MHC-restricted, and it is now clear that minor H antigens are peptides derived from polymorphic or allelically expressed cellular proteins and are presented to T cells in association with self-MHC [52]. The genes encoding minor H antigens are not linked to the MHC locus but are scattered throughout the genome, such as the H-Y male-specific histocompatibility antigens located on the Y chromosome, MTF antigens on mitochondrial chromosomes, and other antigens on autosomal chromosomes [53]. When grafts are exchanged between MHC-identical siblings (but not identical twins), multiple minor differences are presented, but the T-cell response is limited to a small number of immunodominant peptide epitopes [54,55]. The reason for this peptide immunodominance is unclear, although it is probably due to these particular minor peptides binding with greater affinity to MHC molecules, thus increasing the avidity of the T-cell interaction [53].

A. Human Minor Antigens and GVHD

The male-specific H-Y antigen is broadly expressed on human cells, and two peptides have been identified derived from SMCY, a protein encoded on the Y chromosome [56]. One of these peptides is presented in association with HLA-B7 and the other in association with HLA-A2 (both class I MHC molecules).

Another minor H antigen has been identified that is recognized by an HLA-A2.1–restricted cytotoxic T-cell clone and is named HA-2 [57]. This peptide is derived from the class I myosin protein family. In addition to HA-2, four other minor H antigens recognized by T cells in association with HLA-A1 and HLA-A2 have been investigated for association with GVHD in the context of bone marrow transplantation. Mismatch at one or more of these loci was significantly associated with GVHD when compared with donor-recipient pairs that were matched for all four of these antigens [58]. Thus consideration of minor antigenic differences is important in bone marrow transplantation and may influence donor selection in the future.

VI. SELF-TOLERANCE

In order to understand how tolerance to allogenic tissue may be induced it is helpful to consider the mechanisms that underlie tolerance to self. Tolerance to self may be divided into central (i.e., thymic) tolerance and peripheral tolerance. It is via these pathways that deleterious autoreactive cells are prevented from causing autoimmune disease in the host.

A. Central Tolerance

The principal mechanism underlying central tolerance is intrathymic negative selection of differentiating self-reactive T cells by clonal deletion [59]. This has been demonstrated in two ways. The first visualization of thymic deletion was achieved using monoclonal antibodies specific for TCR Vβ families. In response to mouse mammary tumor virus–encoded superantigens, wholesale deletion of thymocytes bearing particular Vβ elements was seen [59]. More recently, thymic negative selection has been studied using TCR-transgenic mice. For example, mice transgenic for a TCR specific for an H-Y peptide presented by the MHC class I molecule H2-K^b were generated. In female H-2^b mice, most of the T cells selected in the thymus carried the transgene-encoded TCR. However, in male transgenic mice, almost all the thymocytes expressing the H-Y specific TCR were deleted because of negative selection [60].

Both positive and negative selection in the thymus requires recognition of peptides in association with self-MHC; therefore, how can signals transduced through the same TCR lead to such diametrically opposed outcomes? One possibility is that the cell type displaying the peptide-MHC complex may be important in determining the outcome of TCR engagement. In general, thymic epithelial cells are relatively inefficient at deleting thymocytes as compared with bone marrow–derived dendritic cells [61].

The process of thymocyte positive selection also appears to be peptide-dependent. Experiments using fetal thymic organ cultures (FTOCs) from mice with mutations interfering with peptide loading or presentation on MHC molecules have shown that peptides play an important role in positive selection when added to these cultures [62–64]. These experiments allowed the definition of peptides capable of selecting a particular TCR. However, conflicting results emerged, depending on the particular TCR and the nature of the peptide used. It would seem, therefore, that positive selection can be a highly promiscuous process. Further experiments with a transgenic mouse model that expresses a single class II MHC molecule occupied by a single peptide show that in this situation, a surprisingly large proportion (>25%) of the normal TCR repertoire can be selected [65]. It appears, therefore, that a single peptide can promote selection of a large population of T cells, but no single peptide is capable of selecting a complete repertoire. Depending on the experimental system and peptide-TCR combination used, positive selection may be highly peptide-specific or exhibit a marked degree of degeneracy.

B. Peripheral Tolerance Mechanisms

It seems highly unlikely that every self peptide can be presented to developing T cells in the thymus, particularly for antigens with peripheral tissue-specific expression. Peripheral tolerance is therefore necessary to avoid autoimmunity. A variety of mechanisms appear to contribute to the induction and the maintenance of peripheral T-cell tolerance, as outlined below.

1. Self-Ignorance

In certain circumstances, the T cell may simply ignore the autoantigen, owing to the absence of noncognate activating signals. Transgenic mice expressing a TCR specific for the immunodominant peptide of myelin basic protein (MBP) fail to develop spontaneous experimental autoimmune encephalomyelitis unless they are removed from a pathogen-free environment or immunized with MBP or pertussis toxin [66]. In other cases, the T cell may be completely ignorant of its specific ligand because it is specific for a cryptic epitope—i.e., a poorly processed and presented peptide. These T cells are not tolerant to their ligand because they have never encountered it in sufficient quantity.

2. Anergy

In order to understand anergy, we must briefly consider normal T-cell activation. MHC-peptide binding to a TCR alone is not sufficient to trigger T-cell activation. It is necessary for the T cell to receive a second signal contemporaneously for

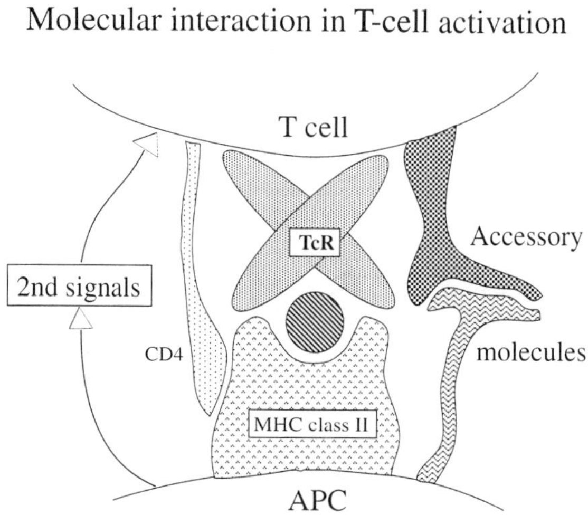

Figure 6 Two-signal model of T-cell activation. Signal 1 is supplied by the cognate interaction of the TCR-CD3 complex with its MHC-peptide ligand. For activation of IL-2 secreting cells there is a requirement for receipt by the T cell of a second, or costimulatory signal. The B7-CD28 interaction is important in the generation of signal 2.

full activation (Figure 6) [67]. If the T cell receives signal 1 (TCR binding MHC-peptide) in the absence of signal 2, then the IL-2 gene is silenced and the T cell becomes refractory to further stimulation [68]. This appears to apply specifically to previously activated T cells rather than to naive T cells and has been observed in vitro using T-cell clones and enriched memory T cells. Anergy is the predominant extrathymic mechanism of inducing self tolerance and has been demonstrated conclusively in a variety of experimental systems [69,70]. The possibility of inducing T-cell anergy provides an opportunity to modulate the immune response to alloantigens, as discussed below.

One of the key molecular interactions required for the generation of signal 2 involves the B7 family of molecules on the APC and their T-cell ligands, CD28 and CTLA-4 [71]. B7-1 and B7-2 are expressed on ''professional'' APCs, such as dendritic cells, activated B cells, and macrophages. Recent evidence suggests that B7 binding to CD28 provides efficient costimulation (i.e., signal 2 in the presence of signal 1), whereas CTLA-4, which is present only at the T-cell surface upon activation, inhibits T-cell activation [72]. It can thus be seen that a balance between activation and inhibition will determine the ultimate outcome of a T-cell recognizing its ligand.

The type of APC that displays the antigen to the T cell may help to explain some features of peripheral tolerance. Many parenchymal cell types can be induced to express MHC class II molecules, particularly under the influence of interferon-γ. If these cells then present peptide antigen in association with the class II molecules to circulating memory T cells (as naive T cells do not enter tissues), then the outcome of this encounter is likely to result in T-cell anergy. This phenomenon has been demonstrated convincingly in vitro [73–75]. The "two signal" model of T-cell activation does not explain all mechanisms of anergy induction, however, as evidenced by work using altered peptide ligands (APLs). If single-residue substitutions are made at certain crucial positions in an antigenic peptide, then, despite a full complement of costimulatory molecules on the APC, the T cell may be anergized [76] or induced to produce anti-inflammatory cytokines in the absence of proliferation [77].

3. Deletion/Exhaustion

Peripheral deletion of mature T cells, or the related phenomenon of clonal exhaustion, has been demonstrated in a number of experimental systems utilizing TCR transgenic mice [78–80]. The key variable highlighted by these models is that of antigen dose. At persistently high doses of antigen, T cells are either deleted or anergized. Clonal exhaustion may also occur due to TCR interaction with superantigen. Exotoxins produced by certain bacterial strains are capable of activating all T cells bearing particular TCR Vβ regions irrespective of their ligand specificity. Superantigens can influence the T cell repertoire by causing intrathymic deletion of entire Vβ families [81], or they may interact with peripheral T cells, causing activation followed by deletion and anergy [82].

4. Suppression

Another mechanism whereby self tolerance may be maintained is through suppression of autoreactive cells. This has been demonstrated by adoptive transfer studies in which T cells from tolerant animals were able to transfer tolerance to naive recipients when coinjected with specific antigen [83–85] (Figure 7). This suppression may be mediated by cytokines such as IL-4 or IL-10 or via competition for local cytokines by the suppressive T cells. The effect of competition for cytokines has been demonstrated *in vitro* using anergic T-cell clones that inhibited antigen-specific and allospecific T-cell proliferation by competing for the APC surface and for locally produced IL-2 [86]. There are other data to suggest that potentially autoreactive T cells that have escaped thymic deletion may be suppressed by regulatory T-cell subsets [87,88]. In many rodent models, the regulatory cells appear to be of a Th2 phenotype (they produce IL-4, IL-5, IL-10 and induce B-cell differentiation) [89]. This may be of significance in bone marrow transplantation as it has been suggested that successful outcome after grafting is correlated with the development of a Th2-type response [90].

In summary, deletion of autoreactive T cells in the thymus is the major

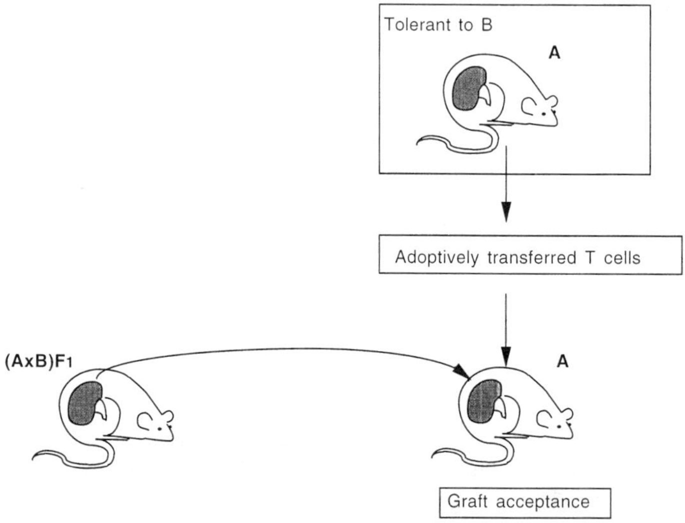

Figure 7 Adoptive transfer of tolerance. T cells from a tolerant animal are able to transfer specific tolerance to a naive animal when injected together with alloantigen. If T cells are taken from an animal of strain A, which is tolerant to a renal allograft of strain B, then a graft from an (A $\times$ B) F_1 donor is not rejected even in the absence of immunosuppression.

mechanism for the establishment of self tolerance, but there are additional peripheral mechanisms that are important for the maintenance of tolerance. Knowledge of the mechanisms that underlie self tolerance in mature peripheral T cells is crucial to the understanding of how the immune system may be manipulated to induce tolerance to allografts.

VII. ALLOGRAFT TOLERANCE

Since the introduction of more effective immunosuppressive drugs, there has been a marked improvement in allograft survival. Despite this, the rate of allograft rejection remains relatively high, with the loss of 10–20% of kidney grafts in the first year alone [91]. Additionally, immunosuppressive therapy is relatively nonspecific and is associated with a number of complications, such as infection and malignancy. Thus there is a search for strategies to favor specific allograft tolerance to improve this situation.

As mentioned above, the mechanisms of self tolerance provide a useful model to understand tolerance to allografts. However, there are several important differences between the two. Unlike a self antigen present throughout T-cell ontogeny, an allograft presents an abrupt challenge to the immune system. Furthermore, the number of potentially alloreactive T cells in the normal repertoire is much greater than conventional antigen-specific T-cell numbers, as discussed above.

A. Central Mechanisms

Central mechanisms of tolerance play less of a role in allotolerance as compared with self tolerance. There are occasions, however, where transplantation tolerance may result from intrathymic clonal deletion. This is demonstrated in the situation of allogeneic bone marrow chimeras formed by reconstituting lethally irradiated rodents with allogeneic bone marrow [92]. In such models, these allogeneic chimeras are tolerant to both donor and recipient antigens *in vitro* and *in vivo*. Resistance to bone marrow engraftment, which is largely T-cell mediated, is overcome by total-body irradiation, and depleting the marrow of T cells prior to transplantation prevents GVHD. There are probably two mechanisms of tolerance induction in this model. First, donor bone marrow cells repopulate the thymus and induce intrathymic deletion of T cells reactive to donor antigens. Second, tolerance to recipient antigens must be mediated by thymic epithelial cells, and this may involve the induction of anergy [93]. A problem that arises in systems of this type is that, since T cells are selected in the thymus for self-MHC restriction, once the T cells are exported, they will then recognize only foreign antigen efficiently when presented by recipient APCs. However, the majority of peripheral APCs in allogeneic bone marrow chimeras will be of donor origin. Therefore, in these chimeras, peripheral APC–T cell interactions are poor and the host is immunologically compromised [94].

This last problem seems to have been overcome by reconstituting the recipient with a mixture of recipient and donor bone marrow to create a mixed bone marrow chimera [95]. This permits recipient APCs to remain in the periphery and abrogate problems with T cell–APC interactions. Donor-specific marrow infusion has been reported to improve renal allograft survival rates from a 1-year survival rate of 71 to 90% [96] and rejection-free graft survival appeared to correlate with the presence of allogeneic chimerism [97].

A more direct route to induce tolerance via thymic clonal deletion is to inject donor cells directly into the recipient thymus during a period of transient immunosuppression. This has been used successfully with pancreatic islet transplants [98], although tolerance was incomplete, as the islet recipients could reject a skin graft from the same donor, which then caused rejection of the transplanted islets [99].

B. Peripheral Mechanisms

Although intrathymic presentation of alloantigen seems to be an important feature of bone marrow transplants, it is less likely to be the main mechanism whereby allotolerance may be induced. However, it is possible for donor antigens to be shed and to travel to the thymus either via the circulation or in association with recipient APCs. Indeed there has been the suggestion that graft acceptance depends on a state of mixed chimerism in the recipient and the graft mediated by mutual host-graft leukocyte interactions [100]. However, whether this chimerism is the cause of graft acceptance or the consequence of it is difficult to determine.

An important concept to consider is the difference between antigenicity and immunogenicity. Antigenicity means that a graft displays antigens that can be recognized by the host immune system, whereas immunogenicity means that those antigens can elicit an immune response. As discussed above, tolerogenic mechanisms usually require the interaction of TCRs with MHC-peptide, so that donor-specific tolerance requires an antigenic stimulus. However, allogeneic MHC molecules, while being antigenic, are not necessarily immunogenic, as has been discussed in the context of the two-signal model of T-cell activation. One approach to inducing donor-specific tolerance is therefore to reduce the immunogenicity of the graft in some way so as to induce a state of alloreactive T-cell anergy.

One strategy to reduce immunogenicity of an allograft is to remove donor-derived professional APCs, as previously discussed. This can be achieved by a period of *in vitro* or *in vivo* culture prior to transplantation. Once transplanted, the host T cells would encounter only alloantigens presented by graft parenchymal cells, which—lacking costimulatory molecules, such as B7—would anergize these T cells. This effect has been demonstrated in murine thyroid [39] and islet-cell grafts [101]. Additionally, in a rat model, renal allografts that are transplanted under immunosuppressive cover are not rejected after cessation of immunosuppression. These grafts may then be retransplanted into a syngeneic naive recipient without immunosuppression in certain strain combinations (Figure 8) [102]. While the graft is ''parked'' in the original recipient, donor passenger leukocytes are replaced by those from the recipient. Attempts to translate these findings into clinical transplantation by depletion of dendritic cells using monoclonal antibodies have so far been disappointing [103].

Another way to induce anergy or nonresponsiveness in alloreactive T cells is to block the delivery of costimulation by APCs. Several studies have shown that blocking the interactions of adhesion molecules at the time of grafting can induce graft-specific unresponsiveness [104]. Additionally, antibodies to CD4 can prolong the survival of allografts [105], either by inducing T-cell anergy or by favoring the development of Th2-type T cells.

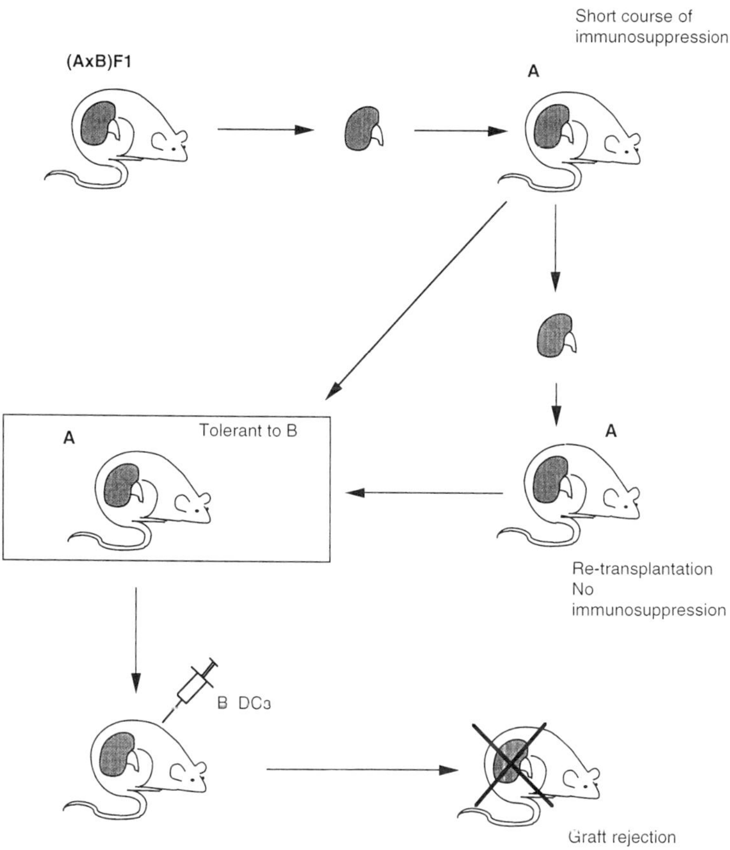

Figure 8 Renal allografts transplanted under a short course of immunosuppression are not rejected after immunosuppression is withdrawn. After retransplantation into a naive syngeneic recipient in the absence of further immunosuppression, the allograft is not rejected because passenger leukocytes within the graft have been replaced by those from the first recipient. Furthermore, infusion of allogeneic dendritic cells (DCs) into the recipient of a retransplanted allograft causes prompt rejection of the allograft.

As the importance of the B7/CD28 interaction has become more apparent, blocking of this receptor-ligand pair with the soluble recombinant fusion protein CTLA4-Ig has been shown to induce allospecific tolerance in a variety of experimental systems [106,107]. Furthermore, simultaneous blocking of another important costimulatory pathway, the CD40-CD40L interaction, has been able to prolong the survival of cardiac allografts indefinitely in mice [108].

VIII. CONCLUSION

In summary, it is well established that alloantigens evoke vigorous immune responses from the host. The molecular basis of allorecognition has been discussed with reference to both major and minor histocompatibility antigens. The greater understanding of self tolerance and the induction of tolerance to allografts should allow for more precisely targeted immunosuppression, with concomitant reduction of unwanted and sometimes fatal side effects.

REFERENCES

1. Ford D, Burger D. Precursor frequency of antigen-specific T cells: effects of sensitization in vivo and in vitro. Cell Immunol 1983; 79:334–344.
2. Lindahl KF, Wilson DB. Histocompatibility antigen-activated cytotoxic T lymphocytes: II. Estimates of the frequency and specificity of precursors. J Exp Med 1977; 145:508–522.
3. Zinkernagel RM, Callahan GN, Althage A, Cooper S, Klein PA, Klein J. On the thymus in the differentiation of "H-2 self-recognition" by T cells: evidence for dual recognition? J Exp Med 1978; 147:882–896.
4. Zinkernagel RM, Doherty PC. The discovery of MHC restriction. Immunol Today 1997; 18:14–17.
5. Zinkernagel RM, Doherty PC. Immunological surveillance against altered self components by sensitised T lymphocytes in lymphocytic choriomeningitis. Nature 1974; 251:547–548.
6. Bevan MJ. High determinant density may explain the phenomenon of alloreactivity. Immunol Today 1984; 5:128–130.
7. Matzinger P, Bevan MJ. Hypothesis: why do so many lymphocytes respond to major histocompatibility antigens? Cell Immunol 1977; 29:1–5.
8. Ajitkumar P, Geier SS, Kesari KV, Borriello F, Nakagawa M, Bluestone JA, Saper MA, Wiley DC, Nathenson SG. Evidence that multiple residues on both the alpha-helices of the class I MHC molecule are simultaneously recognized by the T cell receptor. Cell 1988; 54:47–56.
9. Clayberger C, Rosen M, Parham P, Krensky AM. Recognition of an HLA public determinant (Bw4) by human allogeneic cytotoxic T lymphocytes. J Immunol 1990; 144:4172–4176.
10. Hogan KT, Clayberger C, Bernhard EJ, Walk SF, Ridge JP, Parham P, Krensky AM, Engelhard VH. A panel of unique HLA-A2 mutant molecules define epitopes recognized by HLA-A2-specific antibodies and cytotoxic T lymphocytes. J Immunol 1989; 142:2097–2104.
11. Grandea AG IIIrd, Bevan MJ. Single-residue changes in class I major histocompatibility complex molecules stimulate responses to self peptides. Proc Natl Acad Sci USA 1992; 89:2794–2798.
12. Parham P, Clayberger C, Zorn SL, Ludwig DS, Schoolnik GK, Krensky AM. Inhi-

bition of alloreactive cytotoxic T lymphocytes by peptides from the alpha 2 domain of HLA-A2. Nature 1987; 325:625–628.
13. Schneck J, Maloy WL, Coligan JE, Margulies DH. Inhibition of an allospecfic T cell hybridoma by soluble class I proteins and peptides: estimation of the affinity of a T cell receptor for MHC. Cell 1989; 56:47–55.
14. Lombardi G, Barber L, Sidhu S, Batchelor JR, Lechler RI. The specificity of alloreactive T cells is determined by MHC polymorphisms which contact the T cell receptor and which influence peptide binding. Int Immunol 1991; 3:769–775.
15. Elliott TJ, Eisen HN. Cytotoxic T lymphocytes recognize a reconstituted class I histocompatibility antigen (HLA-A2) as an allogeneic target molecule. Proc Natl Acad Sci USA 1990; 87:5213–5217.
16. Heath WR, Kane KP, Mescher MF, Sherman LA. Alloreactive T cells discriminate among a diverse set of endogenous peptides. Proc Natl Acad Sci USA 1991; 88: 5101–5105.
17. Townsend A, Ohlen C, Bastin J, Ljunggren HG, Foster L, Karre K. Association of class I major histocompatibility heavy and light chains induced by viral peptides. Nature 1989; 340:443–448.
18. Engelhard VH. Structure of peptides associated with class I and class II MHC molecules. Annu Rev Immunol 1994; 12:181–207.
19. Eckels DD, Gorski J, Rothbard J, Lamb JR. Peptide-mediated modulation of T-cell allorecognition. Proc Natl Acad Sci USA 1988; 85:8191–8195.
20. Rock KL, Benacerraf B. Selective modification of a private I-A allo-stimulating determinant(s) upon association of antigen with an antigen-presenting cell. J Exp Med 1984; 159:1238–1252.
21. Schendel DJ. On the peptide model of allorecognition: cytotoxic T lymphocytes recognize an alloantigen encoded by two HLA-linked genes. Hum Immunol 1990; 27:229–239.
22. Sherman LA. Mutationally derived H-2 antigenic differences as defined by cytolytic T lymphocyte clones. J Immunol 1981; 127:1259–1260.
23. Essaket S, Fabron J, de Preval C, Thomsen M. Corecognition of HLA-A1 and HLA-DPw3 by a human CD4+ alloreactive T lymphocyte clone. J Exp Med 1990; 172:387–390.
24. Lombardi G, Sidhu S, Batchelor JR, Lechler RI. Allorecognition of DR1 by T cells from a DR4/DRw13 responder mimics self-restricted recognition of endogenous peptides [published erratum appears in Proc Natl Acad Sci USA 1989; 86:10074]. Proc Natl Acad Sci USA 1989; 86:4190–4194.
25. Dellabona P, Wei BY, Gervois N, Benoist C, Mathis D. A single amino acid substitution in the A^k molecule fortuitously provokes an alloresponse. Eur J Immunol 1991; 21:209–213.
26. Hunt HD, Pullen JK, Dick RF, Bluestone JA, Pease LR. Structural basis of Kbm8 alloreactivity: amino acid substitutions on the beta-pleated floor of the antigen recognition site. J Immunol 1990; 145:1456–1462.
27. Mattson DH, Shimojo N, Cowan EP, Baskin JJ, Turner RV, Shvetsky BD, Coligan JE, Maloy WL, Biddison WE. Differential effects of amino acid substitutions in the beta-sheet floor and alpha-2 helix of HLA-A2 on recognition by alloreactive viral peptide-specific cytotoxic T lymphocytes. J Immunol 1989; 143:1101–1107.

28. Bernhard EJ, Le AX, Yannelli JR, Holterman MJ, Hogan KT, Parham P, Engelhard VH. The ability of cytotoxic T cells to recognize HLA-A2.1 or HLA-B7 antigens expressed on murine cells correlates with their epitope specificity. J Immunol 1987; 139:3614–3621.
29. Heath WR, Sherman LA. Cell-type-specific recognition of allogeneic cells by alloreactive cytotoxic T cells: a consequence of peptide-dependent allorecognition. Eur J Immunol 1991; 21:153–159.
30. Koller TD, Clayberger C, Maryanski JL, Krensky AM. Human allospecific cytolytic T lymphocyte lysis of a murine cell transfected with HLA-A2. J Immunol 1987; 138:2044–2049.
31. Lombardi G, Sidhu S, Lamb JR, Batchelor JR, Lechler RI. Co-recognition of endogenous antigens with HLA-DR1 by alloreactive human T cell clones. J Immunol 1989; 142:753–759.
32. Heath WR, Hurd ME, Carbone FR, Sherman LA. Peptide-dependent recognition of H-2K^b by alloreactive cytotoxic T lymphocytes. Nature 1989; 341:749–752.
33. Weber DA, Terrell NK, Zhang Y, Strindberg G, Martin J, Rudensky A, Braunstein NS. Requirement for peptide in alloreactive CD4+ T cell recognition of class II MHC molecules. J Immunol 1995; 154:5153–5164.
34. Lechler R, Lombardi G. Structural aspects of allorecognition. Curr Opin Immunol 1991; 3:715–721.
35. Kisielow P, von Boehmer H. Development and selection of T cells: facts and puzzles. Adv Immunol 1995; 58:87–209.
36. George A, Dazzi F, Lynch J, Sidhu S, Marelli F, Batchelor RJ, Lombardi G, Lechler RI. Biased TCR gene usage in alloreactive T cells specific for a structurally dissimilar MHC alloantigen. Int Immunol 1994; 6:1785–1790.
37. Shoskes DA, Wood KJ. Indirect presentation of MHC antigens in transplantation. Immunol Today 1994; 15:32–38.
38. Lechler RI, Batchelor JR. Restoration of immunogenicity to passenger cell-depleted kidney allografts by the addition of donor strain dendritic cells. J Exp Med 1982; 155:31–41.
39. Lafferty KJ, Cooley MA, Woolnough J, Walker KZ. Thyroid allograft immunogenicity is reduced after a period in organ culture. Science 1975; 188:259–261.
40. Lafferty KJ, Bootes A, Dart G, Talmage DW. Effect of organ culture on the survival of thyroid allografts in mice. Transplantation 1976; 22:138–149.
41. Auchincloss H Jr, Sultan H. Antigen processing and presentation in transplantation. Curr Opin Immunol 1996; 8:681–687.
42. Auchincloss H, Jr., Lee R, Shea S, Markowitz JS, Grusby MJ, Glimcher LH. The role of ''indirect'' recognition in initiating rejection of skin grafts from major histocompatibility complex class II-deficient mice. Proc Natl Acad Sci USA 1993; 90: 3373–3377.
43. Sayegh MH, Perico N, Gallon L, Imberti O, Hancock WW, Remuzzi G, Carpenter CB. Mechanisms of acquired thymic unresponsiveness to renal allografts: thymic recognition of immunodominant allo-MHC peptides induces peripheral T cell anergy. Transplantation 1994; 58:125–132.
44. Bailey DW. Genetics of histocompatibility in mice: I. New loci and congenic lines. Immunogenetics 1975; 2:249–256.
45. van Els CA, Bakker A, Zwinderman AH, Zwaan FE, van Rood JJ, Goulmy E.

Effector mechanisms in graft-versus-host disease in response to minor histocompatibility antigens: I. Absence of correlation with cytotoxic effector cells. Transplantation 1990; 50:62–66.

46. van Els CA, Bakker A, Zwinderman AH, Zwaan FE, van Rood JJ, Goulmy E. Effector mechanisms in graft-versus-host disease in response to minor histocompatibility antigens: II. Evidence of a possible involvement of proliferative T cells. Transplantation 1990; 50:67–71.
47. Bevan MJ. The major histocompatibility complex determines susceptibility to cytotoxic T cells directed against minor histocompatibility antigens. J Exp Med 1975; 142:1349–1364.
48. Gordon RD, Simpson E, Samelson LE. In vitro cell-mediated immune responses to the male specific(H-Y) antigen in mice. J Exp Med 1975; 142:1108–1120.
49. Loveland BE, Simpson E. The non-MHC transplantation antigens reviewed: neither weak nor minor. Immunol Today 1986; 7:223–229.
50. Antoniou A, McCormick D, Scott D, Yeoman H, Chandler P, Mellor A, Dyson J. T cell tolerance and activation to a transgene-encoded tumor antigen. Eur J Immunol 1996; 26:1094–1102.
51. Hederer RA, Chandler PR, Dyson PJ, Antoniou AN, Millrain MM, Mellor AL, Simpson E, Robinson PJ. Acceptance of skin grafts between mice bearing different allelic forms of beta 2-microglobulin. Transplantation 1996; 61:299–304.
52. Rotzschke O, Falk K, Wallny HJ, Faath S, Rammensee HG. Characterization of naturally occurring minor histocompatibility peptides including H-4 and H-Y. Science 1990; 249:283–287.
53. Simpson E, Roopenian D. Minor histocompatibility antigens. Curr Opin Immunol 1997; 9:655–661.
54. Pion S, Fontaine P, Desaulniers M, Jutras J, Filep JG, Perreault C. On the mechanisms of immunodominance in cytotoxic T lymphocyte responses to minor histocompatibility antigens. Eur J Immunol 1997; 27:421–430.
55. Nevala WK, Wettstein PJ. The preferential cytolytic T lymphocyte response to immunodominant minor histocompatibility antigen peptides. Transplantation 1996; 62:283–291.
56. Wang W, Meadows LR, den Haan JM, Sherman NE, Chen Y, Blokland E, Shabanowitz J, Agulnik AI, Hendrickson RC, Bishop CE, Hunt DF, Goulmy E, Engelhard VH. Human H-Y: a male-specific histocompatibility antigen derived from the SMCY protein. Science 1995; 269:1588–1590.
57. den Haan JM, Sherman NE, Blokland E, Huczko E, Koning F, Drijfhout JW, Skipper J, Shabanowitz J, Hunt DF, Engelhard VH, Goulmy E. Identification of a graft versus host disease-associated human minor histocompatibility antigen. Science 1995; 268:1476–1480.
58. Goulmy E, Schipper R, Pool J, Blokland E, Falkenburg JH, Vossen J, Grathwohl A, Vogelsang GB, van Houwelingen HC, van Rood JJ. Mismatches of minor histocompatibility antigens between HLA-identical donors and recipients and the development of graft-versus-host disease after bone marrow transplantation. N Engl J Med 1996; 334:281–285.
59. Kappler JW, Roehm N, Marrack P. T cell tolerance by clonal elimination in the thymus. Cell 1987; 49:273–280.
60. Kisielow P, Bluthmann H, Staerz UD, Steinmetz M, von Boehmer H. Tolerance

in T-cell-receptor transgenic mice involves deletion of nonmature CD4+8+ thymocytes. Nature 1988; 333:742–746.
61. Marrack P, Lo D, Brinster R, Palmiter R, Burkly L, Flavell RH, Kappler J. The effect of thymus environment on T cell development and tolerance. Cell 1988; 53: 627–634.
62. Ashton Rickardt PG, Bandeira A, Delaney JR, Van Kaer L, Pircher HP, Zinkernagel RM, Tonegawa S. Evidence for a differential avidity model of T cell selection in the thymus. Cell 1994; 76:651–663.
63. Hogquist KA, Jameson SC, Heath WR, Howard JL, Bevan MJ, Carbone FR. T cell receptor antagonist peptides induce positive selection. Cell 1994; 76:17–27.
64. Sebzda E, Wallace VA, Mayer J, Yeung RS, Mak TW, Ohashi PS. Positive and negative thymocyte selection induced by different concentrations of a single peptide. Science 1994; 263:1615–1618.
65. Liu CP, Parker D, Kappler J, Marrack P. Selection of antigen-specific T cells by a single IE^k peptide combination. J Exp Med 1997; 186:1441–1450.
66. Goverman J, Woods A, Larson L, Weiner LP, Hood L, Zaller DM. Transgenic mice that express a myelin basic protein-specific T cell receptor develop spontaneous autoimmunity. Cell 1993; 72:551–560.
67. Jenkins MK, Pardoll DM, Mizuguchi J, Chused TM, Schwartz RH. Molecular events in the induction of a nonresponsive state in interleukin 2–producing helper T-lymphocyte clones. Proc Natl Acad Sci USA 1987; 84:5409–5413.
68. Jenkins MK, Schwartz RH. Antigen presentation by chemically modified splenocytes induces antigen-specific T cell unresponsiveness in vitro and in vivo. J Exp Med 1987; 165:302–319.
69. Lo D, Burkly LC, Flavell RA, Palmiter RD, Brinster RL. Antigen presentation in MHC class II transgenic mice: stimulation versus tolerization. Immunol Rev 1990; 117:121–134.
70. Bal V, McIndoe A, Denton G, Hudson D, Lombardi G, Lamb J, Lechler R. Antigen presentation by keratinocytes induces tolerance in human T cells. Eur J Immunol 1990; 20:1893–1897.
71. Van Gool SW, Vandenberghe P, de Boer M, Ceuppens JL. CD80, CD86 and CD40 provide accessory signals in a multiple-step T-cell activation model. Immunol Rev 1996; 153:47–83.
72. Perkins D, Wang Z, Donovan C, He H, Mark D, Guan G, Wang Y, Walunas T, Bluestone J, Listman J, Finn PW. Regulation of CTLA-4 expression during T cell activation. J Immunol 1996; 156:4154–4159.
73. Marelli Berg FM, Hargreaves RE, Carmichael P, Dorling A, Lombardi G, Lechler RI. Major histocompatibility complex class II-expressing endothelial cells induce allospecific nonresponsiveness in naive T cells. J Exp Med 1996; 183:1603–1612.
74. Lombardi G, Arnold K, Uren J, Marelli Berg F, Hargreaves R, Imami N, Weetman A, Lechler R. Antigen presentation by interferon-gamma-treated thyroid follicular cells inhibits interleukin-2 (IL-2) and supports IL-4 production by B7-dependent human T cells. Eur J Immunol 1997; 27:62–71.
75. Croft M, Bradley LM, Swain SL. Naive versus memory CD4 T cell response to antigen: memory cells are less dependent on accessory cell costimulation and can respond to many antigen-presenting cell types including resting B cells. J Immunol 1994; 152:2675–2685.

76. Sloan Lancaster J, Evavold BD, Allen PM. Induction of T-cell anergy by altered T-cell-receptor ligand on live antigen-presenting cells. Nature 1993; 363:156–159.
77. Evavold BD, Allen PM. Separation of IL-4 production from Th cell proliferation by an altered T cell receptor ligand. Science 1991; 252:1308–1310.
78. Moskophidis D, Lechner F, Pircher H, Zinkernagel RM. Virus persistence in acutely infected immunocompetent mice by exhaustion of antiviral cytotoxic effector T cells. Nature 1993; 362:758–761.
79. Rocha B, Grandien A, Freitas AA. Anergy and exhaustion are independent mechanisms of peripheral T cell tolerance. J Exp Med 1995; 181:993–1003.
80. Bertolino P, Heath WR, Hardy CL, Morahan G, Miller JF. Peripheral deletion of autoreactive CD8+ T cells in transgenic mice expressing H-2K^b in the liver. Eur J Immunol 1995; 25:1932–1942.
81. White J, Herman A, Pullen AM, Kubo R, Kappler JW, Marrack P. The V beta-specific superantigen staphylococcal enterotoxin B: stimulation of mature T cells and clonal deletion in neonatal mice. Cell 1989; 56:27–35.
82. Hewitt CR, Lamb JR, Hayball J, Hill M, Owen MJ, O'Hehir RE. Major histocompatibility complex independent clonal T cell anergy by direct interaction of Staphylococcus aureus enterotoxin B with the T cell antigen receptor. J Exp Med 1992; 175:1493–1499.
83. Batchelor JR, Phillips BE, Grennan D. Suppressor cells and their role in the survival of immunologically enhanced rat kidney allografts. Transplantation 1984; 37:43–46.
84. Kilshaw PJ, Brent L, Pinto M. Suppressor T cells in mice made unresponsive to skin allografts. Nature 1975; 255:489–491.
85. Tilney NL, Graves MJ, Strom TB. Prolongation of organ allograft survival by syngeneic lymphoid cells. J Immunol 1978; 121:1480–1482.
86. Lombardi G, Sidhu S, Batchelor R, Lechler R. Anergic T cells as suppressor cells in vitro. Science 1994; 264:1587–1589.
87. Tung KS. Mechanism of self-tolerance and events leading to autoimmune disease and autoantibody response. Clin Immunol Immunopathol 1994; 73:275–282.
88. Asano M, Toda M, Sakaguchi N, Sakaguchi S. Autoimmune disease as a consequence of developmental abnormality of a T cell subpopulation. J Exp Med 1996; 184:387–396.
89. Fowell D, Mason D. Evidence that the T cell repertoire of normal rats contains cells with the potential to cause diabetes: characterization of the CD4+ T cell subset that inhibits this autoimmune potential. J Exp Med 1993; 177:627–636.
90. Imami N, Brookes PA, Lombardi G, Hakooz B, Johns M, Goldman JM, Batchelor JR, Lechler RI, Ritter MA. Association between IL-4 producing T lymphocyte frequencies and reduced risk of graft-versus-host disease. Transplantation. 1998; 65: 979–988.
91. Lechler R, Gallagher RB, Auchincloss H. Hard graft? Future challenges in transplantation. Immunol Today 1991; 12:214–216.
92. Rayfield LS, Brent L. Tolerance, immunocompetence, and secondary disease in fully allogeneic radiation chimeras. Transplantation 1983; 36:183–189.
93. Schonrich G, Momburg F, Hammerling GJ, Arnold B. Anergy induced by thymic medullary epithelium. Eur J Immunol 1992; 22:1687–1691.
94. Zinkernagel RM, Althage A, Callahan G, Welsh RM Jr. On the immunocompetence

of H-2 incompatible irradiation bone marrow chimeras. J Immunol 1980; 124: 2356–2365.
95. Ildstad ST, Sachs DH. Reconstitution with syngeneic plus allogeneic or xenogeneic bone marrow leads to specific acceptance of allografts or xenografts. Nature 1984; 307:168–170.
96. Barber WH, Mankin JA, Laskow DA, Deierhoi MH, Julian BA, Curtis JJ, Diethelm AG. Long-term results of a controlled prospective study with transfusion of donor-specific bone marrow in 57 cadaveric renal allograft recipients. Transplantation 1991; 51:70–75.
97. McDaniel DO, Naftilan J, Hulvey K, Shaneyfelt S, Lemons JA, Lagoo Deenadayalan S, Hudson S, Diethelm AG, Barber WH. Peripheral blood chimerism in renal allograft recipients transfused with donor bone marrow. Transplantation 1994; 57: 852–856.
98. Posselt AM, Barker CF, Tomaszewski JE, Markmann JF, Choti MA, Naji A. Induction of donor-specific unresponsiveness by intrathymic islet transplantation. Science 1990; 249:1293–1295.
99. Posselt AM, Naji A, Roark JH, Markmann JF, Barker CF. Intrathymic islet transplantation in the spontaneously diabetic BB rat. Ann Surg 1991; 214:363–371.
100. Starzl TE, Demetris AJ, Murase N, Thomson AW, Trucco M, Ricordi C. Donor cell chimerism permitted by immunosuppressive drugs: a new view of organ transplantation. Immunol Today 1993; 14:326–332.
101. Lacy PE, Davie JM, Finke EH. Prolongation of islet allograft survival following in vitro culture (24 degrees C) and a single injection of ALS. Science 1979; 204: 312–313.
102. Batchelor JR, Welsh KI, Maynard A, Burgos H. Failure of long surviving, passively enhanced kidney allografts to provoke T-dependent alloimmunity: I. Retransplantation of (AS X AUG)F1 kidneys into secondary AS recipients. J Exp Med 1979; 150:455–464.
103. Brewer Y, Palmer A, Taube D, Welsh K, Bewick M, Bindon C, Hale G, Waldmann H, Dische F, Parsons V, Snowden S. Effect of graft perfusion with two CD45 monoclonal antibodies on incidence of kidney allograft rejection. Lancet 1989; 2: 935–937.
104. Isobe M, Yagita H, Okumura K, Ihara A. Specific acceptance of cardiac allograft after treatment with antibodies to ICAM-1 and LFA-1. Science 1992; 255:1125–1127.
105. Alters SE, Shizuru JA, Ackerman J, Grossman D, Seydel KB, Fathman CG. Anti-CD4 mediates clonal anergy during transplantation tolerance induction. J Exp Med 1991; 173:491–494.
106. Baliga P, Chavin KD, Qin L, Woodward J, Lin J, Linsley PS, Bromberg JS. CTLA4Ig prolongs allograft survival while suppressing cell-mediated immunity. Transplantation 1994; 58:1082–1090.
107. George AJ, Ritter MA, Lechler RI. Disease susceptibility, transplantation and the MHC. Immunol Today 1995; 16:209–211.
108. Larsen CP, Elwood ET, Alexander DZ, Ritchie SC, Hendrix R, Tucker Burden C, Cho HR, Aruffo A, Hollenbaugh D, Linsley PS, Winn KJ, Pearson TC. Long-term acceptance of skin and cardiac allografts after blocking CD40 and CD28 pathways. Nature 1996; 381:434–438.

3
Experimental Animal Models in the Study of GVL Reactions

Robert L. Truitt and Bryon D. Johnson
Medical College of Wisconsin
Milwaukee, Wisconsin

Robert Korngold and Robert Townsend
Jefferson Medical College
Philadelphia, Pennsylvania

Bruce R. Blazar
University of Minnesota
Minneapolis, Minnesota

I. INTRODUCTION: THE CAPACITY OF THE DONOR TO DESTROY RESIDUAL LEUKEMIA CELLS BY THE REACTION OF IMMUNITY—AND PERHAPS ALSO THE HOST

The hypothesis that bone marrow transplantation (BMT) can provide an effective antileukemia reaction was tested in experimental models during the very earliest days of BMT research. Barnes and coworkers [1], in their 1956 paper entitled "Treatment of Murine Leukaemia with X Rays and Homologous Bone Marrow," described the potential and problems of using allogeneic BMT for the treatment of leukemia in this way:

> When mice are given an otherwise lethal dose of x rays to the whole body they can recover if injected intravenously with homologous [allogeneic] myeloid cells. . . . This suggests that leukemia of the mouse might be successfully treated. On the one hand, the dose of x rays which is sufficiently lethal to normal cells of the bone marrow and lymphatic tissues to cause death of

> the animal might well be completely lethal to leukemic cells. . . . On the other hand, if the dose of x rays sufficient to kill the animal is not 100% lethal to leukemic cells, the malignant condition would in these circumstances recur by growth from the surviving cells, since neither host not graft has the ability to resist; but, if homologous bone marrow from a different strain of mouse were given, the colonizing cells might retain the capacity of the donor to destroy by the reaction of immunity these residual leukemic cells—and perhaps also the host.

The immunological antitumor component of allogeneic BMT came to be known as the ''graft-versus-leukemia'' (GVL) effect, but as predicted by Barnes and colleagues, allogeneic BMT was often associated with a lethal ''secondary syndrome,'' which we now know as ''graft-versus-host disease'' (GVHD). In some animal models, the GVL effect could not be distinguished from the GVH reaction, while in others the two were separable. It was postulated that either distinct and, therefore, separable effector cells were responsible for GVL and GVH reactions or that the same effector cells with differing thresholds of reactivity against leukemic and normal host cells mediated the preferential killing of leukemia [2,3]. If distinct effector cells are responsible for GVL and GVH reactions, then the reactions are potentially separable. If the same effector cells are involved in both but exhibit differing thresholds of reactivity against normal and malignant cells, then alternative strategies are necessary to separate GVL and GVH reactivity.

Only recently, with the advent of new technologies for manipulating antihost and antitumor immune reactions in vivo and ex vivo, has the successful clinical use of GVL reactivity become a reality. Experimental animal models contributed significantly to this success and will continue to be valuable tools for exploring new approaches and establishing biological principles. For this chapter, investigators from three laboratories, whose work has been instrumental in establishing and testing the principles of GVL and GVH reactivity, were asked to review their work using animal models to study GVL reactions.

II. MANIPULATION OF GVH REACTIVITY TO OBTAIN A GVL EFFECT AFTER MHC-MATCHED ALLOGENEIC BONE MARROW TRANSPLANTATION

A. Introduction

For the past two decades, our laboratory has investigated the relationship between the GVL and GVH reactions in murine models of allogeneic BMT. This relationship continues to be controversial. However, with dissection of clinical GVHD at the cellular and molecular levels and emergence of new technologies, strategies to modulate the syndrome without loss of the beneficial GVL reaction have evolved. In the first section of this chapter, we present an overview of experimental strategies that we have used in various attempts to prevent GVHD without loss of the GVL effect in a murine model of MHC-matched allogeneic BMT. Figure 1 summarizes the effector mechanisms leading to GVHD in this model and some of the strategies that we have evaluated.

B. Tumor Model: Acute T-Cell Lymphoblastic Leukemia in AKR Mice

The tumor model used in these studies is the acute T-lymphoblastic leukemia (AKR-L) which develops spontaneously in AKR ($H2^k$) mice at approximately 8 months of age [4]. Recombination between endogenous ecotropic and xenotropic murine leukemia viruses (MuLV) leads to the production of a duotropic retrovirus that is leukemogenic. Spontaneously arising AKR leukemia develops as a thymoma and is weakly immunogenic. AKR mice, as well as other high-leukemia-incidence strains of the $H2^k$ haplotype, develop little or no antiviral CTL activity [5,6]. Quantitative reductions of the MHC-restriction elements as well as qualitative alterations of other cell-surface molecules are thought to impair T-cell reactivity against spontaneous AKR leukemias [7]. AKR-L is a useful tumor model for the study of GVL effects that are dominated by reactivity against minor histocompatibility antigens (miHA) rather than MuLV or leukemia-associated antigens.

C. B10.BR → AKR Chimeras as a Model for MHC-Matched, Unrelated Allogeneic BMT

1. Role of CD4 and CD8 T cells in GVHD and GVL Reactivity

Donor B10.BR and host AKR mice differ at multiple miHA as well as MHC class IB molecules encoded within the Tla/Qa region. MLR reactivity is one-way in the GVH (B10.BR anti-AKR) direction and strongly influenced by the $Mls\text{-}1^a$ superantigen expressed by AKR mice. The incidence and intensity of GVHD in B10.BR → AKR chimeras depends upon the number of mature T cells transplanted with the donor marrow inoculum, but other factors such as the conditioning regimen also affect the outcome [8]. The severity of GVHD is directly proportional to number of CD4+ T cells present in the marrow inoculum [2]. T cells expressing the Vβ6 TCR dominate the antihost reactive donor T-cell population in this donor/host combination. CD8+ B10.BR cells contribute to GVHD in AKR hosts, but they are dependent on CD4+ T cells to provide help. Depletion of CD4+ T cells alone is sufficient to eliminate lethal GVHD in this model [2]. Presensitization of the B10.BR donor to AKR alloantigen, however, results in activation of CD8+ T-cell clones capable of causing GVHD indepen-

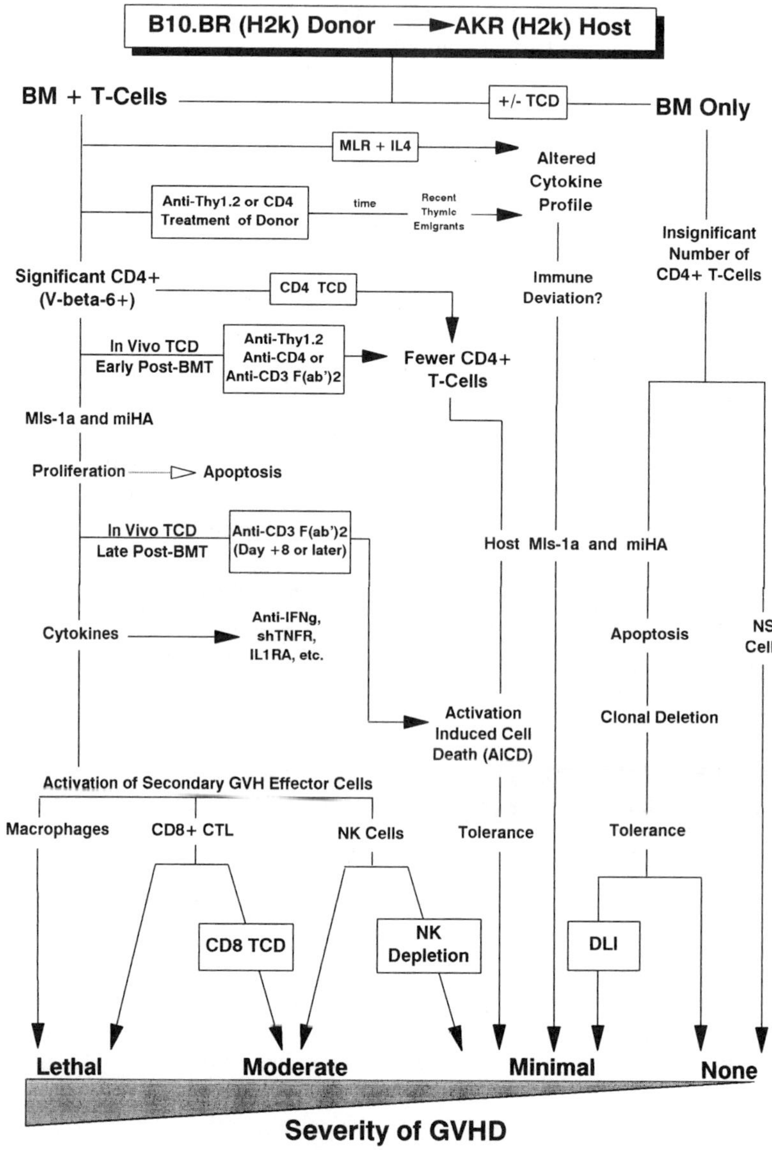
B10.BR (H2k) Donor → AKR (H2k) Host
BM + T-Cells
+/- TCD
BM Only
MLR + IL4
Altered Cytokine Profile
Anti-Thy1.2 or CD4 Treatment of Donor
time
Recent Thymic Emigrants
Insignificant Number of CD4+ T-Cells
Significant CD4+ (V-beta-6+)
CD4 TCD
Immune Deviation?
In Vivo TCD Early Post-BMT
Anti-Thy1.2 Anti-CD4 or Anti-CD3 F(ab')2
Fewer CD4+ T-Cells
Mls-1a and miHA
Proliferation
Apoptosis
In Vivo TCD Late Post-BMT
Anti-CD3 F(ab')2 (Day +8 or later)
Host Mls-1a and miHA
Cytokines
Anti-IFNg, shTNFR, IL1RA, etc.
Apoptosis
NS Cells
Activation Induced Cell Death (AICD)
Clonal Deletion
Activation of Secondary GVH Effector Cells
Macrophages
CD8+ CTL
NK Cells
Tolerance
Tolerance
CD8 TCD
NK Depletion
DLI
Lethal
Moderate
Minimal
None
Severity of GVHD

dent of CD4 help [2]. Using MoAb to deplete CD4 and CD8 subsets in vivo, we found that the early phase of GVH reactivity is CD4-mediated, while later phase appears to be CD8-mediated [2]. CD8+ T cells are essential for elimination of residual host cells and for establishment of complete donor chimerism in this model [8,9]. In the absence of CD8+ T cells, the transplanted mice become stable mixed donor/host T-cell chimeras.

Optimal GVL reactivity in B10.BR/AKR chimeras is dependent on the presence of both CD4 and CD8 T cells [9]. The antileukemic reaction is directed toward host miHA and class IB MHC molecules [10]. Presensitization of donors to host alloantigens (alloimmunization) can enhance the antileukemic effect by increasing the CTL precursor frequency [10]. Cloned CTL reactive to AKR miHA [10] and to Qal^b molecules [11] can mediate a GVL effect in vivo. GVHD was induced in AKR mice after injection of a single H2K-restricted miHA-specific CTL clone, indicating that clonal activation of donor T cells to a single immunodominant miHA can lead to lethal GVHD [10]. The miHA-specific CTL provided a GVL effect, but with GVHD as a complication. Cytolytic activity of host-specific T-cell clones in vitro did not correlate with induction of GVHD after adoptive transfer in vivo, suggesting that other functional properties of the T cells (probably cytokine secretion) are critical for induction of the GVH syndrome [11].

2. NK Cells in GVHD and GVL Reactivity

We have also shown that donor NK cells can be both helpful and harmful to the host. Donor NK cells contribute to ''early'' GVL reactivity, whereas GVL reactivity at a ''later'' stage post-BMT is dominated by T cells, and depletion of NK

Figure 1 Schematic representation of the effector mechanisms responsible for GVHD in a murine model of MHC-matched, miHA-mismatched BMT (B10.BR → AKR) and strategies that have been evaluated in attempts to minimize GVHD without loss of the beneficial GVL reactivity. In this model, the incidence and intensity of GVHD is dependent on the number of donor CD4 T cells in the marrow inoculum. Other GVH effector cells and cytokines play secondary roles. Strategies that have been tested and are discussed in the first section of this chapter include (A) pan T–cell depletion of the donor marrow; (B) CD4 T–subset depletion; (C) CD8 T–subset depletion; (D) depletion of donor NK cells; (E) immune deviation through the use of RTE in vivo or IL-4 in vitro to polarize donor T-helper cells; (F) use of T cell–specific MoAbs in vivo to prevent or treat GVHD and induce tolerance; and (G) donor leukocyte infusions (DLI) post-BMT. Strategies to block macrophages and/or inflammatory cytokines are not discussed here, but have been studied by others.

cells has little effect on GVL reactivity [2]. Depletion of donor NK cells significantly increases the survival rate of hosts with mild-to-moderate GVHD without compromising either donor T-cell engraftment [12] or late GVL reactivity [2]. We attribute the improved survival rate to elimination of NK-mediated immunodeficiency, which manifests itself clinically as GVH-associated mortality. NK cells may also suppress GVL reactivity. Using the B10.BR/AKR model, we found that depletion of CD4 T cells resulted in loss of GVL reactivity despite the presence of alloreactive CD8 T cells (Figure 2). When we increased the number of transplanted CD4-depleted, CD8-replete spleen cells, we did not observe an increase in leukemia-free survival [13]. However, when donor NK cells were depleted, there was a significant increase in leukemia-free survival in MHC-matched chimeras given CD4-depleted cells (Figure 2). Thus, NK cells are duplicitous. They provide beneficial GVL reactivity during the early stages after BMT, but they subsequently suppress GVL reactivity and contribute to GVH pathology. It is not clear whether separate NK subsets are responsible for these distinct effects in vivo.

Collectively, our results support a three-compartment model of GVL/GVH reactivity in B10.BR/AKR chimeras in which CD4+, CD8+ and NK cells are highly interactive. In addition to being multicompartmental, GVL/GVH reactiv-

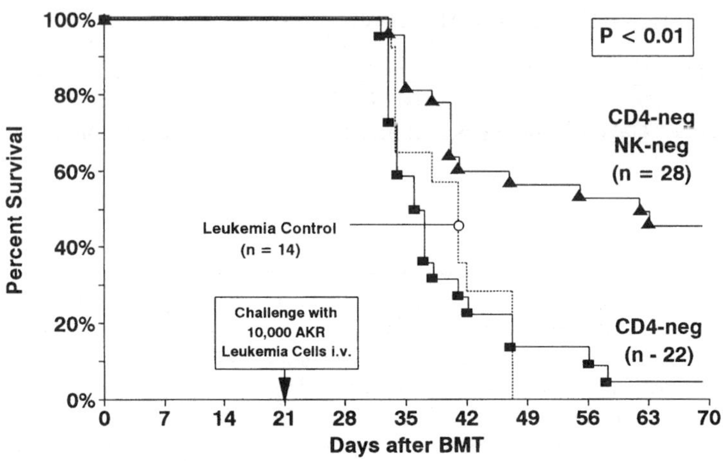

Figure 2 GVL reactivity of donor CD8+ T-cells in MHC-matched B10.BR → AKR chimeras is negatively regulated by donor NK cells in the absence of CD4+ T-helper cells. B10.BR donor mice were depleted of CD4+ T cells alone (CD4-neg) or along with NK1.1+ cells (CD4-neg, NK-neg) by injection of MoAb in vivo. Chimeras were given BM plus 25 × 10^6 spleen cells on day +0 and then challenged with a supralethal dose of AKR leukemia on day +21. Leukemia controls are normal AKR hosts.

ity in this donor/host combination is dynamic with effector cells and their functions changing over time.

3. Macrophages, Inflammatory Cytokines, and GVHD

We have not specifically examined the role of macrophages in the pathology of GVHD in our chimeras. However, Ferrara and colleagues [14,15] using another MHC-matched BMT model, B10.BR → CBA, have shown that macrophages and proinflammatory cytokines, especially IL-1 and TNF-α, contribute significantly to the GVH syndrome. A direct role for macrophages in antileukemic reactivity has not been documented, but they may influence GVL reactivity (positively or negatively) by altering the immunological milieu in which the leukemia must survive.

4. Immune Deviation to Prevent GVHD Without Loss of GVL Reactivity

During the course of studies on the role of CD4+ T cells in GVHD, we observed that spleen cells taken from donors that had been CD4-depleted (CD4 TCD) with MoAb in vivo and then allowed to repopulate their spleens for a short time with newly emigrating thymocytes (RTE or recent thymic emigrants), did not cause GVHD when transplanted into susceptible hosts [2]. More importantly, there was a significantly higher GVL effect when the spleen cells were taken from donors that had been allowed to repopulate for a limited time as compared to CD4-depleted donors that had not yet repopulated their spleens (55 versus 22% leukemia-free survival, $p = 0.03$) [2].

The RTE found in the spleen arose de novo in the donor thymus, since thymectomized B10.BR donors failed to repopulate their spleens [16]. The CD4+ RTE were hyporesponsive to alloantigen stimulation with MHC or miHA disparate cells; however, they proliferated and secreted cytokines in response to TCR cross-linking with immobilized anti-CD3 MoAb [16]. CD4+ RTE exhibited diminished expression of CD45RB. With time, the splenic CD4+ T cells reacquired alloreactivity, and there was a temporal relationship between re-expression of CD45RB and restoration of alloreactivity. The CD8+ T cells in these CD4 TCD/repopulated spleen cells donors were normal, but they proliferated in vitro only when the CD4+ T cells were functional (i.e., capable of secreting IL-2) [16].

CD4+ RTE may be anergic by virtue of their maturational state or they may be highly susceptible to induction of tolerance once in the periphery. Charlton et al. [17] found that single positive CD4+ RTE taken from the thymus are capable of causing GVHD. We also found that single positive CD4+ T cells taken from the repopulating thymus of CD4 TCD donors were responsive to alloantigen; however, single positive CD4+ T cells taken from the spleen of the same donor did not respond to host antigen in vitro. This suggests that a peripheral mechanism may be involved in inducing anergy in CD4+ RTE as suggested by Alters et al. [18].

CD4+ RTE cells are thought to be Th0-type cells capable of secreting large amounts of IL-4, IL-5, γ-IFN, and IL-10 [19]. In the periphery they differentiate into Th1-type cells in the absence of IL-4, but exposure to IL-4 is thought to drive their differentiation toward the type 2 cytokine pathway. We speculate that IL-4 in the BMT recipient is responsible for the diminished GVH reactivity of CD4+ RTE cells. The source of IL-4 in the host following BMT is not yet known, but we are testing the hypothesis that donor-derived NK-1.1+ CD3+ T cells are responsible. NK-1.1+ T cells produce large quantities of IL-4 (as well as γ-IFN, IL-5, and IL-10 but little or no IL-2) [20], have been shown to promptly produce IL-4 in response to in vivo challenge with anti-CD3 MoAb, and are $CD45RB^{dull}$ [21]. IL-4 skews the functional activity of peripheral T-helper and T-cytotoxic subsets, a phenomenon referred to variously as ''immune deviation'' or ''polarization.'' Ferrara and colleagues [22] report that GVHD is significantly diminished when donor T cells are polarized toward type 2 cytokines, and Fowler et al. [23,24] exploited this phenomenon to prevent GVH reactivity while retaining GVL reactivity of donor T cells. Thus, immune deviation in some form may prove to be a useful strategy for separating GVHD from GVL reactivity.

5. Tolerance Induction with MoAb In Vivo

Ex vivo depletion of donor T cells is an effective way to prevent GVHD, although its impact on clinical GVL reactivity has been variable [25,26]. Therefore, we decided to examine the use of monoclonal antibodies (MoAbs) specific for Thy-1.2, CD4, CD8, and CD3 in vivo post-BMT to prevent and to treat GVHD [2]. Pan T–cell depletion with anti-Thy-1.2 MoAb was effective at preventing acute GVHD in B10.BR/AKR chimeras, but T subset–specific MoAbs had only transient effects. Anti-CD3 MoAb (clone 145 2C11, a hamster IgG which recognizes the ε chain of the murine TCR complex [27]) effectively prevented acute GVHD, but it induced an acute and lethal T cell–dependent ''cytokine syndrome'' in both syngeneic (AKR → AKR) and allogeneic (B10.BR → AKR) chimeras. Therefore, all experiments were done with nonmitogenic anti-CD3 $F(ab')_2$ fragments. Others have demonstrated that anti-CD3 $F(ab')_2$ fragments induce a selective T-helper dysfunction in vivo [28] and modulate GVHD after MHC-mismatched murine BMT [29,30], but no one had evaluated the in vivo effect of anti-CD3 $F(ab')_2$ antibody on GVL reactivity.

Anti-CD3 $F(ab')_2$ MoAb prevented lethal GVHD in MHC-matched B10.BR → AKR chimeras in a dose- and time-dependent manner [31]. Injection of antibody every 2 days for 20 days completely abrogated clinical symptoms of GVHD, and treated chimeras could not be distinguished from BM controls.

A "short course" of anti-CD3 $F(ab')_2$ (five infusions) was sufficient to prevent lethal GVHD. Fewer infusions with the same total amount of antibody resulted in diminished capacity to prevent GVHD, indicating that duration of treatment was more important than dose of antibody once a threshold was passed. Anti-Thy MoAb also was effective at preventing GVHD [2], but it was less effective at reversing established GVHD (i.e., when given several days after transplantation) [13].

Antibody-treated mice became complete donor T cell chimeras, whereas untreated chimeras given BM alone were mixed donor/host T-cell chimeras. MLR activity and TCR cross linking with immobilized MoAb were used to assess tolerance induction after antibody treatment [2]. Responses to Vβ6 MoAb are informative because Vβ6+ T cells respond to the Mls 1^a superantigen on AKR cells, and GVHD in this model correlates with the number of Vβ6+ cells given.

Cells from chimeras given BM only (GVH-negative controls) showed a transient response to Vβ6 cross linking 2–8 weeks posttransplant, but no clinical GVHD. Mature donor-educated Vβ6+ cells in the periphery were eventually exhausted, and T cells produced de novo in the host thymus failed to respond to Vβ6 crosslinking or to AKR alloantigens in MLR. BM-only chimeras have little GVL reactivity and showed mixed donor-host chimerism in the spleen [8,9]. There was a correlation between the response to immobilized Vβ6 MoAb and resistance to leukemia challenge. However, to detect this low level of GVL reactivity, the dose of leukemia had to be reduced to a minimal level, i.e., the magnitude of the GVL effect was small. When the Vβ6-responsive T cells were exhausted, the BM-only chimeras were no longer able to mount an effective response against the leukemia. Clonal exhaustion of GVL reactive T-cell populations, whether specific for the leukemia or host miHA, may account for late relapse if the host is not "cured" before this occurs. Some leukemias have been shown to persist in a sustained dormant state (e.g., Ref. 32), and we have shown that even strong GVL reactivity can be lost over time [33]. Reemergence of leukemia late after transplant may be influenced in part by loss of antileukemic reactive cells. However, strategies to deal with late relapse, such as donor leukocyte infusions (DLI), have been developed and used in experimental models and clinical settings to treat late relapse. These are described in more detail later in this chapter. A critical issue in the success of such strategies is the susceptibility of the leukemia to GVL effector T cells.

Anti-CD3 $F(ab')_2$ treated B10.BR/AKR chimeras given BM plus spleen cells and tested >8 weeks post-BMT responded to Vβ6 cross linking, indicating that Vβ6+ donor T cells were not clonally deleted. However, the duration of anti-CD3 $F(ab')_2$ treatment influenced the extent of Vβ6 deletion. Chimeras given a "short course" of anti-CD3 $F(ab')_2$ (5 infusions) responded to Vβ6 MoAb, while chimeras given a "long course" (14 infusions) did not.

Tolerance induction with MoAb prevents GVHD, but such strategies must be evaluated in terms of their impact on GVL reactivity as well. We examined the effect of tolerance-induction with anti-CD3 $F(ab')_2$ antibody on GVL reactivity directed against miHA antigens (i.e., allospecific GVL) in B10.BR/AKR chimeras [31]. Leukemia-bearing AKR mice were given B10.BR BM plus spleen cells and 50 μg of anti-CD3 $F(ab')_2$ antibody as either a single intraperitoneal (IP) injection on day 0 or as 3 or 5 injections given every other day. Leukemic mice given the least immunosuppressive regimen (50 μg × 1) survived leukemia-free, but analysis of individual chimeras showed that they had experienced GVHD based on splenic atrophy with few B cells [31]. In contrast, chimeras given the same amount of anti-CD3 $F(ab')_2$ antibody over an 8-day period (10 μg × 5) did not show significant clinical symptoms of GVHD but relapsed with leukemia. The third group of chimeras given three infusions of antibody did not develop clinically evident GVHD and survived leukemia-free. Flow cytometric analysis of their spleens indicated that they were complete donor T cell chimeras with normal sized spleens and B-cell content. These experiments demonstrate that GVHD can be regulated without loss of the GVL effect through the use of MoAb administered after allogeneic BMT. However, they also show that excessive or ill-timed MoAb administration can eliminate GVL reactivity.

In an effort to enhance the GVL reactivity following a tolerance-inducing regimen of anti-CD3 $F(ab')_2$ MoAb, we delayed infusion for 8 days [31]. We hypothesized that donor T cells allowed to recognize and react to alloantigens on normal and leukemic AKR tissues for 8 days would be more effective in mediating the GVL effect, but that GVHD could still be treated. In the antibody-treated groups, none of the mice developed GVHD, but 83% of the mice relapsed within 50 days of transplant. In contrast, none of the mice treated with anti-CD3 $F(ab')_2$ between 8 and 16 days relapsed. Quantitative analysis of the GVL response in leukemia dose–response assays established that delayed administration of anti-CD3 $F(ab')_2$ MoAb resulted in a 150% increase in the minimum lethal dose (MLD) of leukemia over that which could be eliminated when antibody was given prophylactically [31]. The GVL reaction in anti-CD3 $F(ab')_2$-treated chimeras was at least two orders of magnitude above that of chimeras given antibody and BM only. However, the MLD was below that of untreated chimeras, indicating that the GVL response was diminished but not abolished by anti-CD3 $F(ab')_2$ treatment.

Of significant note in these studies of MoAb-induced donor/host tolerance were the sites of leukemia relapse and the phenotype of the tumors that recurred. Relapsing antibody-treated chimeras often developed lymphomas in extra-lymphoid tissues, including the liver, limbs, neck, face, and along the spine in various animals. Almost all of the animals that relapsed were complete donor T-cell chimeras, and some had no evidence of leukemia in their spleens when tested by PCR/SSOPH using leukemia-specific primers and probes. While the tumors grew slowly and in discrete nodules in the B10.BR/AKR chimeras, they grew rapidly and were widely distributed after transfer to normal AKR mice. Some recurrent tumors in antibody-treated chimeras were infiltrated with donor CD4 and CD8 T cells (up to 23% in one chimera). These results suggest that the GVL reaction in extralymphoid tissues may not be sufficient to eliminate all tumor cells and that tumoristatic mechanisms limit progression of the tumors in the tolerant chimeras. Leukemia cells from antibody-treated (tolerant) chimeras often showed phenotypic changes, including loss of CD4 and, in some cases, CD3 expression. Thy 1.1 and $H2^k$ expression usually remained stable. These phenotypic changes were associated with the transplantation of donor T cells and did not occur in chimeras given BM alone. Alloactivated donor T cells may have created an immunological milieu in these chimeras that fostered change or immunoselection of leukemia variants. The changes were maintained when the cells were transferred to normal AKR hosts. Detection of the Y chromosome by PCR/SSOPH analysis confirmed that the cells were derived from the injected (male) leukemia and did not arise de novo in the transplanted (female) mice. Whether the altered cell-surface properties render the leukemia cells more resistant to GVL effector cells remains to be determined.

6. Donor Leukocyte Infusions Post-BMT

Early experimental data suggested that GVHD was less severe when the donor T cells were infused at later times after BMT (reviewed in Ref. 34). Because of early success with clinical application of DLI therapy [35], we used our B10.BR $\rightarrow$ AKR murine model of MHC-matched BMT to test strategies for avoiding GVHD while still providing a GVL effect by late infusion of donor leukocytes [34,36,37]. AKR hosts given B10.BR BM plus 30×10^6 spleen cells at the time of BMT developed lethal GVHD; hosts given BM only did not develop GVHD but did not show any significant GVL reactivity. When the spleen cells infusion was delayed until at least 21 days after BMT, few mice showed signs of clinical GVHD and 96% survived long-term. Importantly, the mice that developed into complete donor T-cell chimeras were able to resist a leukemia challenge. Infusion of cells before 21 days was associated with increased likelihood of GVHD, but multiple doses and incremental doses of spleen cells could be given without evidence of GVHD if infused beyond 21 days. DLI with spleen cells from donors that were presensitized to host alloantigens caused chronic rather than acute GVHD.

The frequency of anti–host specific cytotoxic (CTL) and IL-2-secreting T-helper cells in chimeras infused with spleen cells 21 days post-BMT was quantified by LDA assays and compared with that of controls given BM alone or BM plus the same spleen inoculum on day +0 [37]. The frequency of T-helper cells in chimeras given DLI was significantly lower than that for BM and spleen cells on day +0, but within the 95% confidence intervals of estimates for controls given BM only. CTL frequencies were intermediate between controls given BM only or BM plus spleen cells on day +0. Thus, delayed infusion of donor spleen cells appeared to minimize the effect of T-helper cells without suppression of CTL activity. We have confirmed the hyporesponsiveness of CD4+ T cells to IL-2 and host alloantigen in DLI chimeras using quantitative flow cytometry [38]. The mechanism by which anergy was induced in infused CD4+ T cells remains to be determined; however, recent experiments using an MHC-mismatched DLI model (C57BL/6 into AKR) suggest a role for donor-derived Thy-1+ suppressor cells [39].

In contrast to the anergic T cells in BM-only chimeras, T cells from DLI chimeras responded to TCR cross-linking with immobilized anti-Vβ6 MoAb and to host alloantigen in MLR assays [37], suggesting that graft-host tolerance was broken by DLI. More importantly, the persistence of anti–host-reactive donor T cells correlated with a long-term GVL effect that was still present at 100 days post-BMT despite a decrease in GVHD. GVL reactivity was higher with multiple spleen cells infusions and with greater donor-host genetic disparity (i.e., haplotype mismatch) [34,36,37].

In a recent study, we evaluated the use of DLI as a means to restore the GVL reactivity lost as a consequence of using anti-CD3 $F(ab')_2$ to induce tolerance and prevent GVHD in B10.BR/AKR chimeras [3]. Induction of donor-host tolerance was confirmed by loss of response to Vβ6 TCR cross linking and anti-host MLR reactivity. Antibody-treated chimeras were given no further treatment (negative controls) or infused with an additional 20×10^6 donor spleen cells on day +21, and all groups were challenged with 1,000 AKR-M2 leukemia cells on day +28. Antibody-treated chimeras that were not given DLI all died with leukemia; however, 54% of the antibody-treated chimeras given DLI survived >100 days after leukemia challenge ($p < 0.05$). These experimental results indicate that it is possible to induce tolerance in order to avoid lethal GVHD and to restore GVL reactivity using DLI therapy in the event of leukemia relapse at a later time.

D. Summary

The GVL effect is often associated with GVHD in both acute and chronic leukemias. However, the presence of GVHD does not guarantee an antileukemic effect and the absence of GVHD does not necessarily mean the absence of a GVL effect. GVL/GVH reactivity is influenced by the immunogenetic relationship between the BM donor and recipient as well as by the immunobiology of the leukemia itself. Strategies designed to prevent or modulate GVHD must be carefully assessed for their impact on leukemia relapse. Mixed chimerism and donor-host tolerance are manifestations of immunological reactivity between donor and host that can significantly affect relapse after BMT. Whether an effective (curative), ineffective (relapse), or inefficient (cytostatic) GVL reaction develops in the presence or absence of GVHD may depend partly on the number and nature of GVL/GVH effector and regulatory systems activated post-BMT. DLI in both the clinical and experimental setting has provided the most dramatic example of successful manipulation of GVL/GVH reactivity, but it is not without complications. It is critical that we understand the immunological cells and cytokines involved, how they interact, and how they are affected by pre- and post-BMT manipulations if we are to continue to improve long-term disease-free survival in leukemia patients.

III. PRECLINICAL STUDIES OF DONOR LEUKOCYTE INFUSIONS (DLI) FOR THE TREATMENT OF ACUTE MYELOGENOUS LEUKEMIA (AML) AFTER BMT

A. Introduction

Although relapse rates after histocompatible sibling donor BMT for AML are 10–30% for patients transplanted in first complete remission, relapse rates range from 36–57% in patients transplanted in relapse or in second remission (reviewed in Refs. 40–42). Intensive chemotherapy regimens typically used to induce AML patients into complete remission are likely to be poorly tolerated, especially early after BMT. Alternative therapies for AML patients who relapse post-BMT are clearly needed.

One such approach relies upon the recognition of antigens present on AML cells by donor immune effector cells. The administration of IL-2 has been used to prolong remission following relapse, indicating that immune effector cells are capable of reducing AML tumor burden [43]. After autologous or allogeneic BMT, IL-2 infusions have been given to as consolidative therapy to prevent AML relapse [44–49]. Direct evidence for a cellular immune response to AML after allogeneic BMT is evident when comparing the relapse rates of patients receiving allogeneic to syngeneic donor BM (18 versus 59% relapse rates, respectively) [50]. Relapse rates also are significantly lower in patients that have acute and/or chronic GVHD as compared to those with no GVHD [25,51,52]. Collectively, these data indicate that immune responses to AML could be used as therapy for AML relapse or possibly as an adjunct preventive measure to reduce AML relapse post-BMT.

In another approach that exploits the susceptibility of AML cells to immune effector cells, DLI has been used to provide a GVL response to AML patients who relapse post-BMT. Complete remission rates are approximately 30% if DLI are given after prior chemotherapy induction and only 15% if no prior chemotherapy is used for remission induction [42,53–55]. In contrast to the higher remission rates and long-standing duration of such remissions typically observed in chronic myelogenous leukemia (CML) patients given DLI post-BMT, complete remissions in AML often do not exceed 2–3 years. For AML patients who relapse post-BMT, approaches designed to improve the extent and duration of remission induction are needed. To determine which factors limit the efficacy of adoptive immune therapy for AML treatment post-BMT, preclinical BMT model systems were required and have been established. Following a summary of the characterization of the immune response of AML cells in non-BMT mice, findings relevant to allogeneic or syngeneic BMT settings are discussed.

B. Tumor Model: Acute Myelogenous Leukemia in C57BL/6 Mice

As a representative example of some types of AML in humans, we chose to focus our studies on the immune response of mice to C1498 cells, a cell line that arose spontaneously in C57BL/6 (B6) mice in the 1940s. C1498 is reverse transcriptase–negative and does not express detectable amounts of cell surface p15 envelope protein [56]; therefore immune responses to C1498 are not likely to be related to endogenous retroviruses prevalent in the mouse but not the human genome. After intravenous (IV) injection, C1498 widely metastasizes in B6 mice [56]. Like human AML, C1498 infiltrates the marrow, liver, spleen, lymph nodes, kidney, ovary, skin, and central nervous system. Leukemia-induced mortality is dose-dependent: 10^6 (100% lethal by 1 month); 10^5 (100% lethal by 2 months); 10^4 (30% lethal); 10^3 (0% lethal). Immunohistochemistry and flow-cytometric analysis of C1498 has shown this tumor to be of myelomonocytic origin. C1498 is MHC class I+, II− and expresses several adhesion antigens including LFA-1 (CD11a), ICAM-1 (CD54), ICAM-2 (CD102), Mac-1 (CD11b), and Mac-3 (CD107b). Activated NK cells and CD8+ T cells are each capable of lysing C1498 tumor targets in vitro. Low doses of C1498 cells given in vivo are susceptible to NK-mediated resistance. As also observed in vitro, the in vivo blockade of LFA-1 interaction with C1498 cells is detrimental to immune recognition of C1498, such that mice given anti-LFA1 antibody are more susceptible to C1498 lethality than controls.

C. Effect of IL-2 and IL-2 Gene Transduction on CTL Response to AML

B6 mice exposed to higher doses of C1498 cells mount a poor anti-C1498 CTL response [56]. As compared with naive B6 controls, 3 weeks following IV administration of live C1498 cells, splenic pCTL frequencies to C1498 were noted to increase more than twofold despite the absence of morphologically or flow cytometry–detectable tumor cells. pCTL frequency to C1498 cells is increased sixfold and tumorigenicity is significantly reduced when IL-2 is provided as a paracrine growth factor by transducing C1498 with an IL-2 expressing retrovirus vector (65 versus 0% survival for control transductants) [56]. Based upon C1498 dose titration studies, tumorigenicity is reduced by approximately 10-fold by IL-2 gene transduction. Consistent with the pCTL data, depletion of CD8+ T cells significantly lowered resistance to C1498/IL-2 transductants. The IL-2 facilitated induction of pCTL was strong enough to partially cross-protect parental type C1498 cells: The co-administration of a lethal dose of IL-2 transduced C1498 with a lethal dose of control transductants conferred an improved survival compared to the infusion of control transduced C1498 cells alone (25 versus 0% survival, respectively). In contrast, the daily infusion of IL-2 delivered in a liposome vehicle at a dose of 25,000 units/day for 15 days did not significantly increase actuarial survival rates in these same studies. These data suggest that tumor delivery of IL-2 may provide higher levels or a more prolonged bioavailability of IL-2 at the site of immune response than achievable with relatively high doses of exogenous IL-2 given for 2 weeks.

Our data with IL-2 infusion in naive mice suggested that this mode of therapy would not drive a tumor-specific immune response sufficient to prevent tumor recurrence after syngeneic BMT. More impressive results for protecting mice against C1498 were obtained following immunization with irradiated tumor cells [56]. A potent CTL response to C1498 was demonstrated in mice that received subcutaneous (SQ) immunization with high doses (10^7) of irradiated C1498 cells. Splenic pCTL frequencies to C1498 cells often increase >15-fold and 90–100% of immunized mice will resist a lethal dose of C1498 cells (10^5) given 2 weeks after the first immunization. The immune response can be very long-lived (memory cell) such that 38% of immunized mice are completely resistant to challenge with a lethal dose (10^5) of live C1498 cells given over 1 year after initial immunization. From these studies, we hypothesize that the presence of sufficient numbers of C1498-reactive CTL could prevent tumor recurrence after syngeneic BMT.

D. Role of Costimulatory Molecules in CTL Response to AML

The occurrence of AML in patients prior to BMT indicates that the malignant AML blasts have successfully escaped immune surveillance mechanism(s) in the patient. The immune dysfunction early post-BMT, coupled with the relatively poor antitumor response observed in naive mice given IL-2 infusions stimulated us to investigate cellular infusional approaches to directly provide tumor-reactive CTL to BMT recipients. As proof in principle that early post-BMT adoptive immunotherapy could prevent AML induced lethality, C1498-reactive CD8+ CTL lines were generated for the purpose of adoptive transfer into syngeneic BMT recipients. Three weeks after SQ immunization with 10^6 live C1498 cells, draining lymph nodes were isolated as a source of C1498-reactive CTLs [57].

To facilitate induction of CTL formation, one group of mice was given C1498 cells that had been transduced with a retroviral vector which produces B7-1 (CD80) ligand. B7-1 binds to CD28, constitutively expressed on mouse T cells. MHC class I molecules, presumably containing tumor peptides, that are present on C1498 cells, ligate the T-cell receptor causing the triggering of a cascade of events including transcription of cytokine mRNA in the T cell. Productive T-cell responses require a second (costimulatory) signal, which can be delivered by the binding of B7 ligands on target cells or antigen-presenting cells to CD28 expressed on virtually all murine T cells. Because C1498 does not express B7 ligands, T cells encountering C1498 may not be optimally stimulated to generate a productive response, including CTL reactivity toward C1498. To determine whether the lack of B7-1 expression may be responsible in part for the relatively poor immune response to live C1498 cells, which was observed 3 weeks after initial inoculation as described above, C1498 were transduced with a B7-1 retroviral vector [57]. C1498 is of myelomonocytic origin. We have found that this cell line has the capacity to present antigens to T-cells. For example, C1498 can present tryptic digests of ovalbumin to an ovalbumin-reactive CD8+ CTL line that is dependent upon antigen-presenting cells (APCs) to present relevant antigens/peptides to maintain in vitro growth. Because of the APC capacity of this cell line, C1498 is an ideal tumor cell line for B7-1 transduction since the expression of B7-1 could permit C1498 to function as a bona fide APC for costimulation of C1498-specific CTL responses. After B7-1 retroviral-mediated gene transfer, a high level of B7-1 expression was achieved. C1498 B7-1 transductants had a >10-fold reduced tumorigenicity. Consistent with these data, Matulonis et al. [58,59] have also shown that the AML cell line, 32cDc113, when transformed with the p210 BCR/ABL oncogene and B7-1, can protect mice against wild-type tumor challenge and eradicate minimal residual disease.

Our data suggest that B7-1 transductants might serve as superior immunogens for the generation of CTL lines. Arceci and coworkers [60] have shown that irradiated B7-1 transductants of a radiation-induced AML cell line can confer long-lasting protective immunity when used as immunogens. When used as an immunogen for SQ immunization of B6 mice, B7-1 transductants but not parental cells permitted the generation of C1498-reactive CTL lines that could be propagated in bulk culture for an extended period of time [57]. Two of these three lines were cytolytic and one (termed T15) was selected for in-depth analysis. T15 preferentially lysed parental C1498 and C1498 B7-1 transductants but not other syngeneic tumor cells, including two hematopoietic lines FBL3 (erythroleukemia) and EL4 (T cell leukemia/lymphoma). As with T cells obtained from naive mice, the cytolysis of C1498 by these CTL lines was dependent upon the expression of both CD8 and LFA-1 antigens. Interestingly, T15 did not recognize lectin (concanavalin A) stimulated splenic blasts or CFU-GM progenitor cells from B6 mice, suggesting that T15 might be recognizing a very early hematopoietic differentiation antigen or a bona fide leukemia antigen.

E. GVL Responses to AML in Vivo

1. Syngeneic GVL Responses

To assess the capacity of C1498-reactive CTL cells to prevent AML recurrence in vivo after syngeneic BMT, lethally irradiated B6 recipients were infused IV with syngeneic BM seeded with C1498 cells at doses of 0.2, 0.6, or 2.0×10^5 cells [57]. All mice receiving no adoptive immune therapy died by 1 month post-BMT. A cohort of mice given T15 CTL cells on days 1, 8, and 15 post-BMT all survived for the 4-month observation period, while a cohort of mice receiving B6 spleen cells at the same daily dose of T15 CTL cells uniformly died by 5 weeks post-BMT. C1498 dose titration experiments showed that as few as 2×10^3 cells resulted in 66% lethality. All mice receiving C1498 cells at doses ranging from $2 \times 10^4 - 2 \times 10^6$ cells died by 5 weeks post-BMT. The administration of T15 CTL completely prevented C1498 induced lethality when 2×10^5 cells were infused and was 56% effective in preventing lethality following a dose of 2×10^6 C1498 cells. In contrast, T15 cell infusions were entirely ineffective in preventing the lethality induced by either FBL3 or EL4, consistent with the lack of cytolytic responses by T15 cells against either of these B6-derived hematopoietic tumor cells lines. A cohort of syngeneic BMT mice given 2×10^6 C1498 cells followed by the infusion of an ovalbumin-specific CD8+ CTL line derived from B6 mice (GX1) at the same dose and schedule as T15 CTL did not show an increase in actuarial survival rate. Together, these data indicate that the administration of AML-reactive CTL cells could be used as a means of preventing AML recurrence post-syngeneic BMT. Additional studies are needed to develop efficient strategies for the ex vivo generation of AML-reactive CTLs that are applicable to clinical trials.

2. Allogeneic GVL Response to AML and DLI Therapy to Avoid GVHD

AML cells are sensitive to CTL effector cells induced in vivo or infused after syngeneic BMT. In both instances, leukemia-reactive CTL cells are syngeneic to the AML cell line. For allogeneic BMT recipients, immune effector mechanism(s) are allogeneic to AML cells. In addition to the recognition of possible leukemia-specific antigens/peptides or hematopoietic differentiation antigens present on AML blasts allo-immune responses can be directed against miHA or MHC antigens present on AML cells. Falkenberg and colleagues have shown that AML reactive CTL can be generated in vivo against alloantigens (miHA antigens) and in some cases against putative leukemia-specific antigens or hematopoietically restricted differentiation antigens present on human AML cells [61–64].

Because C1498 is susceptible to CTL effector cells in vivo and complete remissions from DLI in AML are inferior to those in CML, we established an allogeneic DLI model system to further investigate the biology of the DLI-induced GVL response to allogeneic AML cells. The model is a modification of the one designed by Johnson and Truitt [36,37]. Lethally irradiated B6 recipients are given T cell–depleted MHC class I + II disparate B10.BR donor BM cells. On day 21 post-BMT, recipients are infused with donor splenocytes and one week later challenged with a supralethal dose of C1498 cells [65]. Recipients given C1498 (10^5) without donor splenocytes had a 3% survival rate, with 95% of deaths occurring within approximately 1 month after C1498 inoculation. AML was documented in 97% of recipients examined at the time of death. Recipients receiving donor splenocytes (50×10^6) on day 21 post-BMT followed by C1498 cells had a 45% actuarial survival rate at 6 months post-BMT. Only 16% of mice examined at the time of death had evidence of AML cells; the majority of the remaining mice had clinically significant GVHD. A third cohort of mice received a lower dose of donor splenocytes (15×10^6) on day 0 of BMT and were not subsequently challenged with C1498 cells. All of these mice died from GVHD. Collectively, these data indicated (1) that DLI can prevent death from AML post-BMT, albeit at the expense of GVHD-induced death in approximately one-half of treated mice and (2) that DLI are tolerated at far higher doses when administered 3 weeks post-BMT as compared to immediately post-BMT.

Patients that relapse post-BMT had existing disease at the time of DLI. It is possible that DLI needed to be administered for 1 week prior to C1498 challenge to permit sufficient in vivo activation of donor splenocytes for an effective anti-AML response. Experiments were performed to determine whether DLI could be given after C1498 challenge to simulate a setting of minimal residual disease such as occurs after BMT or consolidation chemotherapy in patients that relapse post-BMT. Recipients given C1498 cells on day 20 (or on day 17) before a day 21 post-BMT infusion of donor splenocytes had a significant survival benefit from the GVL effect of DLI. DLI treatment reduced the tumorigenicity of C1498 by > 10-fold such that 50% of DLI-treated recipients of 2×10^5 cells survived >3 months post-BMT versus only 10% of non-DLI treated recipients of 2×10^4 cells on day 20 post-BMT. These data indicate that effector cells do not need to be primed prior to AML challenge to mediate a significant GVL effect.

Because the relapse rates were only 16% in DLI treated recipients, this model system did not simulate the human clinical response. The model was modified by administering fewer splenocytes (25×10^6) and more C1498 cells (2×10^5), thereby reducing the effector: target ratio by fourfold. Recipients given

C1498 cells all succumbed with AML cells by 2 months post-BMT. DLI treatment resulted in a 23% actuarial survival rate at 8.5 months and 70% of recipients had AML cells at the time of death or elective sacrifice. Recipients given splenocytes without C1498 had a comparable actuarial survival rate as those not given C1498 indicating that the GVH side effects of DLI were considerable. T cell–subset depletion studies revealed that the GVL effector cells in this model are CD8+ T cells and that an optimum GVL effect required both CD4+ and CD8+ T cells.

CD4+ T cells cannot directly recognize C1498 which is MHC class II–negative. It is more likely that CD4+ T cells supported the expansion of alloreactive and/or C1498-reactive CD8+ T effector cells by recognition of host MHC class II–positive cells (e.g., residual host hematopoietic cells; activated endothelial cells). The target antigens in this situation are not known and include either alloantigens present on host tissue (or C1498 cells) or putative tumor antigens. Host MHC class II–positive target cells might include dendritic cells or activated B cells, both of which could serve as a source of host antigen for direct allorecognition. Donor CD4+ T cells could be stimulated to recognize C1498 peptide presented by donor BM-derived APC. In either instance, the costimulation of donor T cells by the target cells would facilitate a vigorous T-cell response.

F. Influence of CD28/B7 Interactions on GVL Response to AML in Vivo

Because CD28/B7 interaction is known to support T-cell expansion and generation of pCTL cells, experiments were performed to determine whether blockade of CD28/B7 interaction would interfere with the GVL effect to C1498. In earlier studies, we showed that the in vivo administration of anti-B7 MoAb is highly effective in preventing GVHD mediated by either CD4+ or CD8+ T cells, presumably by efficiently outcompeting CD28 for B7 ligands [66]. Anti-B7 MoAb given to DLI-treated recipients challenged with C1498 cells completely prevented the GVH side effect of donor splenocytes [65]. However, the GVL response was also entirely suppressed such that anti-B7 MoAb treated recipients all relapsed in a similar time course as anti-CD4+ CD8 MoAb treated recipients. These data show (1) that CD28/B7 binding facilitates the DLI mediated GVL effect against AML cells in this model and (2) that blockade of CD28/B7 interaction prevents the GVH side effect of DLI.

Despite the fact that DLI significantly reduced actuarial relapse rates, 70% of treated recipients eventually succumbed with AML. Moreover, there was no memory cell response in DLI treated recipients such that all mice rechallenged with C1498 after successfully completing DLI therapy developed AML within 80 days after rechallenge. We have previously shown that the transduction of C1498 with a B7-1 retroviral vector markedly reduced tumorigenicity and permitted the generation of CTL lines with reactivity against parental C1498 [57]. To determine whether the expression of B7-1 by AML cells would increase the likelihood of generating a productive DLI mediated immune response, C1498 B7-1 transductants were used instead of parental C1498 cells in the DLI model [65]. Under the same conditions which lead to a 70% incidence of AML at 8 months post-BMT in DLI treated recipients challenged with parental C1498 cells, none of the DLI treated recipients of C1498 B7-1 transductants had detectable AML cells present 11 months post-BMT. T cells were required for the GVL response against C1498 B7-1 transductants since anti-CD4+ anti-CD8 MoAb depleted DLI treated recipients all had detectable C1498 cells at the time of death. In contrast to results obtained in DLI treated recipients of parental cells, anti-CD8 MoAb treated recipients survived at least 300 days without AML cells. Despite the APC capacity of C1498 B7-1 transductants, the fact that CD4+ T cells were required for optimal GVL effect against C1498 B7-1 transductants implicates APCs as important facilitators of the GVL response. As was observed with parental C1498 cells, DLI treated recipients of C1498 B7-1 transductants had no memory cell response to C1498 cells upon rechallenge.

G. GVL Responses to Acute Lymphoblastic Leukemia (ALL)

ALL patients who relapse post-BMT have had a lower response rate to DLI therapy than patients with either acute or chronic myeloid leukemia. To determine whether T-ALL was susceptible to DLI, we used the same strain combination and conditions as for the C1498 studies. Recipients of high-dose DLI (50×10^6 cells) were given EL4, a T-ALL/lymphoma cell line syngeneic to B6 recipients, IP at various cell doses ranging from $3 \times 10^3 - 3 \times 10^6$ cells [65]. As few as 3×10^3 cells was lethal to 90% of untreated recipients. Although a GVL effect could be documented by statistical analysis at all EL4 doses tested, long-term survival did not exceed 10% except in DLI-treated recipients of the lowest dose of EL4 cells tested in this setting (3×10^4). These data are compatible with human clinical results and suggest that only under situations of minimal tumor burden are DLIs an effective form of therapy for recipients with ALL relapsing post-BMT.

The success of DLI therapy for the treatment of recipients of C1498 B7-1 transductants prompted the examination of EL4 B7 transductants in the DLI model system. DLI-treated (50×10^6 splenocytes) recipients of parental EL4 cells (3×10^6) had only a modest prolongation of actuarial survival rates as compared with controls, with recipients having detectable tumor by 2.5 months post-BMT. Recipients of EL4 B7-1 transductants had a low (6%) relapse rate. Ex vivo T-cell depletion of donor splenocytes did not adversely affect relapse rates after DLI. The immune response in naive B6 mice to this EL4 B7-1 transductant required mature donor T-cell infusion. Thus, our data are most consistent with the possibilities that the small numbers of residual T cells remaining after depletion could expand to sufficient levels to mediate a potent GVL effect. Alternatively, the low relapse rate was a consequence of in vivo immune effector cells present at the time of EL4 inoculation. In subsequent experiments, recipients were given DLI (25×10^6 cells), followed 12 days later by EL4 B7-1 transductants in doses ranging from $3 \times 10^4 - 3 \times 10^7$ cells [65]. Despite the lower DLI dose used in this studies, the relapse curves were consistent with a $\geq 3 \log_{10}$ cell elimination of EL4 B7-1 transductants by DLI. CD8+ T cells, but neither CD4+ T cells nor NK cells, were required for the GVL effect. Cumulatively, these data indicate that the expression of B7-1 on ALL cells markedly reduces tumorigenicity even in BMT recipients. The transduction of ALL cells with B7-1 could provide an important means of facilitating a GVL-mediated immune response to ALL cells after BMT.

H. GVHD as a Complication of DLI Therapy

The GVH related side effects of DLI in humans and rodents can be a significant cause of morbidity and mortality [35,53–55]. An important aspect of preclinical studies and clinical trials will be to identify approaches that inhibit the GVH side effect of DLI without impairing the GVL effect. The infusion of anti-B7 MoAb inhibits the costimulation of donor T cells capable of causing GVH as well as those capable of causing GVL [65]. Therefore, although anti-B7 MoAb was shown to prevent DLI-induced weight loss, anti-B7 MoAb-treated mice uniformly relapsed. Some pharmacological agents are also capable of inhibiting the generation of intracellular signaling events necessary for a productive T-cell response. One such agent is rapamycin (RAPA), a macrocylic lactone that inhibits T-cell function by blocking T-cell responses to lymphokines. RAPA is highly effective in reducing murine GVHD lethality in several donor-recipient strain combinations [67,68]. RAPA is currently being tested in patients for GVHD therapy post-BMT. The effect of RAPA on DLI-mediated GVL is unknown.

In recent studies, we have found that RAPA preferentially inhibits the expansion and GVH effects of two T-cell populations typically associated with CTL activity (CD8+ and TCR $\gamma\delta$+ T cells) although RAPA is less effective in inhibiting GVHD mediated by CD4+ T cells [69]. RAPA administration was associated with a profound reduction in the in vivo generation of donor T cells with a T helper type 1 (Th1)/T cytotoxic type I (Tc1) cell phenotype during a GVH response [69]. In the DLI model for AML, RAPA administration given at the time of DLI was highly beneficial in preventing the GVH side effect of DLI [69]. However, the GVL effects of DLI against C1498 cells were abolished. The RAPA-induced suppression of the GVL may be related to a shift away from a Th1/Tc1 phenotype (immune deviation). Alternatively, the fact that donor CD8+ T-cell expansion is especially sensitive to the inhibitory effects of RAPA may provide an explanation for the elimination of the DLI-mediated GVL effect against C1498 cells. These data are consistent with those of Fowler and Gress, who have shown that Tc1-mediated GVL is more potent than the Tc2-mediated GVL effect against myeloid leukemia in mice [24,70].

I. Summary

In summary, T-cell immune responses generated against AML cells can prevent tumor recurrence after either syngeneic or allogeneic BMT. Our experience to date shows that increasing CD28/B7 interaction is a potent means of generating a GVL response after BMT. Conversely, blocking CD28/B7 interactions reduces the GVH side-effects of allogeneic DLI but at the expense of relapse. New agents such as RAPA, which inhibit lymphokine mediated signaling events, abolish the GVH side effects of DLI but also eliminate the GVL effect. Preclinical studies in rodents will be important in the exploration of novel approaches to facilitate GVL responses and to address the limitations of allogeneic DLI therapy for the treatment of AML and other leukemias.

IV. SYNGENEIC AND ALLOGENEIC GVL RESPONSES TO ACUTE MYELOGENOUS LEUKEMIA

A. Tumor Model: MMB3.19 Myeloid Leukemia in C57BL/6 Mice

Murine models for the study of GVL responses to AML have been limited because of the few virus-induced stable AML lines available and the problems of associated live viral replication. Therefore, we sought to establish a model of myelogenous leukemia that would better reflect the immunogenicity of spontaneously arising leukemias which do not express viral proteins. We took advantage of a mouse retrovirus construct (pEVX-mycXH) recently developed by Baumbach et al. [71] that could efficiently transfer the c-*myc* protooncogene into myeloid series cells and thereby generate leukemia lines. The original construct involved the placement of the c-*myc* coding exons between two Moloney-MuLV LTRs in a plasmid configuration that allowed synthesis of a packageable, but defective, mouse retroviral RNA. This construct was then transfected into the j2 murine fibroblast cell line, which contained a nonpackageable helper MMLV provirus genome, forming the new j2myc8 cell line. This cell line in culture produces and releases into the supernatant ecotropic virus particles containing the pEVX-mycXH encoded RNA, which can then be converted to cDNA and integrated into the DNA of myeloid cells from bone marrow preparations in vitro [71]. Alternatively, the viral vector can be injected into mice IP with the potential to generate myeloid leukemias 2–5 months later, depending upon the strain of mice [72]. These myeloid leukemia cells have the pEVX-mycXH proviral genome, constitutively express c-*myc* but most notably do not produce any other detectable retrovirus components and cannot replicate the retroviral vector autonomously.

The MMB3.19 myeloid leukemia line was generated in C57BL/6 (B6) mice using this transfection approach, and the line was subsequently subcloned and carried in culture and/or by in vivo passage [73]. This adherent cell line is phenotypically composed of mature monocyte/macrophage-like cells that express Mac-1, Mac-2, F4/80, LFA-1, MHC class I and class II (I-A^b) but is negative for the B220 B-cell marker. Class II expression, which is constitutively low, can be upregulated by exposure to IFN-γ. In addition, MMB3.19 apparently expresses relevant B6 minor histocompatibility antigens (miHA), as these target cells can be lysed by C3H.SW anti-B6–specific (MHC-matched, miHA allogeneic) CTLs in vitro. The MMB3.19 leukemia line thus seemed suitable for further GVL studies.

It should be noted that in terms of establishing a model system, our intention was to investigate the potential of generating specific GVL activity to myeloid leukemias in the setting of either syngeneic or allogeneic bone marrow transplantation (BMT). The use of c-*myc* transformation or other oncogenes like *raf* [74] to generate a murine myeloid leukemia is likely to be similar to a spontaneous occurrence, particularly in relation to secondary and tertiary transformation events resulting in leukemogenesis [74–76]. It is these subsequent events involving inappropriate expression of normal genes that may lead to the expression of "leukemia antigens" that may be recognized by GVL-reactive T cells. Another interesting advantage of the c-*myc* myeloid leukemias is that they are heterogeneous in the phenotypes of myeloid cells generated. For example, in the A/J strain, it was found that c-*myc* myeloid lines, although all of mature phenotype, displayed different abilities to process Ag and had different levels of class II expression [72]. This heterogeneity provides the opportunity to study GVL responses under a variety of myeloid cell conditions that have never before been explored.

B. Syngeneic GVL Reactivity to MMB3.19 Myeloid Leukemia

Initially, dose titration experiments established that the intraperitoneal injection of 10^5 MMB3.19 cells into irradiated (850 cGy) B6 mice one day after transplantation with 2×10^6 syngeneic B6 T cell–depleted bone marrow cells (ATBM) yielded 100% mortality with a median survival time (MST) of 28 days. This time frame allowed for the development of GVL activity, and this dose of MMB3.19 cells was selected for use in all subsequent BMT experiments. In contrast to irradiated recipients, normal B6 mice were more resistant to the challenge of MMB3.19 cells. Greater than 5×10^6 cells were required to obtain high mortality with a median survival time (MST) of 34 days. The observation suggested that in normal mice there might be a radiosensitive immune component responsible for resistance.

To investigate the immunotherapeutic potential of syngeneic donor GVL activity (analogous to the use of autologous BMT), irradiated (850 cGy) B6 mice were transplanted with an inoculum of 2×10^6 syngeneic B6 ATBM, alone, or along with increasing dosages of a pooled population of B6 spleen and LN cells. The recipients were challenged a day later with 10^5 MMB3.19 cells, and it was found that a significant increase in survival (60%) could be achieved with the mice transplanted with $\geq 2.5 \times 10^7$ lymphocytes. Lymphocyte subset depletion experiments were performed to determine which subpopulations of cells were effective in the syngeneic GVL response. Donor spleen and LN cells were pretreated in vitro with MoAb specific for Thy1.2, CD4, or CD8 in the presence of complement (C). In addition, enriched T-cell populations were prepared by depleting B cells via panning techniques over goat-antimouse Ig-coated plates. Mice in the positive control ATBM group challenged with leukemia succumbed within 31 days post-transplant (MST of 19 days); the transplant of 2.5×10^7 untreated spleen and LN cells exhibited better survival (40%) with a significantly prolonged MST of 35 days ($p < 0.01$). Pretreatment of donor lymphocytes with anti-Thy1.2 MoAb plus C eliminated most of the resistance to leukemia challenge with 100% mortality and an MST of 26 days; however, some GVL activity was still observed. This GVL activity may be due to residual T cells or other non–T cell populations such as B cells, NK cells, and/or macrophages. Pretreatment of the donor cells with anti-CD4 MoAb plus C resulted in a significant prolongation of survival ($p < 0.01$) with an MST of 33 days, but there was still 100% fatality and the MST was significantly shorter than the mice injected with the untreated lymphocyte control ($p < 0.01$). Mice injected with donor lymphocytes, depleted of either CD8+ T cells or B cells, exhibited nearly as effective a resistance to leukemic challenge as those mice given the untreated lymphocytes, with MST values of 35 days (20% survival) and 33 days (30% survival), respectively. In summary, this experiment suggested that T cells were important for GVL activity, and that both CD4+ and CD8+ subsets could play a role in resistance, although CD4+ cells appeared more potent [73].

To confirm the role of T cells in GVL activity, titrated dosages of T cell–enriched B6 donor lymphocyte preparations were transplanted into the irradiated B6 recipients, and the hosts were challenged with 10^5 MMB3.19 leukemia cells. Mice given 2.5×10^7 B6 T cells exhibited substantial GVL activity with 60% of the mice surviving [73]. Lower doses of 1.25×10^7 and 2.5×10^6 T cells resulted in less survival (50 and 40%, respectively); 5×10^5 T cells had no significant effect on leukemia-free survival. Clearly, naive T cells could mediate GVL activity, but high numbers of T cells were needed to obtain the protective effect.

C. Enhancement of Syngeneic GVL Reactivity by Presensitization to Leukemia

GVL immunotherapeutic activity of donor T cells was significantly improved if the donor B6 mice were presensitized with an IP injection of 10^7 irradiated (3000 cGy) MMB3.19 cells 3 weeks before transplantation [73]. By day 65 posttransplant, the transfer of as few as 5×10^5 presensitized T cells along with ATBM resulted in 82% survival of the MMB3.19-challenged irradiated syngeneic recipients, and the fivefold higher dose of 2.5×10^6 T cells resulted in 100% survival (Figure 3). Results of gross autopsies of surviving mice also correlated with the dose of T cells transferred in that approximately 60% of the recipients of the two higher doses were completely tumor-free. The remaining mice exhibited small to medium-sized solid tumors localized to the site of injection. In contrast, all of the surviving mice given the lowest T-cell dose (5×10^5 T cells) had large tumor masses that spread throughout the peritoneum. From a practical point of view, obtaining efficient GVL activity with presensitized T cells at doses 10-fold lower than naive T cells facilitated characterization of the T-cell subsets involved in the GVL response.

Although naive CD4+ T cells had previously exhibited GVL potential when greater than 1.25×10^7 cells were used, CD4+ T cells from MMB3.19-presensitized B6 donor mice had significantly enhanced GVL activity. As few as 10^6 presensitized CD4+ T cells added to ATBM resulted in 60% long-term

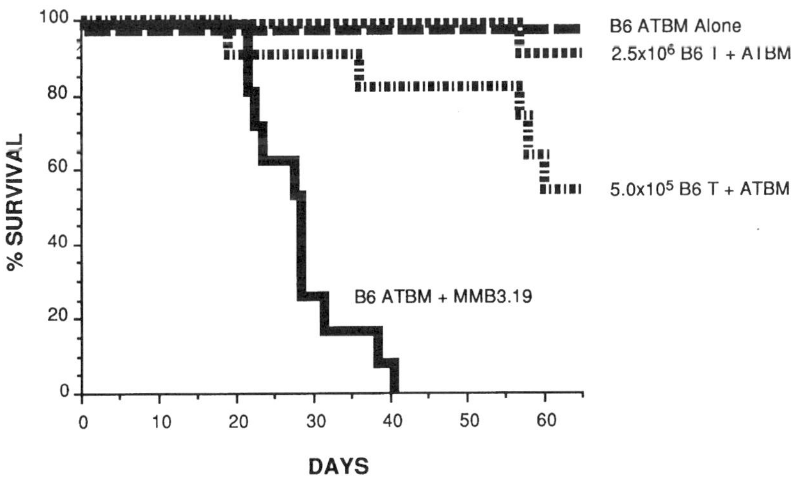

Figure 3 GVL responses against MMB3.19 myeloid leukemia with presensitized syngeneic donor T cells and ATBM transplantation.

(>80 days) survival of irradiated syngeneic recipients, and 2×10^6 cells resulted in 100% survival. The mechanism by which these presensitized donor CD4+ T cells mediate GVL activity is of significant interest and hypothetically could involve either direct cytolytic effects upon the MMB3.19 leukemia cells (e.g., perforin or granzyme release), cytostatic or tumoricidal effects of released cytokines (e.g., TNF-α), or activation of secondary effector cells (e.g., NK cells). In regard to the latter point, the potential role of NK cells in the GVL activity was investigated by depleting NK cells from the recipients on a continuing basis in the posttransplant period. It was observed that administration of anti-NK1.1 MoAb to the mice weekly following BMT showed no diminution of the protective effect of the donor CD4+ T cells, suggesting that NK cells were not necessary for protection.

The role of cytolytic CD4+ or CD8+ T cells in GVHD and antitumor responses has been demonstrated by others [77–79]. In most cases, the cytolytic activity of these cells has been closely linked to the expression of Fas ligand and/or perforin in the effector populations of most CTLs. Perforin-deficient and Fas ligand–deficient knockout mice have been used to study the effector mechanisms involved in GVHD and several antitumor responses. It has been demonstrated that both pathways are involved in the development of various aspects of GVHD. Antitumor responses against various tumors have also been investigated utilizing these knockout mice and both of these mechanisms appear to have an important role. Thus, the knockout mice make ideal tools for studying the role of both the Fas ligand–and perforin-mediated cytolytic activity in the development of GVL activity in our murine BMT model. These studies are currently in progress and will hopefully advance our understanding of the GVL response mechanism.

D. Molecular Analysis of GVL Reactive Syngeneic T Cells

To further define the cells involved in protection, leukemia-reactive T cells were isolated from syngeneic mice (C57BL/6) that had been presensitized against the MMB3.19 tumor and submitted for phenotypic and functional analyses. To investigate the nature of the GVL response and the level of TCR diversity utilized against the MMB3.19, leukemia-reactive T cells were divided into either CD4+ and CD8+ T-cell subsets and Vβ CDR3-size spectratype analysis was performed on each subset. Spectratype analysis utilizes PCR to detect CDR3 size polymorphisms in the VDJ regions of each Vβ subset [80]. A typical "non-reactive" Vβ population maintains a gaussian distribution when the PCR product is separated by size on a 6% polyacrylamide, 6 M urea denaturing gel. If a particular Vβ population has reacted to antigen and expanded, relative to the unresponsive T cells, a gaussian distribution will not likely be found upon separation and the distribution pattern will appear skewed. Preliminary results suggested that the

TCR-Vβ utilization of both leukemia-reactive T-cell subsets had a restricted oligoclonal Vβ repertoire. The CD4+ T-cell GVL response seemed to involve specificities in the Vβ7, 13, and 20 families, whereas the CD8+ T-cell response was defined by the Vβ11 and to a lesser extent Vβ 5, 7, 13, and 18 families (Table 1). Currently, we are cloning the sequence of dominant specificities within each responsive Vβ family for both T-cell subsets. With a full understanding of the GVL T-cell repertoire, it is theoretically possible to positively select for donor GVL-reactive cells by Vβ sorting and use this population in vivo to protect recipients from the leukemia challenge. In the case of CD8+ T cells, further analysis can determine if a particular Vβ family is also involved in GVHD; if not, donor cells of GVL-reactive Vβ families can be utilized to mediate protection without concomitant GVHD.

An analysis of cytokine production by leukemia-reactive T cells was performed by the Elispot assay [81]. The Elispot assay can yield a phenotypic description of the immune response involved in the GVL protection (i.e., Th1 versus

Table 1 TCR Vβ Utilization as Analyzed by CDR3 Size Spectratyping of TDL from MMB3.19-Primed C57BL/6 Mice[a]

	CD4+ T cells	CD8+ T cells
Vβ 1	—	—
Vβ 2	—	—
Vβ 3	—	—
Vβ 4	ND	ND
Vβ $5_{1,2}$	—	+
Vβ 6	—	—
Vβ 7	++	+
Vβ $8_{1,2,3}$	—	—
Vβ 9	—	—
Vβ 10	—	—
Vβ 11	—	++
Vβ 12	—	—
Vβ 13	+++	+
Vβ 14	—	—
Vβ 15	—	—
Vβ 16	—	—
Vβ 18	—	+
Vβ 20	++	—

[a] ND = no data; +/++/+++ = increasing level of detectable change in CDR3 size spectratype; — = no detectable change in CDR3 size spectratype.

Th2), as well as indicate the frequency of the responding T cells within the total population. Preliminary results suggest that upon presensitization of B6 mice with irradiated MMB3.19 cells, isolated CD4+ T cells exhibit an increased frequency of both the IL-4–and IL-2–producing cells. The IL-2–producing frequency increases nearly threefold and the IL-4–producing frequency increases nearly fivefold. It also appears that the relative frequency of IL-4–producing cells is much higher than the IL-2–producing cells. These results suggest that both a Th1- and a Th2-type of response is occurring against the leukemia, albeit, the Th2 response appears to be more substantial.

E. Allogeneic GVL Response to Myeloid Leukemia and GVHD

Since autologous or syngeneic BMT for clinical treatment of myelogenous leukemia clearly has less advantage in regard to GVL activity than allogeneic BMT [82,83], we adapted the MMB3.19 model to the allogeneic MHC-matched C3H.SW ($H2^b$) → B6 ($H2^b$) strain combination. Here, the important question to investigate was whether effective GVL responses can be generated without concomitant GVHD. Our approach was to take advantage of the T-cell subsets that were involved in each reaction. In C3H.SW → B6 chimeras, CD8+ T cells are largely responsible for the development of GVHD, whereas CD4+ T cells do not cause lethality or any observable GVHD pathology [84]. We therefore hypothesized that the depletion of CD8+ T cells from the inoculum, leaving allogeneic donor CD4+ T cells alone, could mediate a GVL response in the recipients without GVHD. To test this notion, C3H.SW ATBM cells (2×10^6) were transplanted into irradiated (850 cGy) B6 mice along with 2.5×10^7 C3H.SW lymphocytes that were depleted of CD8+, CD4+, or Thy1+ T cells using specific MoAbs and C. Recipient mice were challenged a day later with 10^5 MMB3.19 leukemia cells. Although the transplantation of untreated or either T-cell subset-depleted donor lymphocytes significantly prolonged the survival of recipients in comparision to T-cell depletion or ATBM+ MMB3.19 alone, the transplant of CD8+ T cell–depleted cells resulted in the best survival at 35%, with no evidence of GVHD [73]. This CD8+ T cell–depleted group exhibited significantly greater survival than either the untreated or the CD4+ T cell–depleted groups, both of which had clinical and pathological signs of GVHD.

F. Effect of Leukemia Presensitization on GVL/GVH Reactivity After Allogeneic BMT

As previously observed with the syngeneic model, presensitization of C3H.SW donor mice with an IP injection of 10^7 irradiated (3000 cGy) MMB3.19 cells, 3 weeks prior to transplantation of 1.25×10^7 T cells and ATBM to irradiated B6 recipients, led to dramatically improved survival against an MMB3.19 leukemia challenge. Again using T-cell subset depletion of the presensitized donor lymphocytes, all groups exhibited enhanced survival, but it was clear that the untreated and CD8+ T cell–enriched groups were undergoing GVHD with symptoms of hair loss, scleroderma, diarrhea, and weight loss, whereas the CD4+ T cell–enriched group appeared healthy. The results of this experiment strongly supported the hypothesis that minor H antigen allogeneic C3H.SW CD4+ T cells are capable of mediating a GVL effect against the MMB3.19 myeloid leukemia in the absence of GVHD and that the model will be viable for future studies. The results also indicate that there are also GVL-reactive allogeneic donor CD8+ T cells that are either recognizing host miHA or leukemia-specific antigens on the MMB3.19 cells.

In an effort to separate the GVHD-inducing alloresponses from the leukemia-specific responses of the adoptively transferred CD8+ T cells, attempts were made to remove the alloreactive T cells from the donor inoculum by an in vivo negative selection technique. Donor (C3H.SW) T cells were isolated and injected intravenously into lethally irradiated mice of the host strain (C57BL/6). Lymph was collected 24 h later from these mice by thoracic duct cannulation. Based on previous studies, this thoracic duct lymph is likely to contain the circulating donor T cells devoid of any alloreactive cells. The alloreactive cells that were undergoing the process of activation in the lymphoid system remain in the tissues for an additional day or two before the clonally expanded populations begin to migrate in mass. Preliminary studies with the negatively selected T cells from the thoracic duct suggest that this process results in a T-cell population still capable of protecting against leukemia growth without inducing GVHD. This finding supports the notion that the antileukemia response and the GVHD response can be physically separated.

G. Leukemia-Specific Antigens and GVL Reactivity to Myeloid Leukemia

One of the ultimate goals of our laboratory effort is to identify the leukemia-specific antigens that are recognized by the T cells mediating the GVL response. Expression cloning techniques have been utilized in the past to identify and isolate genes that encode tumor antigens. To achieve our goal, cDNA libraries are being generated from mRNA isolated from the MMB3.19 cell line and the exhaustive chore of expression cloning to isolate the T cell–reactive antigens can be undertaken. Identification of the leukemia antigens and their source may help us to better understand the potential immunogenicity of myeloid leukemias in general. These putative tumor antigens may then be utilized for vaccine development to immunize donor mice and boost their GVL activity or to allow in vitro stimulation techniques to generate leukemia-specific T cells for periodic infusion into recipients.

An important question regarding the identity of these leukemia-specific antigens is whether or not different myelogenous leukemias share some of the same tumor antigens. To address this issue, several different myelogenous leukemia cell lines have been generated in B6 mice; the MMB1.10, MMB2.18, and MMB3.19 lines. B6 mice were irradiated and transplanted with ATBM and anti-MMB3.19 presensitized syngeneic T cells. Mice were subsequently challenged with either MMB3.19, MMB1.10, or MMB2.18 and followed for survival. Our preliminary results suggest that MMB3.19-primed T cells can give added protection to mice challenged with the MMB1.10 tumor but not the MMB2.18 tumor. This suggests that some of the myelogenous leukemias (MMB3.19 and MMB1.10) share antigens that are capable of stimulating or being targets of a protective immune response while others do not (MMB2.18). Additional work is needed to further define these antigens and the T cells that respond to them.

H. Summary

In summary, using this murine model of myeloid leukemia, we have demonstrated that it is possible to separate out T-cell GVL responses from allogeneic donor cells that mediate GVHD. Leukemia-specific responses are capable of efficient protection in both the syngeneic and allogeneic settings. Further elucidation of these T-cell responses and target antigens on myeloid leukemias will enable the development of approaches to enhance these targeted GVL responses after bone marrow transplantation.

ACKNOWLEDGEMENTS

This work was supported by U.S. Public Health Service Grants CA39854 (RLT), CA72669 (BRB), and CA60630 (RK) from the National Cancer Institute.

REFERENCES

1. Barnes DWH, Corp MJ, Loutit JF, Neal FE. Treatment of murine leukemia with x-rays and homologous bone marrow. Br Med J 1956; 2:626–627.
2. Truitt RL, Johnson BJ, McCabe C, Weiler MB. Graft-versus-leukemia. In: Burakoff S, Ferrara JLM, eds. Graft-vs-Host Disease. 2nd ed. New York: Marcel Dekker, 1996:385–423.
3. Truitt RL, Johnson BD. Principles of graft-vs-leukemia reactivity. Biol Blood Marrow Transplant 1995; 1:61–68.

4. Bortin MM, Truitt RL. AKR T cell acute lymphoblastic leukemia: a model for human T cell leukemia-lymphoma. Biomedicine 1977; 26:309–311.
5. Green WR. Genetic control of the induction of cytolytic T lymphocyte responses to AKR/gross viral leukemias: I. H-2-encoded dominant gene control. J Immunol 1984; 132:2658–2664.
6. Green WR. Genetic control of the induction of cytolytic T lymphocyte responses to AKR/gross viral leukemais: II. Negative control by the Fv-1 locus in AKR mice of responder H-2 haplotype. J Immunol 1984; 132:2665–2671.
7. Schäfer A, Schmidt W. Resistance to cellular immune response in AKR leukemias. Eur J Immunol 1986; 16:753–759.
8. Truitt RL, Atasoylu AA. Impact of pretransplant conditioning and donor T cells on chimerism, graft-versus-host disease, graft-versus-leukemia reactivity, and tolerance after bone marrow transplantation. Blood 1991; 77:2515–2523.
9. Truitt RL, Atasoylu AA. Contribution of CD4+ and CD8+ T cells to graft-vs-host disease and graft-vs-leukemia reactivity after transplantation of MHC-compatible bone marrow. Bone Marrow Transplant 1991; 8:51–58.
10. Truitt RL, LeFever AV, Shih CY, Jeske J, Martin TM. Graft-vs-leukemia effect. In: Burakoff SJ, Deeg HJ, Ferrara JLM, Atkinson K, eds. Graft-vs-Host Disease: Immunology, Pathophysiology, and Treatment. New York: Marcel Dekker, 1990: 177–204.
11. LeFever AV, Truitt RL, Shih CY. Reactivity of in vitro expanded alloimmune CTL and Qa-1 specific CTL against AKR leukemia in vivo. Transplantation 1985; 40: 531–537.
12. Johnson BJ, Truitt RL. Selective depletion of donor NK cells in vivo decreases graft-vs-host disease without loss of graft-vs-leukemia reactivity after MHC-matched bone marrow transplantation. Transplantation 1992; 54:104–112.
13. Truitt RL. Unpublished data.
14. Hill GR, Crawford JM, Cooke KR, Brinson YS, Pan L, Ferrara JL. Total body irradiation and acute graft-versus-host disease: the role of gastrointestinal damage and inflammatory cytokines. Blood 1997; 90:3204–3213.
15. Abhyankar S, Gilliland DG, Ferrara JL. Interleukin-1 is a critical effector molecule during cytokine dysregulation in graft-versus-host disease to minor histocompatibility antigens. Transplantation 1993; 56:1518–1523.
16. Garlie N. Personal communication, 1996.
17. Charlton B, Meltzer J, Fathman CG. CD4+ heat-stable antigen+ thymocytes cause graft-versus-host disease across non-major histocompatibility complex incompatibilities. Eur J Immunol 1994; 24:1706–1709.
18. Alters SE, Song HK, Fathman CG. Evidence that clonal anergy is induced in thymic migrant cells after anti-CD4-mediated transplantation tolerance. Transplantation 1993; 56:633–638.
19. Bendelac A, Schwartz RH. Th0 cells in the thymus: the question of T-helper lineages. Immunol Rev 1991; 123:169–188.
20. Vicari AP, Zlotnik A. Mouse NK1.1+ T cells: a new family of T cells. Immunol Today 1996; 17:71–76.
21. Yoshimoto T, Paul WE. CD4+, NK1.1+ T cells promptly produce interleukin 4 in response to in vivo challenge with anti-CD3. J Exp Med 1994; 179:1285–1295.

22. Krenger W, Snyder KM, Byon JCH, Galzarano G, Ferrara JLM. Polarized type 2 alloreactive CD4+ and CD8+ donor T cells fail to induce experimental acute graft-versus-host disease. J Immunol 1995; 155:585–593.
23. Fowler DH, Kurasawa K, Husebekk A, Cohen PA, Gress RE. Cells of Th2 cytokine phenotype prevent LPS-induced lethality during murine GVH reactions. J Immunol 1994; 152:1004–1013.
24. Fowler DH, Breglio J, Nagel G, Eckhaus MA, Gress RA. Allospecific CD8+ Tc1 and Tc2 populations in graft-versus-leukemia effect and graft-versus-host disease. J Immunol 1996; 157:4811–4821.
25. Horowitz MM, Gale RP, Sondel PM, Goldman JM, Kersey J, Kolb HJ, Rimm AA, Ringden O, Rozman C, Speck B, Truitt RL, Zwaan F, Bortin MM. Graft-versus-leukemia reactions after bone marrow transplantation. Blood 1990; 75:555–562.
26. Marmont AM, Horowitz MM, Gale RP, Sobocinski K, Ash RC, van Bekkum DW, Champlin RE, Dicke KA, Goldman JM, Good RA, Herzig RH, Hong R, Masaoka T, Rimm AA, Ringdén O, Speck B, Weiner RS, Bortin MM. T-cell depletion of HLA-identical transplants in leukemia. Blood 1991; 78:2120–2130.
27. Leo O, Foo M, Sachs DH, Samelson LE, Bluestone JA. Identification of a MoAb specific for a murine T3 polypeptide. Proc Natl Acad Sci USA 1987; 84:1374.
28. Hirsch R, Archibald J, Gress RE. Differential T cell hyporesponsiveness induced by in vivo administration of intact or $F(ab')_2$ fragments of anti-CD3 MoAb: F(ab′) fragments induce a selective T helper dysfunction. J Immunol 1991; 147:2088–2093.
29. Blazar BR, Taylor PA, Vallera DA. In vivo or in vitro anti-CD3ϵ chain MoAb therapy for the prevention of lethal murine GVHD across the MHC barrier in mice. J Immunol 1994; 152:3665–3674.
30. Blazar BR, Taylor PA, Snover CD, Bluestone JA, Vallera DA. Nonmitogenic anti-CD3$F(ab')_2$ fragments inhibit lethal murine graft-versus-host disease induced across the major histocompatibility barrier. J Immunol 1993; 150:265–277.
31. Johnson BJ, McCabe C, Hanke CA, Truitt RL. Use of anti-CD3ϵ $F(ab')_2$ fragments in vivo to modulate graft-versus-host disease without loss of graft-versus-leukemia reactivity after MHC-matched bone marrow transplantation. J Immunol 1995; 154: 5542–5554.
32. Vitetta ES, Tucker TF, Racila E, Huang YW, Marches R, Lane N, Scheuermann RH, Street NE, Watanabe T, Uhr JW. Tumor dormancy and cell signaling: V. Regrowth of the BCL1 tumor after dormancy is established. Blood 1997; 89:4425–4436.
33. Truitt RL, Horowitz MM, Atasoylu AA, Drobyski WR, Johnson BJ, LeFever AV. Graft-vs-leukemia effect of allogeneic bone marrow transplantation: clinical and experimental aspects of late leukemia relapse. In: Stewart THM, ed. Cellular Immune Mechanisms and Tumor Dormancy. Boca Raton, FL: CRC Press, 1992:111–128.
34. Johnson BD, Hanke CA, Truitt RL. The graft-versus-leukemia effect of post-transplant donor leukocyte infusion. Leuk Lymph 1996; 23:1–9.
35. Kolb H-J, Mittermuller J, Clemm C, Holler E, Ledederose G, Brehm G, Heim M, Wilmanns W. Donor leukocyte transfusions for treatment of recurrent chronic myelogenous leukemia in marrow transplant patients. Blood 1990; 76:2462–2465.

36. Johnson BJ, Drobyski WR, Truitt RL. Delayed infusion of normal donor cells after MHC-matched bone marrow transplantation provides an antileukemia reaction without graft-vs-host disease. Bone Marrow Transplant 1993; 11:329–336.
37. Johnson BJ, Truitt RL. Delayed infusion of immunocompetent donor cells after bone marrow transplantation breaks graft-host tolerance and allows for persistent antileukemic reactivity without severe graft-vs-host disease. Blood 1995; 85:3302–3312.
38. Johnson BD. Unpublished data.
39. Johnson B, Becker E, Truitt R. Donor-derived Thy1+ cells suppress GVHD after DLI. Annual Meeting, American Society for Blood and Marrow Transplantation, Miami, March 1998.
40. Long GD, Blume KG. Allogeneic bone marrow transplantation for acute myeloid leukemia. In: Forman SJ, Blume KG, Thomas ED, eds. Bone Marrow Transplantation. Boston: Blackwell, 1994:607–617.
41. Clift RA, Buckner CD, Appelbaum FR, Schoch G, Petersen FB, Bensinger WI, Sanders J, Sullivan K, Storb R, Singer J, Hansen JA, Thomas ED. Allogeneic marrow transplantation during untreated first relapse of acute myeloid leukemia. J Clin Oncol 1992; 10:1723–1729.
42. Barrett AJ. Allogeneic stem cell transplantation for AML. Hematology 1997, pp. 121–137.
43. Meloni G, Foa R, Vignetti M, Guarini A, Fenu S, Tosti S, Tos AG, Mandelli F. Interleukin-2 may induce prolonged remissions in advanced acute myelogenous leukemia. Blood 1994; 84:2158–2163.
44. Soiffer RJ, Murray C, Cochran K, Cameron C, Wang E, Schow PW, Daley JF, Ritz J. Clinical and immunologic effects of prolonged infusion of low-dose reconbinant interleukin-2 after autologous and T cell-depleted allogeneic bone marrow transplantation. Blood 1992; 79:517–526.
45. Benyunes MC, Massumoto C, York A, Higuchi CM, Buckner CD, Thompson JA, Petersen FB, Fefer A. Interleukin-2 with or without lymphokine-activated killer cells as consolidative immunotherapy after autologous bone marrow transplantation for acute myelogenous leukemia. Bone Marrow Transplant 1993; 12:159–163.
46. Hamon MD, Prentice HG, Gottlieb DJ, MacDonald ID, Cunningham JM, Smith OP, Gilmore M, Gandhi L, Collis C. Immunotherapy with interleukin 2 after ABMT in AML. Bone Marrow Transplant 1993; 11:399–401.
47. Massumoto C, Benyunes MC, Sale G, Beauchamp C, York A, Thompson JA, Buckner CD, Fefer A. Close simulation of acute graft-versus-host disease by interleukin-2 administered after autologous bone marrow transplantation for hematologic malignancy. Bone Marrow Transplant 1996; 17:351–356.
48. Soiffer RJ, Murray C, Gonin R, Ritz J. Effect of low-dose interleukin-2 on disease relapse after T cell-depleted allogeneic bone marrow transplantation. Blood 1994; 84:964–971.
49. Robinson N, Sanders JE, Benyunes MC, Beach K, Lindgren C, Thompson JA, Appelbaum FR, Fefer A. Phase I trial of interleukin-2 after unmodified HLS-matched sibling bone marrow transplantation for children with acute leukemia. Blood 1996; 87:1249–1254.
50. Gale RP, Champlin R. How does bone marrow transplantation cure leukaemia? Lancet 1984; 2:28–30.

51. Fefer A, Sullivan KM, Weiden P, Buckner CD, Schoch G, Storb R, Thomas ED. Graft versus leukemia effect in man: the relapse rate of acute leukemia is lower after allogeneic than after syngeneic marrow transplantation. Prog Clin Biol Res 1987; 244:401–408.
52. Sullivan KM, Weiden PL, Storb R, Witherspoon RP, Fefer A, Fisher L, Buckner CD, Anasetti C, Appelbaum FR, Badger C, Beatty P, Berenson R, Bigelow C, Cheever MA, Clift R, Deeg HJ, Doney K, Greenberg P, Hansen JA, Hill R, Loughran T, Martin D, Neiman P, Petersen FB, Sanders J, Singer J, Stewart P, Thomas ED. Influence of acute and chronic graft-versus-host disease on relapse and survival after bone marrow transplantation from HLA-identical siblings as treatment of acute and chronic leukemia. Blood 1989; 73:1720–1728.
53. Giralt SA, Champlin RE. Leukemia relapse after allogeneic bone marrow transplantation: a review. Blood 1994; 84:3603–3612.
54. Kolb H-J, Schattenberg A, Goldman JM, Hertenstein B, Jacobsen N, Arcese W, Ljungman P, Ferrant A, Verdonck L, Niederwieser D, vanRhee F, Mittermueller J, deWitte T, Holler E, Ansari H. Graft-versus-leukemia effect of donor lymphocyte transfusions in marrow grafted patients. Blood 1995; 86:2041–2050.
55. Collins RH, Shpilberg O, Drobyski WR, Porter DL, Giralt S, Champlin R, Goodman SA, Wolff SN, Hu W, Verfaillie C, List A, Dalton W, Ognoskie N, Chetrit A, Antin JH, Nemunaitis J. Donor leukocyte infusions in 140 patients with relapsed malignancy after allogeneic bone marrow transplantation. J Clin Oncol 1997; 15:433–444.
56. Boyer MW, Orchard PJ, Gorden K, Anderson PM, McIvor RS, Blazar BR. Dependency upon intracellular adhesion molecule (ICAM) recognition and local IL-2 provision in generation of an in vivo CD8+ T cell immune response to murine myeloid leukemia. Blood 1995; 85:2498–2506.
57. Boyer MW, Vallera DA, Taylor PA, Gray GS, Katsanis E, Gorden K, Orchard PJ, Blazar BR. The role of B7 costimulation by murine acute myeloid leukemia in the generation and function of a CD8+ T-cell line with potent in vivo graft-versus-leukemia properties. Blood 1997; 89:3477–3485.
58. Matulonis UA, Dosiou C, Lamont C, Freeman GJ, Mauch P, Nadler LM, Griffin JD. Role of B7-1 in mediating an immune response to myeloid leukemia cells. Blood 1995; 85:2507–2515.
59. Matulonis UA, Dosiou C, Freeman GJ, Lamont C, Mauch P, Nadler LM, Griffin JD. B7-1 is superior to B7-2 costimulation in the induction and maintenance of T cell-mediated antileukemia immunity: further evidence that B7-1 and B7-2 are functionally distinct. J Immunol 1996; 156:1126–1131.
60. Dunussi-Joannopoulos K, Weinstein HJ, Nickerson PW, Strom TB, Burafkoff SJ, Croop JM, Arceci RJ. Irradiated B7-1 transduced primary acute myelogenous leukemia (AML) cells can be used as therapeutic vaccines in murine AML. Blood 1996; 87:2938–2946.
61. Falkenburg JH, Goselink HM, van der Harst D, van Luxemburg-Heijs A, Kooy-Winkelaar YM, Faber LM, de Kroon j, Brand A, Fibbe WE, Willemze R, Goulmy E. Growth inhibition of clonogenic leukemic precursor cells by minor histocompatibility antigen-specific cytotoxic T lymphocytes. J Exp Med 1991; 174:27–33.
62. Faber LM, van Luxemburg-Heijs SA, Willemze R, Falkenburg JH. Generation of

leukemia-reactive cytotoxic T lymphocyte clones from the HLA-identical bone marrow donor of a patient with leukemia. J Exp Med 1992; 176:1283–1289.

63. van der Harst D, Goulmy E, Falkenburg JHF, Kooij-Winkelaar YMC, van Luxemburg-Heijs SAP, Goselink HM, Brand A. Recognition of minor histocompatibility antigens on lymphocytic and myeloid leukemic cells by cytotoxic T-cell clones. Blood 1994; 83:1060–1066.
64. Mutis T, Schrama E, van Luxemburg-Heijs SA, Falkenburg JH, Melief CJ, Goulmy E. HLA class II restricted T cell reactivity to a developmentally regulated antigen shared by leukemic cells and CD34+ early progenitor cells. Blood 1997; 90:1083–1090.
65. Blazar BR, Taylor PA, Boyer MB, Panoskaltsis-Mortari A, Gorden KB, Allison JP, Vallera DA. CD28/B7 interactions are required for sustaining the graft-versus-leukemia effect of delayed post-BMT splenocyte infusion in murine recipients of myeloid or lymphoid leukemia cells. J Immunol 1997; 159:3460–3473.
66. Blazar BR, Sharpe AH, Taylor PA, Panoskaltsis-Mortari A, Gray GS, Korngold R, Vallera DA. The infusion of anti-B7.1 (CD80) and anti-B7-2 (CD86) monoclonal antibodies inhibits murine graft-versus-host disease lethality in part via direct effects on CD4+ and CD8+ T cells. J Immunol 1996; 157:3250–3259.
67. Blazar BR, Taylor PA, Snover DC, Sehgal SN, Vallera DA. Murine recipients of fully mismatched donor marrow are protected from lethal graft-versus-host disease by the in vivo administration of rapamycin but develop an autoimmune-like syndrome. J Immunol 1993; 151:5726–5741.
68. Blazar BR, Taylor PA, Panaskoltsis-Mortari A, Sehga S, Vallera DA. The in vivo inhibition of cytokine responsiveness and GVHD mortality by rapamycin leads to a clinical-pathological syndrome discrete from that observed with cyclosporin A. Blood 1996; 87: 4001–4009.
69. Blazar BR, Taylor PA, Panoskaltsis-Mortari A, Vallera DA. Rapamycin inhibits the generation of graft-versus-host disease and graft-versus-leukemia causing T cells by interfering with the production of Th1 or Th1 cytotoxic cytokines. J Immunol 1998; 160:5355–5365.
70. Fowler DH, Breglio J, Nagel G, Hirose C, Gress RE. Allospecific CD4+, Th1/Th2 and CD8+, Tc1/Tc2 populations in murine GVL: type I cells generate GVL and type II cells abrogate GVL. Biol Blood Marrow Transplant 1996; 2:118–125.
71. Baumach WR, Keath EJ, Cole MD. A mouse c-myc retrovirus transforms established fibroblast lines in vitro and induces monocyte-macrophage tumors in vivo. J Virol 1986; 59:276–283.
72. Trannoy E, Manser T, Cole MD, Daley MJ. Monoclonal c-myc transformed macrohage cell lines: I. Heterogeneity in ability to process and present antigen. J Immunol 1993; 151:3042–3056.
73. Korngold R, Leighton C, Manser T. Graft-versus-myeloid leukemia responses following syngeneic and allogeneic bone marrow transplantation. Transplantation 1994; 58:278–287.
74. Rapp UR, Cleveland JL, Fredrickson TN, Holmes KL, Morse HC III, Jansen HW, Patschinsky T, Bister K. Rapid induction of hemopoietic neoplasms in newborn mice by raf(mil)/myc recombinant murine retrovirus. J Virol 1985; 55:23–33.
75. Eccles MR, Baumbach WR, Cole MD. Examination of the role of CSF-1 indepen-

dence in myc retrovirus induced monocyte tumorigenesis. Oncogene 1990; 5:1535–1539.
76. Rabbitts TH. Translocations, master genes, and differences between the origins of acute and chronic leukemias. Cell 1991; 67:641–644.
77. Graubert TA, DiPersio JF, Russell JH, Ley TJ. Perforin/granzyme-dependent and independent mechanisms are both important for the development of graft-versus-host disease after murine bone marrow transplantation. J Clin Invest 1997; 100:904–911.
78. Armstrong JM, Vitetta ES. The roles of fas and perforin in LAK T cell/bispecific antibody-mediated killing of the murine B-lymphoma cells, BCL1. Int J Cancer 1996; 68:822–827.
79. Lee RK, Spielman J, Zhao DY, Olsen KJ, Podack ER. Perforin, fas ligand, and tumor necrosis factor are the major cytotoxic molecules used by lymphokine-activated killer cells. J Immunol 1996; 157:1919–1925.
80. Gorski J, Yassai M, Zhu X, Kissella B, Keever C, Flomenberg N. Circulating T cell repertoire complexity in normal individuals and bone marrow recipients analyzed by CDR3 size spectratyping. J Immunol 1994; 152:5109–5119.
81. Fujihashi K, McGhee JR, Beagley KW, McPherson DT, McPherson SA, Huang CM, Kiyono H. Cytokine-specific ELISPOT assay: single cell analysis of IL-2, IL-4 and IL-6 producing cells. J Immunol Meth 1993; 160:181–189.
82. Gale RP, Grosveld G, Canaani E, Goldman JM. Chronic myelogenous leukemia: biology and therapy. Leukemia 1993; 7:653–658.
83. Antin JH. Graft-versus-leukemia: no longer an epiphenomenon. Blood 1993; 82: 2273–2277.
84. Korngold R, Sprent J. Variable capacity of L3T4+ T cells to cause lethal graft-versus-host disease across minor histocompatibility barriers in mice. J Exp Med 1987; 165:1552–1564.

4

Effector Cells and Mechanisms of the GVL Effect

Yin-Zheng Jiang
Yale New Haven Health
Bridgeport, Connecticut

I. INTRODUCTION

It is now generally accepted that the curative effect of allogeneic bone marrow transplantation (BMT) in hematological malignancies is mediated in part by an alloimmune response termed the graft versus leukemia (GVL) reaction [1–5]. The antitumor effect of bone marrow allografts was only fully appreciated in clinical BMT after the observation of higher leukemia relapse rates after T cell–depleted BMT [6–8] and was strengthened by reports of the reinduction of remission by donor lymphocyte transfusion (DLT) in leukemia relapsing after BMT [9,10]. Although variable in its strength, the GVL effect appears to extend to a variety of malignancies, including acute and chronic myeloid and lymphoid leukemias [9–11], lymphoma [12], myeloma [13,14], and possibly solid tumors [15].

There is accumulating evidence that alloreacting donor lymphocytes are responsible for the GVL effect after BMT and DLT in humans [6–11]. MHC restricted CD4+ T cells [11,16,17], CD8+ T cells [18,19], and natural killer (NK) cells [20–22] have all been implicated in the GVL reaction. The GVL effect has been extensively reviewed. This chapter focuses on the biology of the effector cells and their role in mediating GVL reactions, particularly in chronic myeloid leukemia (CML). Regulation of these effector cells in mediating the GVL effect will also be discussed and, finally, important issues remaining to be resolved are highlighted.

II. BIOLOGY OF T CELLS AND NATURAL KILLER (NK) CELLS

A. Developmental Biology of T Cells and NK Cells

1. Development of T Cells

Differentiation and maturation of T cells requires the thymic environment as demonstrated by total failure by thymectomized mice to generate functional T cells [23,24]. Other tissues such as the gut and skin may also provide the environment for T-cell development. Both the epithelial and mesenchymal cells present in the thymic capsule, vessels and interlobular septae of the thymus are required for T-cell development. They not only provide an architectural structure for thymocyte development but also provide cytokine and/or surface molecules supporting T-cell development.

Like all hematopoietic cells, T cells are derived from pluripotent stem cells. Cells with phenotype of CD34^{high}CD38+Thy1+ from human bone marrow are highly enriched for pluripotent stem cells. They can differentiate into myeloid cells as well as T cells in vitro in the presence of thymus tissue and growth factors, whereas CD34+CD45RA+ Thy1− cells from human adult bone marrow can only be induced to differentiate into T cells, B cells, and NK cells but not myeloid cells [25–27]. This latter phenotype probably represents cells at a multipotential stem-cell stage. It is not clear however at what stage of stem-cell development (pluripotent cell or multipotential progenitor cell or committed T-cell progenitor cell, the T cells migrated into the thymus. Recent data strongly suggests that T cells colonize the thymus at the very early stage of the multipotent stem cell because cells extracted from fetal thymus can be induced into myeloid as well as lymphoid lineage cells [28]. However, because of the minimal number of stem cells (<0.01%) present in the thymus, it is not possible to identify whether the multilineage derivatives were from a common stem cell or from multiple committed progenitor cells migrating into the thymus, since the thymus, like other tissues such as the spleen and liver, is capable of supporting myeloid hemopoiesis.

The earliest thymic precursors are CD34^{high} CD45RA^{+}Thy1^{-} [27] as mentioned above. They also express CD33 but lack CD1, CD5, and CD28. The earliest committed T-cell progenitor cells in the thymus have acquired CD1, CD2, CD5, and cyCD3 but lack CD4 and CD8 and have lost CD33 expression [29]. CD4-molecule expression precedes CD8 in the human and is followed by double positivity for CD4 and CD8. There is evidence from animal studies that the expansion of immature thymocytes and acquisition of CD4 and CD8 requires the T cell–antigen receptor (TCR) β chain. Mutant mice, deficient for the TCR β gene or unable to rearrange their TCR genes due to lack of recombination-activating genes (RAG), have reduced numbers of CD4 and CD8 double-positive (DP) cells [30]. The TCR β gene rearranges before the TCR α gene [31]. After completion of a productive rearrangement, the TCR β protein is expressed on the triple-negative cells (CD3−CD4−CD8−) in conjunction with CD3 proteins [32]. This CD3−TCRβ complex can deliver signals to these early T cells, resulting in expansion of immature thymocytes and appearance of CD4+CD8+ cells. After entrance into the DP stage, the thymocytes acquire the completed CD3/TCR complex. The $CD3^{low}$ DP thymocytes are the main target for immune selection [33]. It is now known that the TCR repertoire is shaped by positive and negative selection events. Positive selection is required for inducing maturation of DP cells into single positive T cells that have the capacity to migrate out of the thymus. Negative selection ensures that those T cells efficiently recognizing self antigens are deleted. Both positive and negative selection involves interaction of the TCR αβ dimer of T cells with the MHC-peptide complex of cells in the thymic microenvironment. In the thymus, developing T cells rearrange and express their TCR and undergo a testing process based on the ability of their TCRs to recognize MHC proteins expressed on thymic epithelial cells. The interaction between developing thymocytes and thymic epithelial cells promotes the survival of thymocytes and also directs their lineage choice. The interaction of the TCR/CD3 with the peptide-MHC complex results in upregulation of CD3 and the activation antigen CD69 [34]. In addition to acquisition of some cell surface antigens and loss of others, mRNA of the cytotoxic protein perforin and various cytokine genes are induced as well [35]. The thymocytes are further matured into single positive thymocytes, losing either CD4 or CD8 [36].

Studies on factors that determine the development of thymocytes towards CD4 or CD8 T lymphocytes have shown that MHC molecules on thymic epithelial cells, as well as expression of Notch-1 gene in thymocytes are the two most influential factors. T cells with TCR recognizing MHC class I molecule will develop as CD8 cells; whereas recognition of class II antigen will ensure a CD4 T-cell development. Expression of an activated form of Notch during thymic development favored CD8 T-cell development while suppressing CD4 T-cell development. In addition, activated Notch permits the development of CD8 lineage cells in the absence of Class I MHC, a ligand that is normally required for CD8 cell development [37]. Mature thymocytes are $CD3^+$, $CD4^+$ or $CD8^+$, CD1−CD27+CD45RA+ when they migrate out of the thymus into the periphery. Based on their functional characteristics, mature CD4+ or CD8+ can be further divided into Th0, Th1, or Th2 and Tc1 or Tc2 subgroups [38].

2. Development of NK Cells

Development of NK cells also requires a special environment although less stringent compared to that required by T cells. Bone marrow probably is the main site for NK-cell development. Several studies have demonstrated that human NK cells can differentiate from immature bone marrow progenitors (CD34+ or CD34− cells) in long term bone marrow cultures in the presence of interleukin-2 (IL-2) and bone marrow stromal cells [39]. There is evidence that the thymic environment may be permissive for NK-cell development. It has been known for a long time that the thymus contains NK cells, which constitute a small fraction of the triple-negative thymocytes. The demonstration of thymus containing bipotential T/NK progenitors, committed NK precursors, and mature NK cells [40,41] indicates that NK differentiation can occur in the thymus. However, the fact that athymic nude mice and patients with DiGeorge syndrome have normal numbers of NK cells in the periphery [42,43] suggests that the thymus is not necessary for NK-cell development. Spleen, liver, or blood may also be the sites for NK-cell development, but more studies are required to define the exact process.

It is increasingly clear that NK-cell progenitors differentiate from a common precursor with T cells. To demonstrate the existence of bipotential T/NK cell precursor, CD34+ cells from human bone marrow were single-sorted and expanded for a short period of time with IL2, IL7, and stem-cell factor (SCF) on a feeder cell layer. After a few cell divisions, cells from each clone were divided into two groups. One group cultured in IL-2, IL-7, and SCF almost 100% of the clones developed into CD56+ NK cells, while the other group cultured in the presence of thymic tissue developed into T cells [41]. Although it is not clear at present, at which stage committed NK progenitors divert from committed T-cell progenitors and what events trigger common precursor cells to develop along either T- or NK-cell pathway, it is assumed that the event of TCR β gene rearrangement just before high-level expression of CD3 molecule may play an important role in determining the development of the bipotential progenitors. Early NK cells without expression of CD56 molecules lack cytotoxic activity against NK-sensitivity target cells. Acquisition of the CD56 molecule signals maturation of NK cells and the capability of cytotoxicity [36]. The majority of mature NK cells have surface markers of CD2+, CD7+, CD16+, CD27+, CD45RA+, LFA1+, VLA4+, CD11b+, and CD56+. However, there are subpopulations of NK cells that are CD3+ or CD57+ or CD16−. Activated NK cells strongly express CD69, CD25, IL2Rp75, CD26, and CD95 receptors as well as HLA class II antigens, while the expression of other antigens such as CD57 is downregulated after activation. Although none of these markers are specific for NK cells and most of them are expressed in other cell populations, some of them (i.e., CD56, CD16, CD57) are mainly expressed in NK cells or even in NK subpopulations. NK cells also display killer inhibitory receptors, such as Ly-49 in mice and p58 in humans, that appear to be inhibitory receptors to interact with MHC class I antigens [44]. The functions of these NK cell subsets are less well defined.

B. Target Recognition and Activation of T Cells and NK Cells

1. T Cells

T lymphocytes are capable of specifically recognizing target antigens and sparing innocent bystanders. The specificity of T cells is determined by the clonotypic T cell receptor (TCR). But in addition to the TCR, T cells express monomorphic receptors such as CD2, CD3, CD4, CD8, LFA1, and many others. The involvement of these receptors in the effector mechanism is evident from the finding that monoclonal antibodies against these receptors generally interfere with the proper function of most effector T cells [45–47]. The first step in the response of any effector T cell is the recognition of its specific target cell, which leads to the rapid binding of the two cells. The physical interaction of the effector cell with its target cell serves two important functions: the activation of the effector mechanism and the directed delivery of secretory proteins from the effector to the target thus ensuring the selectivity and specificity of the response. The molecular basis for the formation of stable cell-cell interactions is provided by the ligation of receptors on the surface of one cell with membrane-bound ligands on the surface of the other cell. It has been proposed and demonstrated that if the affinity of a surface receptor for its ligand and its concentration in the membrane are sufficiently high, then the initial binding of a small number of receptor-ligand pairs will result in the recruitment of additional receptor ligand pairs into this site. A stable cell-cell interaction is generated when a large enough number of such ligated receptor molecules are clustered into the contact site [48]. The most critical step in the initiation of T cell–target cell interaction is mediated by TCR binding to its ligand, the peptide antigen in the groove of MHC molecule. Engagement of the TCR with the corresponding peptide antigen activates protein kinases, which results in not only clustering of CD4 or CD8 and LFA1 molecules into the contact site of T cell but also increased affinity of LFA1 molecule to its ligand-ICAM1 on target cells [49]. Ligation of LFA1 with ICAM1, CD4 with MHC class II or CD8 with class I molecule, CD2 with LFA3 increase the stability of T cell–target cell contact [48], which permits additional TCR and costimulatory molecules CD28, or CD40 ligand to engage with additional peptide/MHC molecules and with B7 or CD40 molecules on the target cells, respectively [50]. Once the threshold numbers of TCR are engaged [51], T-cell activation results.

The capacity of the TCR to transduce signals across the T-cell membrane is mediated by the cytoplasmic domains of the subunits of the CD3 antigen and the ζ chain [52]. The intracellular tails of the CD3 and ζ molecules contain a common motif, EX2YX2L/IX7YX2L/I, termed the immunoglobulin receptor family tyrosine-based activation motif (ITAM). This motif is crucial for TCR coupling to intracellular tyrosine kinases and absolutely required for all subsequent TCR signaling responses. The earliest biochemical response elicited by the TCR is the activation of the protein tyrosine kinases (PTK) [53]. Two PTKs associate with the TCR-CD3 complex: the src family kinase p59fyn and a 70-kDa PTK termed ZAP-70. A second src family PTK p561ck are also critical for TCR function [54,55]. The proposed sequence of events in the TCR-regulated PTK cascade is activation of src kinases, the phosphorylation of ITAMs followed by the recruitment, tyrosine phosphorylation, and activation of ZAP-70 [52]. The association of ZAP-70 with the TCR complex is mediated by SH2 domain interactions with ITAMs. ZAP-70 has two SH2 domains and binds preferentially to a doubly phosphorylated ITAM. Although studies on TCR signaling to date have revealed enormous information along the TCR signal transduction pathway for the past decade, the identity of the downstream targets for the above molecules and detailed biochemical events and functions of many of the protein complexes that are targets for TCR signals remain to be illustrated.

CD4 or CD8 molecules are important for T-cell function. They provide not only help for effector-target cell contact but also additional stimulatory signals for T-cell activation. CD4, a 55-kDa integral membrane glycoprotein, recognizes monomorphic class II MHC determinants. CD8 binds to a conserved region in the alpha 3 domain of the MHC class I heavy chain. It has been shown that both CD4 and CD8 molecules (via a specific region within their cytoplasmic tail) are linked to the PTK p56lck [56,57] which also associates with the TCR/CD3 complex. A shared signaling pathway between TCR/CD3 and CD4 or CD8 may account for the importance of CD4 and CD8 in T-cell activation as well as the occasional observation of CD4 or CD8–independent immune responses, where blocking by anti-CD4 or CD8 antibody had no effect on T-cell effector functions [58]. This likely results from differences in TCR occupancy levels for different T-cell antigen combinations. When TCR occupancy is low, CD4 or CD8 binding to the same MHC molecule may be needed to generate additional signal to the TCR-mediated signal, so that a strong enough signal is delivered to fully activate T cells. When the level of TCR occupancy is very high, CD4 or CD8 binding to MHC molecules may not be necessary [58].

Activation of T cells results in several intracellular events: (1) *Polarization of intracellular proteins*. It has been observed by immunofluorescent microscopy that the cytoskeletal protein talin, a 215-kDa protein, clusters under the membrane of the effector cell along the cell-cell contact area [59]. Talin is associated with LFA1 upon activation of PKC and may be important in establishing and maintaining a stable cell-cell interaction. Talin is also important in promoting localized fusion of secretory vesicles with the effector cell membrane at the target cell contact site [60]. More recently, using fluorescent dextran particles it has been observed that recognition of target cells was accompanied by a transient increase in large dextran accessibility over a broad front near the interface between CTL and target cells. This region narrowed to a smaller area from which pseudopodia were extended toward the target [61]. The direction of extension of the pseudopod may guide precise delivery of cytotoxic agents. (2) *Polarization of intracellular organelles*. Using double immunofluorescence microscopy, the microtubulule organizing center and the Golgi apparatus (GA) were found to be colocalized and reoriented to face the bound target cell [62]. This reorientation is antigen specific. The microtubules play a central role in establishing cell polarity and they are also involved in directing the flow of intracellular vesicles between the cell center and the plasma membrane. The GA is the organelle responsible for the final processing of newly synthesized membrane proteins and secretory proteins. The mature proteins are packaged at the *trans* face of the GA into secretory vesicles that are then delivered toward and fuse with the plasma membrane. (3) *Reorientation of dense granules*. These granules contain proteins such as perforin, granzymes, and proteases, and their relocation may result in their directed release toward the bound target. Indeed fusion of the granules with the T-cell membrane at the cell contact has been observed [63]. (4) *Cytokine synthesis and excretion*. IL2, IL3, IL4, IL5, IL6, IL8, IL9, IL10, IL12, IL13, GM-CSF, INF-γ, and TNF-α, depending on the subtypes of T cells, have been detected in T-cell culture medium and mRNA of these cytokines is detected in the cytoplasm at T-cell activation [64]. (5) *Expression of cell-surface markers*. Activation of T cells results in expression of new markers or elevation of existing markers including CD25, HLA-DR, CD69 and Fas ligand (FasL) [65,66]. FasL was recently cloned and shown to be a 40-kDa type II membrane protein, homologous to members of the TNF family which includes TNF-α and β, nerve growth factor, and the ligands for CD40, CD30, and CD27. It is expressed on activated Th1-CD4+ or CD8+ T cells [65].

It is these intracellular changes that ensure effective T-cell function and the directed delivery of secretory vesicles to fuse with the membrane at the region of the cell contact. New membrane proteins are then inserted at the site of cell contact, and the content of the vesicles are released locally in the intercellular space between the two membranes in contact [67]. It is, however, not understood how effector cells protect themselves from these nonspecific cytotoxic agents while target cells are damaged.

2. NK Cells

NK cells were originally described on a functional basis according to their capability of killing certain tumor cells in the absence of prior sensitization. Since NK cells can lyse target cells that express either syngeneic or allogeneic MHC molecules, and even target cells that lack MHC expression, their cytolytic activity has often been referred to as non-MHC restricted. It is generally accepted that NK cells provide a first line of defense against certain tumors or viral infections [68]. Unlike T cells and B cells, NK cells do not rearrange TCR or immunoglobulin genes although they do accumulate nonfunctional transcripts of the constant regions of the TCR β and δ genes [69]. The ability of NK cells to detect and lyse tumor but not normal cells has been interpreted to reflect the existence of multiple receptors for an altered pattern of ligand molecules on tumor cells. These poorly defined NK cell functions and receptors have generated enormous interest in the past several years.

While NK cell–mediated cytolysis is not MHC-restricted, it is regulated by MHC molecules. The major advance in our understanding of NK-cell interaction with target cells has been the identification of several inhibitory receptors, termed killer-cell inhibitory receptors (KIR), on NK cells for MHC class I molecules (Table 1) [70–81]. KIR are characterized by (1) their ability to interact with a large panel of MHC class I allele products (promiscuous recognition) and (2) their ability to transduce a negative signal which leads to the inhibition of both natural cytotoxicity and ADCC programs. KIR are not NK-cell restricted since they are also expressed on T-cell subsets and can inhibit T-cell activation triggered via the CD3-TCR complexes [82,83]. Therefore two major strategies of MHC class I recognition are used by lymphocytes: one is T cell–specific and includes the CD3-TCR complex in the context of the CD8 dimers, whereas the other one has been described in both T and NK cells and is mediated by KIR. These two pathways which regulate T and NK cytotoxicity are complementary, and permit the elimination of a cell presenting a foreign antigen in the context of MHC class I molecules as well as a cell expressing no MHC class I molecules or altered form of the molecule. Since some virus infected or tumor cells down regulate the expression of class I proteins and escape T-cell surveillance, the NK cells appear to play an important role in host defense by eliminating these MHC-negative cells [68]. It is therefore evident that NK cells appear essential in host immune defense in addition to cytolytic T cells that are triggered by class I proteins presenting foreign peptides.

Human KIR belong to a multigenic and probably multiallelic family of Ig-

Table 1 Human NK-cell Receptors with Known Specificities

Name of KIR	Alternative Names	Specificity	References
p70[a]	NKAT4	HLA-A3	74
p70[b]		HLA-Bw4	73
p58.1 and 2		HLA-Cw4,Cw3	70
NKB1	NKAT3	HLA-Bw4,B27,B51,B58	71,72,75
HP-3E4		HLA-Cw4,Cw15	81
CD94		HLA-Bw4,B7,A1,A3,A11	71,76

[a,b] These two p70 receptors are different in cytoplasmic tails with 95 or 84 aa respectively.

like members. A total of 12 members of the human KIR subfamily have been cloned for which the ligands have not all been characterized [84]. Human KIR present three levels of diversity, corresponding to the extracytoplasmic, the transmembrane, and the intracytoplasmic domains. The extracytoplasmic domain is classically composed of two or three Ig-like domains. The two first KIR identified are the 58-kDa proteins specific for HLA-Cw3 and HLA-Cw4, expressing two Ig-like domains in their extracellular portion. In contrast, the HLA-Bw4 specific NKB1 and HLA-A3 specific NKAT4 receptors are 70-kDa proteins that express in their extracellular portions three Ig-like domains [85]. The intracytoplasmic domain is highly conserved but can be 39, 76, 84, or 95 amino acid long. This intracellular tail contains motifs that are in the category of immunoreceptor tyrosine-based inhibitory motifs (ITIMs) as opposed to ITAMs [86].

Like the target structures recognized by the TCR of T cells, NK cells recognize targets also in the form of MHC and peptide complex. NK cells detect and eliminate target cells that do not express adequate self-MHC molecules—e.g., defective expression of one or more MHC alleles. This situation is typical of some virus-infected or tumor cells that either downregulate certain class I alleles or express an altered peptide pattern presented by MHC class I molecules. In vitro experiments have shown that a single amino acid substitution in the $\alpha 1$ helix of both HLA-A and HLA-C altered the protective effect of class I molecules. This substitution is thought to modify the population of peptides that can bind to the HLA molecule [84]. It can be speculated that the function of these peptides would be to define the autologous cells as normal or abnormal. In the case of viral infection, normal self peptides can be displaced or competed with by an excess of peptides derived from viral proteins synthesized in the infected cells. This would lead to the inability of NK cells to recognize the new MHC-peptide complex and would also imply that infected cells could be interpreted by an NK cell as missing self, even when they do not have an altered quantitative expression of MHC class I molecules. Two possible roles for peptides in NK-cell recognition have been proposed. Peptides could be important simply because they bind and stabilize class I molecules [87], in which case any peptide characterized by a structure motif allowing binding to a given class I molecule would confer protection from NK cells. An alternative model is that only the critical peptides binding to class I molecules and also providing particular structural motifs that allow recognition by NK cells would exert a protective effect. Indeed, it has been shown that simple binding to HLA-B27 molecule by natural ligands is not sufficient for a peptide to provide protection. Only one of the several binding peptides conferred protection [88], thus suggesting that only that particular peptide could provide a self motif sensed by NK cells. Similar results have also been shown in the interaction of HLA-Cw4 with its receptor KIR cl42, where only loading of the nonamer peptide QYDDAVYKL onto HLA-Cw4 can promote binding of soluble KIR cl42 molecules to HLA-Cw4. Substitutions at position 7 and 8 of the peptide abolished Cw4 interaction with KIR cl42, despite similar surface expression of HLA-C [89].

To date, studies regarding the role of MHC antigen in regulating NK-cell activity have concerned mainly MHC class I molecules. A role of MHC class II in regulating NK-cell function has not been directly examined. There is some evidence suggesting that MHC class II antigen may play a similar role to MHC class I antigens in inhibiting NK-mediated cytolysis [90]: MHC class II expressing lymphoma cells are more resistant to NK lysis than class II negative cells, and antibody blocking of class II antigen in cells bearing both class I and II antigens significantly increases target cell susceptibility to NK-cell lysis [91,92]. Furthermore, the Daudi cell line is a well-established NK-resistant target, yet these cells have only class II not class I expression. By transfecting a single MHC class II gene into an MHC class I and II–deficient cell, we were able to study the interaction of NK cells with a single MHC class II molecule in isolation. We showed that HLA-DR1 expression renders the classically NK-sensitive K562 cell line resistant to NK cell-mediated lysis [93]. The role of HLA DR1 in inhibiting NK-mediated lysis was further supported by the partial restoration of NK cytolysis by antibody blocking of HLA-DR. Furthermore, treating target cells prior to exposure to effector cells with brefeldin-A, which blocks endogenous peptides presentation, revealed that the protective effect of HLA-DR1 in our system disappeared after BFA treatment. Chloroquine which blocks exogenous antigen presentation had no effect on the protective effect of HLA-DR1 molecule [93]. These findings indicate that the negative effect of HLA-DR1 on NK cell–mediated lysis was mediated by endogenous peptides bound to HLA-DR1, although the exact peptide involved in this process has not yet been identified. These results suggest that down-regulation of NK mediated lysis by MHC class II uses the same mechanism as that described for MHC class I: the presentation by the MHC molecule of different ''self'' peptides provides a negative signal to NK cells [94,95]. Since both MHC class I and II molecules are absent on K562 cells, transfection of HLA-DR1 may have allowed the expression of endogenous antigens which were recognized by NK cells as ''self.'' Our results are therefore consistent with the hypothesis that downregulation of NK activity against K562DR1 transfectants is due to presentation of an endogenous peptide by transfected HLA-DR1, which renders the target in some way recognizable as ''self'' by NK cells.

Since MHC class II molecules are normally present in conjunction with MHC class I molecules on some of the cell surface, it is important to consider a possible physiological role for NK regulation by both MHC class I and II molecules. Class II molecules can present both endogenous and exogenous antigens [96,97] and present larger peptides than class I molecules [98]. It is possible that some ''nonself'' antigens in tumor cells or infected cells may not bind to class I peptide motifs, but still bind to class II to be presented by HLA-DR molecules.

Thus it is conceivable that cells expressing only "self" peptides via class I would escape NK-cell surveillance, while cells expressing class I and II could be lysed if the "nonself" peptide were presented through MHC class II. In other situations where no "foreign" peptide is presented, the double presentation of class I and II "self" peptides may function synergistically to prevent NK killing of normal cells. Furthermore, since most class II–expressing antigen presenting cells (APCs) are professional APCs, longer survival of this cell type through resistance to NK lysis may prolong the ongoing immune response.

The "missing self" theory of NK-cell recognition does not exclude the possibility that allogeneic normal cells expressing adequate levels of MHC molecules can also be killed by NK cells. In addition, other non-MHC ligands may affect the susceptibility to NK cells. Indeed some MHC-negative cells may be resistant to NK-mediated lysis [84]. In this case target cells probably lack appropriate ligands for adhesion or for triggering the activating NK receptors. It should be borne in mind that killing of autologous cells normally expressing MHC molecules has never been observed. Killing of allogeneic cells by NK cells could be interpreted on the basis of the existence of an NK-cell repertoire. It has been demonstrated that NK clones derived not only from different donors but also from single donors were found to display different patterns of cytolytic activity against a series of normal allogeneic cells. Each group of clones displayed a unique pattern of cytolytic activity against the allogeneic donors [99]. These data suggested the existence of different groups of NK cell clones characterized by different specificities and a functional NK cell repertoire related to the ability to lyse or not lyse allogeneic cells [100]. When one NK-cell clone with a given KIR fails to engage its ligand with an allogeneic target, the activating signal prevails over the inhibitory signal and the allogeneic target is killed. It is known that the KIR show promiscuous recognition of MHC products and can recognize allogeneic MHC as self by sensing particular amino acid sequences in the peptide binding groove of the MHC molecule shared by self MHC. In this case the allogeneic MHC can function as self MHC and protect target cells from NK-cell killing. The direct evidence of the critical role of the amino acid residues in determining the specific recognition of a given NK clone has been provided by experiments of site-directed mutagenesis, including residues 77 and 80 of the HLA-C alleles [101,102]. These results indicate that single amino acid substitutions at position 77 and 80 in Cw3 and Cw4 molecules are sufficient to alter the protection of target cells from lysis by NK clones. Since these residues are important in determining the binding of peptides these results suggested that NK cells may sense the combination of MHC and peptide. In our experiments as mentioned above, the small portion of the HLA-DR1 transfected K562 cells that were protected from allogeneic NK lysis probably had peptide residues that were sensed as self by a small subset of allogeneic NK cells. This results also suggested that only limited numbers of peptides had a protective effect. The large proportion of transfected K562 cells that were killed by allogeneic NK cells probably failed to present peptides recognizable by the KIR of the effector NK cells.

It is strongly believed that all NK cells express at least one type of inhibiting receptor for at least one self-HLA class I allele and that KIRs act independently. This implies that, to avoid autoimmune reaction, the NK-cell system has evolved a mechanism of developmental control, possibly based on positive selection of NK cell progenitors expressing inhibiting receptors for self-MHC alleles. If such interaction takes place, the NK cell will be allowed to undergo further maturation. In contrast, NK cells that do not express self-MHC specific receptors would fail to further differentiate [103].

The ability of NK cells to efficiently kill a majority of MHC-negative target cells implies the existence of activating receptors recognizing non MHC–encoded ligands. Among these, CD16 represents the best-characterized NK receptor. The CD16 (FcγRIIIA) antigen is the low-affinity Fc receptor for complexed IgG with preferential binding for murine IgG2a and IgG3 and human IgG1 and IgG3. Two different subclasses exist, one expressed on granulocytes, which is GPI-anchored to the membrane, and another expressed on monocytes and NK cells, which is a transmembrane glycoprotein [104]. Lymphocytes expressing CD16 mediate ADCC function as well as NK-cell activation. The intracytoplasmic domain of CD16 comprises 24 amino acids, which are dispensable for CD16-mediated NK-cell activation. It is in noncovalent association with CD3ζ and FcεRIγ disulfide-linked dimers. These CD3ζ and FcεRIγ polypeptides express in their intracytoplasmic domain one and three ITAM. As a consequence of the presence of CD3ζ and FcεRIγ polypeptides, engagement of the CD16 initiate a series of ITAM-dependent signaling pathways, which are also used by the TCR as well as by the B-cell receptor (BCR) complex. The early events detectable upon CD16 stimulation include the activation of the p561ck PTK, which induces the tyrosine phosphorylation of CD3ζ and FcεRIγ ITAM, which in turn leads to the recruitment/activation of tandem SH2 domains of ZAP-70 PTK [105,106], as described above in T-cell activation. In addition to triggering NK cytotoxicity, stimulation of NK cells through CD16 results in the release of lymphokines such as IFN-γ and TNF-α and the induction of activation antigens such as CD69 and CD25 without inducing NK proliferation [107]. Cross linking of CD16 induces a rapid rise in intracellular Ca^{2+} levels, activation of the phosphatidyl inositol pathway with generation of IP3 and tyrosine phosphorylation of different proteins. After activation, the CD16 receptor is downregulated from the cell surface, probably to prevent over stimulation of NK cells.

In addition to CD16, NKR-P1, a disulfide-linked homodimer belonging to the C-type lectin family expressed on all rodent NK cells, has been shown to play an important role in NK-cell activation [108]. NKR-P1 is an activating receptor mediating natural killing upon binding in a Ca^{2+}-dependent way to carbohydrate ligands on NK sensitive targets. The production of a soluble form of rat NKR-P1 showed that it binds to NK-sensitive target cells but not to NK-resistant cells. In addition, the soluble NKR-P1 blocked the killing of NK-sensitive targets by freshly isolated polyclonal NK cells. Cross-linking of NKR-P1 triggers the breakdown of phosphoinositides, leading to the generation of inositol-triphosphate and to the subsequent mobilization of Ca^{2+} [109,110]. In the mouse, two major functions of NKR-P1 have been identified. First, NKR-P1 is one of the most effective signals for IFN-γ production by IL-2–activated NK cells. Second, NKR-P1 appears to be involved in the regulation of NK-cell growth, since the cross linking of the molecule induces NK-cell growth inhibition. Finally, in the rat, NKR-P1 triggering induces NK cell–mediated cytotoxicity, and monoclonal antibodies directed against human NKR-P1 partially or completely inhibit P815 target-cell lysis mediated by various human NK-cell clones [108].

Another member of the family of receptors encoded by the NK complex is the CD69 antigen. The CD69 molecule is expressed by hematopoietic cells soon after activation. Anti-CD69 monoclonal antibodies can stimulate lymphocyte proliferation and NK cell–mediated cytotoxicity. The NK activation induced by anti-CD69 antibody is inhibited by the simultaneous antibody-induced cross linking of MHC-specific inhibiting receptors [111], indicating that, as in all the other known activating receptors, the CD69-dependent pathway of NK-cell activation is under the control of MHC-specific inhibiting receptors. Additional surface molecules involved in NK-cell activation have been proposed in recent years. These include CD2, Lag molecule, adhesion molecules, a p38 molecule, a p70 molecule, and a p40 molecule [112,113]. The precise role of all these molecules in the complex mechanisms controlling NK-cell functions remains largely unknown.

C. Mechanisms of Killing by T Cells and NK Cells

There are two main classes of cytolytic lymphocytes differing fundamentally in specificity: cytotoxic T lymphocytes (CTLs) recognize target cells presenting processed antigenic peptides, whereas NK cells lyse target cells without classic restriction by MHC molecules. Nevertheless, the observations that cytotoxic T cells and NK cells form conjugates with their respective target cell, possess cytolytic granules that are secreted during the interaction with the target cell, and induce target cell death indicate that there are common pathways for these two classes of killer cells.

1. CD4+ T Cell–Mediated Cytotoxicity

Traditionally CD4+ T cells were considered to act mainly as helpers for antibody production and regulation of immune responses [114]. It is, however, clear now that cytotoxic CD4 cells exist, particularly in the Th1 subpopulation. The cytotoxicity mediated by CD4 CTLs has distinct characteristics, including MHC class II restriction, early DNA fragmentation, and late cell-membrane leakage in the target cell. These characteristics of target cell damage are attributed to the mechanisms employed by CD4 CTLs [115]. CD4 CTLs use the fas-antigen pathway as their major mechanism for killing and the perforin-granzyme pathway as an alternative mechanism for killing [116].

Interaction of CD4 T cells with Fas antigen on target is mediated by Fas-ligand (Fas-L) on the T cells. It has been demonstrated that purified Fas-L can lyse Fas-expressing cells, and nonlymphoid COS cells expressing human Fas-L exhibit cytocidal activity against Fas-expressing target cells [117]. The gene encoding the Fas-L has been recently cloned [65]. Fas-L is a 40-kDa type II transmembrane protein of the TNF family with the C-terminal region oriented on the extracellular side of the membrane. It is found predominantly in activated T cells, B cells, NK cells, the kidney, the lung, and the immune-privileged sites including testis and the anterior chamber of the eye. TNF and most likely Fas-L are expressed as homotrimeric molecules and thus can induce clustering upon binding to TNF-R and Fas-R, respectively [118].

Fas is a 45-KDa transmembrane-signaling molecule belonging to the family of TNF receptor–like molecules, which includes the TNF receptor, the B-cell antigen CD40, the low-affinity nerve growth factor receptor, and the T-cell antigen OX40 [119]. Differential expression of Fas antigen has been determined in a variety of cells and in tissues including the thymus, liver, ovary, heart, myeloid cells, epithelial cells, fibroblast, and others [120,121]. Interestingly, on myeloid and lymphoid cells, Fas is expressed only after activation. Thus, normal macrophages or resting T cells and B cells are Fas-negative but become Fas-positive upon activation [122]. The Fas molecule consists of three TNFR-like extracellular domains (D1, D2, and D3), a hydrophobic transmembrane region, and a cytoplasmic tail containing a death domain. The death domain binds Fas death domain–binding protein (FADD/MORT1) and the Fas receptor interacting protein (RIP), which links fas to a cascade of IL-1β–converting enzyme (ICE)–like proteolytic enzymes known as caspases [123]. Cross linking of Fas antigen results in programmed cell death (apoptosis) in most cells characterized by DNA fragmentation and then cell death: first the cell's chromatin condenses, its membrane and cytoplasm bleb, and its DNA fragments into oligonucleosone-length (multiples of 170 bp) DNA fragments, thus ensuring genetic death of the target cell. Then cells shrink, the endoplasmic reticulum dilates, and finally the cells fragment, resulting in the formation of sealed membrane fragments (apoptotic bodies). The sealed membrane fragments are an interesting characteristic of apoptosis: they are not inflammatory because the apoptotic bodies are phagocytosed by neighboring cells as soon as DNA damage begins [124–126].

CD4 CTLs express high level of Fas-L upon antigen recognition, receptor-ligand interaction, and activation, as discussed earlier. Involvement of fas antigen in CD4+ CTL mediated cytotoxicity has been extensively demonstrated. First, monoclonal antibody blocking of fas antigen by incubation of target cells with fas antibody prior to mix with CD4+ clone has significantly decreased target cell lysis [127]. Second, transfection of Fas expression vector into target cells that were resistant to CD4 CTL–mediated lysis render these cells susceptible to CD4 CTL–mediated lysis, whereas target cells transfected with the same vector without fas gene remain resistant to CD4 CTL lysis [116–118]. Third, in a transgenic mouse model where an induced *lpr* mutation has disrupted the Fas molecule expression, target cells derived from these mice were resistant to CD4+ T cell–mediated cytotoxicity [120].

CD4+ CTLs can also use the perforin-granzyme pathway. RT-PCR and northern blot analysis in CD4+ Th1-, Th2-, and Th0-type clones had revealed that perforin and granzymes were only expressed in those Th1-type clones. Furthermore, granzyme-A activity was also detected in cell pellets and culture supernatants of stimulated Th1 clones [128,129]. Thus the pattern of perforin and granzyme expression would support the killer activity of CD4 CTLs. Indeed, it has been demonstrated that CD4+ CTLs derived from Fas ligand-deficient *gld* mice lysed target cells regardless of Fas antigen expression on the target cells. Furthermore, knock-out of perforin gene in these effector cells severely interfered with target cell lysis by these CD4 CTLs [130]. The perforin-granzyme cytolytic pathway is Ca^{2+} dependent. Depletion of free Ca^{2+} from the environment by EDTA chelation impairs CTL cytotoxicity. Free Ca^{2+} ion is required for granule exocytosis from CTL and binding of perforin to the target cell membrane [131]. Furthermore, this cytolytic pathway can be blocked by inhibitors of serine esterase and cellular secretion but not by protein synthesis inhibitors, cyclosporine or antibodies to tumor necrosis factor (TNF) [132]. More details concerning this pathway are reviewed below in the CD8+ CTL section.

After an immune response has successfully taken place, the numerous activated now "redundant" T cells could be dangerous through their various capacities such as help, killing, and secretion of many cytokines. It is thus mandatory for the organism to remove such potentially hazardous T cells (also B cells and macrophages), whether they are autoreactive or the remnants of the accomplished immune response. Convincing evidence has now come to light that this safeguard is brought about by Fas-FasL evoked apoptosis. As mentioned above, resting T cells, B cells, and macrophages do not express Fas antigen but become fas-positive after activation. Activated T cells also express FasL. Therefore T cells are able to regulate other cells in the immune response. Cross linking of fas antigen leads activated T cells, B cells, and macrophages to apoptosis [133]. It has therefore been proposed that T cells are removed by suicide and B cells are removed by T cells after immune response [134]. However it is also important that the prosecution of activated cells be not carried out too early before completion of their mission. To prevent premature elimination of activated, and hence fas-expressing T cells, two safety mechanisms may be employed. First, it has been observed that freshly isolated T cells are only sensitive to fas-mediated apoptosis after several days in culture or by treatment with protein synthesis inhibitors, such as cyclohexamide, indicating the presence of internal inhibitors [113]. Second, engagement with Fas does not always induce apoptosis, but can enhance proliferation under certain circumstances [135], raising the possibility that during this apoptosis-resistant phase, Fas-FasL interaction may lead to cell expansion rather than cell death.

2. CD8+ T Cell–Mediated Cytotoxicity

Perforin knockout mice have provided a valuable tool for the evaluation of this molecule's role in CTL cytotoxic activity. Since inactivation of perforin does not impair activation and proliferation of T cells, perforin-deficient mice can be used to study defects on the level of effector mechanisms without complicating indirect effects [131]. These experiments have clearly established the perforin-dependent granule exocytosis pathway as the main cytotoxic pathway, because cytotoxic activity of CD8 T cells from perforin-deficient mice against fibroblast and certain lympho-hematopoietic target cells was completely absent [136]. Most lympho-hematopoietic target cells were lysed by perforin-deficient T cells to a varying degree, but with several-fold reduced efficiency. This low level of cytolytic activity is known to be mediated by the interaction of Fas ligand expressed on activated T cells with Fas on the surface of the target cells [137]. The following evidence supports the existence of only two pathways in CD8 CTL mediated cytotoxicity:

1. Transformed and untransformed primary fibroblasts that do not express Fas are completely resistant to cytotoxicity by perforin-deficient effector cells, whereas Fas-expressing cells after gene transduction are lysed with varying efficiency [138].
2. A Fas-specific monoclonal antibody that is not cytotoxic is able to completely block the lytic activity of perforin-deficient T cells against lymphoma target cells, which are Fas antigen–positive [139].
3. Con-A blast target cells from mice with the *lpr* mutation, which results in inactivation of the Fas molecule, are (in contrast to Con-A blast target cells from normal mice) resistant to perforin-independent cytotoxicity [138].

Thus, dependent on the target cell, CD8 T cells confer lysis by either a perforin-dependent pathway alone or by the concomitant action of the perforin-dependent and the Fas-dependent pathway. The complete absence of cytotoxicity of perforin-deficient T cells in the presence of a blocking Fas-specific antibody or against target cells from Fas-deficient *lpr* mice demonstrates that these two pathways alone account for CD8+ CTL-mediated cytotoxicity without any involvement of additional pathways.

Except for reduced efficiency on most target cells, killing via the Fas-dependent pathway exhibits characteristics similar to those of perforin-dependent cytotoxicity: it is blocked by anti-CD8 antibodies; it is specific for an antigenic peptide bound to MHC class I molecules in the same way as it is in CD4+ T cells.

Besides lysis of the plasma membrane as detected by release of radioactive chromium, CTLs also induce fragmentation of target cell DNA into multiple 200-bp fragments. Whereas ^{51}Cr release is only detected 1 h after mixing effector and target cells, DNA fragmentation is detected more rapidly [140]. In these experiments it was difficult to conclude that membrane disruption by perforin pores directly induces cell death, because disruption of the membrane by complement lysis or chemical compounds does not induce DNA fragmentation [141]. It is now known that granzymes were cosecreted with perforin and enter the target cell through the polyperforin pore to trigger a target-cell internal pathway that results in DNA fragmentation [142].

Perforin is a 70-kDa protein stored in the cytoplasmic granules of CTLs. It is water-soluble and yet capable of insertion into biological membranes and artificial lipid bilayers [131]. Perforin belongs to a family of pore-forming peptides and proteins produced widely in nature by organisms ranging from bacteria to mammals, and part of the perforin molecule has sequence homology with the complement component 9 in the region that might fold into an amphipathic α helix [143]. Perforin has been shown to be able to bind and insert into the target cell membrane, where perforin monomers subsequently aggregate to form a polyperforin pore structure traversing the membrane.

The main role of perforin in lymphocyte-mediated cytolysis can be linked to its pore-forming activity. Following their release from the killer lymphocyte into the intercellular space, perforin monomers bind to and polymerize in the membrane of target cells [144]. This activity, which is Ca^{2+} dependent and most efficient at neutral pH, can also be detected using purified perforin in connection with target cells, artificial lipid vesicles or planar lipid bilayers composed of different types of lipids [131]. These findings suggested that the interaction of perforin with target membrane is unlikely to be mediated by receptors or specific lipid moieties. Electron microscopy and electrophysiological studies have shown that the internal diameter and conductance of a typical perforin pore are in the ranges of 5–20 nm and 0.4–6 nanoSiemens (nS), respectively [145]. These results indicate that perforin pores resemble the complement membrane attack complex. The structural and functional sizes of the perforin pores would allow at least small intracellular molecules, such as ATP and K+ ions to leak from perforin-damaged cells and may perturb the intracellular homeostasis. This could contribute to the death of target cells in addition to granzyme induced cell death.

The class of Granzymes include granzyme A, B, C, D, E, F, and/or G [146,147]. They are serine proteases packed in the cytoplasmic granules of CTLs and NK cells together with perforin [148]. Exocytosis of these granules by CTLs into the effector–target cell interspace results in target cell damage. While perforin makes pores on the ell membrane, granzymes once entered into target cells through these pores can trigger a series of internal disintegration activities and lead to cytolysis and DNA breakdown [149,150]. The role of granzyme in CTL-mediated cytotoxicity has been confirmed by the inability of CTL from mutant granzyme-B gene mice to lyse targets. These mice have normal perforin and fas antigen function. Using the classic lytic assays, the ability of granzyme B–deficient CTL and NK cells to mediate ^{51}Cr or $^{125}IUdR$ release from their target cells was measured. ^{51}Cr labels cytoplasmic components; ^{51}Cr release from target cells attacked by CTL is thought to reflect the leakage of cytoplasmic contents due to target cell membrane damage by perforin. $^{125}IUdR$ labels nuclear DNA and its release measures DNA fragmentation or nucleolytic activity. Target cells attacked by CD8+ CTL from these granzyme B–mutant mice had normal ^{51}Cr release, whereas $^{125}IUdR$ release was significantly lower compared with that mediated by CTL from normal mice [151]. Although there are some studies on the enzymatic properties of lymphocyte granzymes, their physiological function and natural substrates have not been firmly established.

3. NK Cell–Mediated Cytotoxicity

Currently it is believed that NK cells mainly utilize the perforin-granzyme dependent pathway of cytotoxicity in the same way as CD8+ CTLs but also use the Fas-FasL pathway in certain circumstances in the same way as CD4+ CTLs. Morphologically NK cells were originally known as large granular lymphocytes. These granules contain high concentrations of cytotoxic agents [145,148,152]. In perforin-deficient mice, NK-cell cytotoxicity is greatly impaired [127]. It has been shown that NK cells can be induced to express Fas-ligand and thus Fas ligand–mediated cytotoxic activity [153]. Interestingly, sera from large granular lymphocyte (LGL) leukemia patients contain high level of soluble Fas-L, reflecting the constitutive expression of Fas-L on NK leukemia cells. The finding that nonactivated NK cells do not express Fas-L is consistent with the failure to detect soluble Fas-L in normal serum [154,155]. These results indicate that a soluble form of Fas-L may function as a pathological agent in causing tissue injury and that Fas mediated cell death is an important alternative pathway through which NK cells execute their cytotoxicity.

III. EFFECTOR CELLS IN GVL

A. Lymphocytes in GVL

In the early 1980s it was observed that the incidence and severity of clinical GVHD was strongly associated with a decreased risk of leukemia relapse [6–10] and it was well known that immune cells derived from the graft mediated this antihost reactivity. Thus the GVL effect was also mediated by an immune reaction. Further evidence from T-cell depletion of the marrow graft to prevent GVHD resulting in significantly higher leukemia relapse [6–8] confirmed that the GVL effect is mediated by lymphocytes. Perhaps the strongest evidence in support of lymphocyte mediation of the GVL effect come from the clinical results of donor lymphocyte transfusion (DLT) for the treatment of relapsed leukemia after BMT. DLT has now become the standard therapy for some leukemias relapsing after BMT. It offers a durable leukemia-free remission for 82% of patients with CML in cytogenetic relapse, 78% in hematological relapse, and 12% in transformed phase [156]. We originally reported two cases of CML relapse treated with DLT [10]. Both patients had complete remission shortly after DLT treatment and became undectable for the bcr/abl transcript by a highly sensitive polymerase chain reaction (PCR) method. Interestingly in both cases, disappearance of the leukemia cells by PCR was mirrored by an increase of the cytotoxic T-lymphocyte precursor (CTLP) frequency against the original leukemia cells and a burst of NK-cell activity after DLT. Additional support for a role of T cells in GVL can be extracted from the correlationship between T-cell manipulation and the probability of leukemic relapse. It has been reported that administration of low-dose interleukin-2 (IL-2) after BMT can decrease the risk of leukemia relapse [157] and addition of IL-2 receptor antibody [158] or CD3 antibody [159] or B7 costimulation molecules [160] to attenuate T-cell activity to prevent GVHD resulted in an increased leukemia relapse rate. Furthermore it has been demonstrated that discontinuation of cyclosporine immune suppression after transplantation can reverse the course of hematological relapse of CML and AML [5,161]. In vivo evidence in support of the role of lymphocytes in mediating GVL is summarized in Table 2.

There is also ample in vitro evidence that T cells play a central role in the GVL reaction. Both myeloid and lymphocytic leukemic cells are susceptible to HLA class I-restricted lysis by cytotoxic T cells specific for minor antigens. These minor antigen specific T cells also inhibit myeloid leukemia progenitors in colony inhibition assays [162]. CD4 and CD8 T cells with cytotoxicity against leukemia cells circulate after BMT [163,164] and DLT [10,165]. We have shown that CTLP frequency of donor lymphocytes against recipient leukemia cells rose from undetectable levels in the unprimed donor cells to a low level of 1/300,000 after HLA-identical sibling BMT and that these antileukemia CTLs were found for a

Table 2 In Vivo Evidence in Support of Lymphocyte Mediation of a GVL Effect

Procedures	Results	References
T cell depletion	↑ Leukemia relapse	6–8
CD3 Ab to treat GVHD	↑ Leukemia relapse	159
CD25 Ab to treat GVHD	↑ Leukemia relapse	158
CD80/86 Ab to treat GVHD	↑ Leukemia relapse	160
Donor leukocyte transfusion	↓ Leukemia relapse	10,156
Discontinuation of cyclosporine	↓ Leukemia relapse	5,161
Low dose of IL-2 post-BMT	↓ Leukemia relapse	157

Abbreviations: Ab, antibody; GVHD, graft-versus-host disease; BMT; bone marrow transplantation; IL-2, interleukin-2.

prolonged period of time after BMT). Furthermore, the level of post CTLP frequency was associated with the probability of leukemia-free survival [164].

B. CD4+ Versus CD8+ T Cells in GVL

There is growing evidence that CD4+ T cells are central to the GVL alloresponse, first because their helper activity augments the function of other effectors and second because CD4+ cells themselves exert antileukemic effects. The relative contribution of the two major T-cell subsets, CD4+ and CD8+, to GVL reactivity has been investigated both in animal models and in humans. Mice receiving CD8-depleted marrow, or marrow with addition of purified CD4+ T cells, experienced a low incidence of GVHD with high leukemia-free survival [166,167], supporting an important role of CD4 cells in conferring GVL. CD8+ T cells can also mediate GVL reactivity. Mice receiving CD8-depleted donor marrow had a higher leukemia relapse incidence than those receiving CD4-depleted marrow [168]. In experimental mouse transplants, the addition of purified CD8+ T cells to the graft prevented tumor growth, or reduced the level of tumor cells in the blood, and facilitated engraftment without inducing GVHD [18]. The conflicting results from murine models may be due to variations between mouse strains and the degree of histocompatibility between donor and recipient. We can, however, conclude that both CD4+ and CD8+ T-cell subsets are important in GVL reactions [169]. In humans, CD4+ alloreactive cells with antileukemia activity have been generated in vitro by several investigators [162,170,171]. Furthermore CD4+ cells with antileukemic activity increase in frequency after BMT [164,165]. We demonstrated the presence of donor-derived cytotoxic T cells in the blood of CML patients after BMT showing specific reactivity to the patient's leukemia cells. Depletion of CD4+ cells from the responding population significantly reduced the cytotoxic T-lymphocyte precursor (CTLP) frequency against the recipient's leukemia cells, whereas CD8+ depletion had only a modest effect [164]. Perhaps the strongest and most direct evidence supporting a role in the GVL effect for CD4+ T cells derives from clinical trials with CD8-depleted marrow transplants or CD8-depleted peripheral blood leukocytes to treat relapsed leukemia after BMT. Nimer et al. [16] used CD8-depleted marrow for transplantation and observed a significantly lower incidence of GVHD without an increase in the rate of leukemia relapse compared with T-replete transplants. Giralt et al. [17] used CD8-depleted peripheral blood lymphocytes to treat relapsed leukemia post-BMT and observed a 60% response with only a 20% incidence of GVHD. Contrasting with these data are other clinical studies showing that CD4-depleted marrow transplants with an adjusted CD8+ T-cell content significantly reduce GVHD without affecting engraftment and immune reconstitution [19]. Since CD4 and CD8 subsets are both involved in GVHD and GVL reactions it does not appear possible to completely separate GVL from GVHD by transplanting marrow depleted of either one of the two major subsets. Furthermore it is possible that the separation of GVL and GVHD observed so far with T-cell subset depletion may simply be the result of transplanting measured low doses of immunocompetent cells, since comparable results have been obtained using similar doses of unmanipulated T cells [172].

Nevertheless, from what we know of T-cell immunology, CD4+ and CD8+ T cells must exert a GVL effect by different mechanisms. It is known that CD4+ T cells have a wider repertoire than CD8 cells [173]. CD4 cells recognize antigens through MHC class II molecules on antigen presenting cells (APCs) whereas CD8+ T cells recognize antigens presented by MHC class I molecules [174]. The fact that in allogeneic BMT the immune reactions are localized to sites where class-II bearing antigen-presenting cells are harbored (e.g., Langerhans cells and their equivalents in the skin and intestinal mucosa, Kupffer cells in the liver), suggests that CD4+ T cells are necessary to initiate the immune response after BMT [175]. Furthermore, CD4+ T cells are capable of producing a large variety of cytokines, which have a wide spectrum of biological activities: IL-2 and IL-12 recruit NK cells and CD8+ T cells into the immune responses and further augment their antitumor cytotoxicity [176,177]; IFN-γ and TNF-α have an inhibitory effect on leukemia cells [164], and both cytokines upregulate MHC class II [178,179] and fas antigen expression [180,181] conditioning the target cells to be susceptible to CD4+ T-cell attack. It is also known that CD4+ T cells can exert cytotoxicity on their own and have been demonstrated to directly kill leukemia cells in vitro [162,170,171]. Thus it appears that CD4+ T cells alone are sufficient to initiate and execute the GVL process. However since CD4+ and CD8+ T cells are both involved in the GVL reaction, it is likely that an optimal GVL effect only occurs when both subsets participate.

C. NK Cells in GVL

NK cells kill a number of tumor cell lines and activation of lymphocytes with IL-2 can further augment NK-cell cytotoxicity against a wide variety of target cells [182]. The role of NK cells in GVL is becoming increasingly recognized as our understanding of NK cell biology is getting better. In vivo NK cell retention in T-cell depleted marrow graft correlates with a significantly reduced leukemia relapse rate with minimal incidence of graft-versus-host disease (GVHD) in murine models [22] and possibly in humans [183]. After allogeneic BMT for chronic myeloid leukemia (CML), NK activity did not correlate with GVHD status but with leukemia-free survival [184]; and activation of donor-derived NK cells by IL-2 induced antileukemia but not antihost activity [185]. Thus it is possible that NK cells can mediate specific antitumor activity without damaging normal host tissues. Similar results regarding the role of NK cells in antileukemia reactivity in acute myeloid leukemia and in mouse leukemia models have also been reported [186]. NK cytotoxicity and the ability of cytokine production by NK cells measured in vitro correlated with the status of leukemia remission [21,187]. Furthermore, it has been demonstrated that administration of selected NK cells after BMT could have superior ability to eradicate residual leukemia cells without mediating clinical overt GVHD in mice leukemia models [186].

NK cells are among the first of immune cells to recover after BMT [188]. Since NK cells can mediate cytotoxicity without prior sensitization [182], they may be the main effectors of GVL in the early posttransplant period. In order to further define the role of NK cells in GVL, we studied 16 patients with CML receiving allogeneic BMT. We measured NK- and T-cell subsets numbers, and NK/LAK cell function in the first 9 months after BMT and correlated results with development of GVHD and leukemia relapse [20]. We confirmed that NK function measured by spontaneous lysis of K562 cells recovered rapidly after BMT and remained within the normal range throughout the period of study. In contrast, LAK activity showed a slower and incomplete recovery. We also measured recovery of cell counts of NK (CD56+), CD4 T cells, and CD8 T cells following allogeneic BMT. There was an elevation of NK-cell counts and a preponderance of CD8 over CD4 lymphocytes in the first 9 months following BMT. Relapse in the 5/16 patients studied was associated with a significantly lower absolute number of circulating NK cells [20], but not total lymphocyte counts. The involvement of both NK cells and T cells has implications for the GVL effect: since leukemias vary in their expression of critical surface molecules including MHC class I and II [189], costimulatory molecules such as B7 [190], and fas antigen [191], their susceptibility to T cells or NK cells may also differ. The particularly strong GVL responses to CML may be due to susceptibility of the leukemia to both MHC restricted T-cell and NK-cell immune responses. We found no correlation with the occurrence and severity of acute GVHD and recovery of lymphocyte count [20]. This may reflect a more central role for cytokines in the GVHD process [192] operating independently of the immune recovery as measured by subset counts and NK function. Alternatively, since it has been postulated that NK cells are directly responsible for the GVL effect but not for GVHD [20–22], these findings support a central role of NK cells in GVL for CML.

However, there is also evidence that NK cells may be involved in GVHD. In animal models, mice receiving NK cell depleted marrow graft experienced a significantly lower incidence of GVHD compared to mice receiving graft which was depleted either of CD4 or CD8 T cells [193]. Similarly it has been observed that during the acute phase of GVHD the activity of NK cells from intestinal and peripheral blood was markedly augmented [195]. In humans, biopsy of skin GVHD lesion revealed significantly higher NK-cell composition among the infiltrating lymphocytes compared to that in skins from non-GVHD sites [194]. The inconsistency of results concerning the role of NK cells in GVL and GVHD probably indicates that NK cells are important in the pathogenesis of both GVHD and GVL reaction, and depending on the genetic combination of the donor and recipient NK cells may predominantly mediate GVL or GVHD.

IV. MECHANISMS OF T CELL–AND NK CELL–MEDIATED GVL

Although the details remain undefined, we can now assemble a working model of T cell–mediated GVL in humans, at least in the alloresponse to myeloid leukemias such as CML. The immune response can be considered in three phases: initiation of the alloresponse, effector cell expansion, and effector mechanisms.

A. Initiation of the GVL Reaction

The antileukemia immune response starts with the presentation of leukemia-associated antigens to donor lymphocytes. Classically this involves the presentation of leukemia antigens via host- or donor-derived professional antigen presenting cells (e.g., dendritic cells, macrophages). Class I molecules are mainly involved in endogenous antigen presentation to CD8+ T cells. While class II molecules are mainly involved in exogenous antigen presentation to CD4+ T cells, it is now known that they also present endogenous antigens [174]. Therefore leukemia cells could themselves act as endogenous antigen-presenting cells and present antigens to both CD4+ and CD8+ T cells. There is good evidence that Ph+ chromosome positive dendritic cells [196] and Ph+ CD34+ cells [197] present endogenous antigen through MHC class I and II. Furthermore leukemic monocytes in CML are competent APC, capturing, processing and presenting exogenous protein antigens [198]. We have shown that CD33+ cells from CML patients are capable of processing and presenting exogenous antigens to CD4 T-cell clones, and this antigen presentation can be blocked by both brefeldin, an endogenous antigen presentation inhibitor, and chloroquine, an exogenous antigen presentation inhibitor [198]. Proteins derived from leukemia-cell catabolism could thus serve as a source of exogenous antigen for leukemic APCs, processing and presenting originally endogenous antigens through the exogenous class II pathway to CD4+ T cells. More recently we examined the capability of CD34+ cells in antigen processing and presentation and found that CD34+ cells can efficiently stimulate HLA class II matched mixed lymphocyte reaction in both primary and secondary immune responses, which suggested that these cells are able to present endogenous antigens to allogeneic T cells. Furthermore, CD34+ cells are also able to process and present exogenous protein antigens (Figure 1) to CD4+ clones. CD34+ cells use pinocytosis rather than phagocytosis to cap-

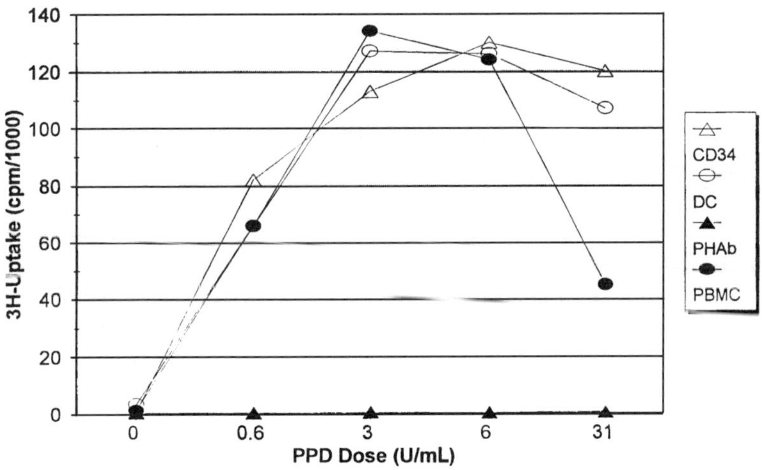

Figure 1 Antigen processing and presentation by CD34+ progenitors. Purified CD34 cells (>97%), flow sorted dendritic cells (DC) derived from CD34+ cells cultured in IL3, GM-CSF, SCF, and TNF, and PHA-stimulated lymphoblast (PHAb) from the same individual were pulsed with ppd-antigen at varying doses for 12 h were tested for antigen processing and presentation. PBMC from a normal donor was used as positive control. Responder cells were from ppd antigen-specific T-cell clone. Responder cells were at 1000 cells per well and stimulator cells at 10_4 cells per well. The cells were cultured total for 66 h. Results show that CD34 cells are efficient APC as compared to DC and PBMC to capture, process, and present protein antigen. PHAb did not present protein antigen. The antigen presentation was HLA-DR1 restricted.

ture soluble antigens. Interestingly CD34+ cells have high levels of HLA-DR expression but do not express costimulatory molecules CD80 (B7.1) and CD86 (B7.2), and the allogeneic immunogenecity of these CD34+ cells as APCs was not affected at all in the absence of B7 molecules (unpublished data). Thus, CD34+ cells are competent APCs and may generate antileukemia immune responses using alternative costimulation other than the B7-CD28 pathway. It therefore seems likely that leukemia cells at the stage of CD33+ and CD34+ along the cellular differentiation are capable of stimulating an immune response.

Since that antigen-presenting capacity of leukemia cells is adequate as discussed above, questions arise as to why the immune system fails to control leukemia growth. The general immune function in leukemia patients, particularly in patients with CML, is in no way deficient. However, there are reports in other types of cancers showing that the cancer-bearing host is immunologically suppressed specifically for the tumor in the absence of a general immunosuppression. In 1992, Mizoguchi et al. [199] reported that splenic T cells, isolated from mice bearing the MCA-38 colon carcinoma, showed an altered pattern of protein tyrosine phosphorylation, and a dramatic reduction or loss of synthesis of the protein tyrosine kinases p56lck and p59fyn. T cells from tumor-bearing mice also lost the ζ chain associated with the CD3/TCR complex; instead they acquired the FcεRγ chain. As CD3ζ and PTKs occupy fundamental positions in the cascade of cytosolic signaling events, it was postulated that such defects contributed to impaired T-cell function and immunological suppression in the tumor-bearing state. These initial observations have been confirmed independently. Thus, tumor-infiltrating lymphocytes (TILs) and peripheral blood lymphocytes (PBLs) isolated from patients with colorectal or renal cell carcinoma, have revealed variable but distinct downregulation of p56lck and/or the CD3ζ chain in T cells, and CD16ζ in NK cells [200,201]. Furthermore, it has been found that the level of CD3ζ and CD16ζ in PBLs of 16 colorectal carcinoma patients correlated with the Duke stage of the disease [202] and expression of CD3ζ and other signal-transducing molecules in T cells correlated with cancer recurrence and survival [203]. However, the loss of signal transducing proteins does not appear to be universal in T cells of cancer bearing hosts. There are also numerous reports that fail to demonstrate any defect of the signal transduction pathway [204]. Thus, the role of autologous T-cell immune-surveillance dysfunction in tumor patients remains to be further examined.

Whether similar defects exist in T cells from patients with leukemia is not known. We and others have previously failed to detect any autologous antileukemia activity of T cells in patients with CML [205]. The fact that a GVL effect does exist in leukemia patients receiving identical twin BMT [206] and is stronger than that observed in autologous BMT suggests that there might be some defects with T cells in leukemia patients. If it is true, this may impose challenges to the strategy of immunotherapy by tumor vaccine to elicit autologous immune response against leukemia. However, this speculation remains to be studied at the molecular level.

Nevertheless, in allogeneic BMT, T cells from normal donor are competent immune cells and able to mount normal immune responses. Therefore, with the capability of APCs from leukemia patients to stimulate, and for normal T cells from allogeneic donor to respond, a strong GVL is likely to occur.

B. Clonal Expansion

Measurement of cytotoxic T-cell precursor frequency (CTLPf) with antileukemia reactivity in BMT recipients gives some clues to the time required for expansion of leukemia-reactive clones. After BMT and in patients treated for relapse by DLT treatment, several months are required for a log expansion in antileukemic CTLP. Interestingly the majority of this GVL effect appeared to be mediated by CD4+ cells [11,165]. Clinical observations indicate that the response of the leukemia to DLT varies from weeks to months. Leukemia regression associated with GVHD tends to be more rapid than that seen in patients not developing GVHD, suggesting that the precursor frequency of CTLP with antileukemia specificity is lower than those CTLP with broader specificity. However many factors, including the susceptibility of the leukemia to immune regulation, may play a role in the time required for a functional GVL response. At present we have only a superficial understanding of these events.

C. Effector Mechanisms

Three cytotoxic mechanisms in GVL have been defined: cell lysis via the perforin or fas pathways and cytokine suppression of leukemia growth. Several investigators have successfully generated leukemia-reactive CD4+ and CD8+ T-cell clones, derived from responders to HLA identical, or closely identical, CML cells [162,170,207]. Such clones have been used to study the antileukemic effect. An important observation is that cytotoxicity is directed most against the leukemic progenitors in CML, as revealed by colony inhibition assay [162]. Chromium- or dye-release assays are less biologically relevant and less sensitive ways of measuring antileukemic cytotoxicity. Hematopoietic progenitor cells in CML have higher fas antigen expression than normal myeloid progenitor cells [101]. In recent experiments with cytotoxic CD4+ clones recognizing CD33+ CML cells presenting exogenous antigen, we demonstrated that the main cytotoxic mechanism was fas-mediated death of the targets [198].

Cytokine production is another mechanism whereby T cells mediate a GVL effect. In addition to cytokines produced by T cells that can exert an autocrine and paracrine function to recruit effectors and enhance effector cell cytotoxicity, it appears that cytokines from antileukemic CD4+ cell clones can directly regulate normal and leukemic hematopoiesis. We have previously shown that allogeneic CD4+ clones directly inhibited leukemia colony growth [170] and produce a diverse spectrum of cytokines: one type of clone produced IFN-γ and TNF-α and inhibited hematopoiesis, and the inhibitory effect was blocked by addition of neutralizing antibodies to the culture [170]. Another type of clone produced GM-CSF and IL-3 that had a stimulatory effect. This stimulatory effect was abolished by anti-IL3 and GM-CSF antibodies [170]. In vitro studies have shown that leukemia cells were more sensitive to the inhibitory cytokines than normal progenitor cells; whereas normal progenitor cells were more responsive to the stimulatory cytokines than leukemia cells [208,209]. We obtained similar results (Figure 2). These studies support a preferential GVL effect, mediated by CD4+

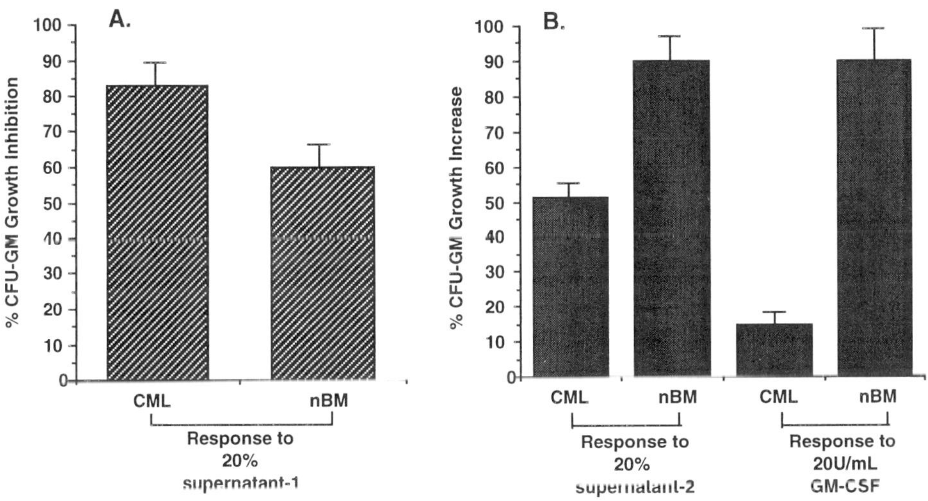

Figure 2 Differential sensitivity of CML and normal bone marrow (nBM) cells to cytokines. Cells from CML patients and normal donors were cultured for CFU-GM growth in 0.3% agar in the presence of (A) 20% T cell–clone culture supernatant-1 + 20 U/mL GM-CSF or (B) supernatant-2 or 20 U/mL GM-CSF. 10^5 BM cells were plated in the culture and the colonies were counted after 14 days. Cultures without supernatant were used as 100% growth. Results showed that supernatant-1 had inhibitory effect and-2 had stimulatory effect on colony growth. CFU-GM counts from CML cells had >80% reduction whereas from nBM had <6-% reduction by supernatant-1. On the other hand, CFU-GM count from CML cells had 50% increase whereas from nBM had 90% increase by supernatant-2. Similarly, CML cells had 15% increase in CFU-GM growth and nBM had 90% increase by GM-CSF. Further studies revealed that supernatant-1 contained TNF-α and IFN-γ and supernatant-2 contained GM-CSF and IL3.

cells, due to differential sensitivity of leukemia cells and normal hematoopoietic progenitors to the stimulatory and inhibitory effect of cytokines. The mechanisms underlying this differential sensitivity of leukemia and normal cells may be due to differential expression of receptors for cytokines on the leukemia or normal progenitor cell surface: For example, fas antigen is expressed on a large number of leukemia cells but not on normal CD34+ cells [191]. TNF-α triggering cells to apoptosis through the fas pathway could therefore preferentially inhibit leukemia cell growth.

V. REGULATION OF THE GVL REACTION

Clinical experience has shown that the potency of the GVL response varies with the type of leukemia treated. Chronic myelogenous leukemia (CML) in chronic phase is most susceptible, acute myelogenous leukemia (AML) has intermediate susceptibility, and acute lymphoblastic leukemia is the least susceptible, showing high relapse rates after allogeneic BMT and infrequent responses to treatment for relapse following BMT with DLT [3]. This suggests that the behavior of the malignant cell as stimulator and target of the alloresponse plays a central part in determining the strength and nature of the GVL effect. As a model to understand the role of key molecules which control the alloresponse, we transfected the MHC class I and II deficient K562 leukemia cell line with HLA-DR1. As previously mentioned, the susceptibility of K562 cells to NK-mediated cytotoxicity was abrogated in K562 cells expressing HLA-DR1. Our experiments indicated that NK cells received a negative signal from the MHC class II transfected cell, possibly mediated by recognition of a self peptide presented by HLA-DR1 [93]. To determine whether the in vitro changes produced by HLA-DR transfection of K562 cells translated into an altered susceptibility to alloreacting lymphocytes in vivo, we established K562 cell tumors in SCID-NOD mice and tested the ability of adoptively transferred human peripheral blood mononuclear cells (PBMC) to control tumor growth [210].

By expressing HLA-DR1 in the MHC class I and II deficient NK-sensitive K562 cell, it was possible to study in isolation the interaction of NK cells and T cells with a single MHC class II molecule. We showed that the expression of HLA-DR1 protected K562 cells from a PBMC mediated antitumor effect in vivo. Furthermore, HLA-DR1 expression inhibits NK cell proliferation while inducing a predominant CD4+ T-cell response. The in vitro resistance to NK lysis by the K562DR1 line was manifest in the SCID/NOD mouse as resistance to the antitumor effect of adoptively transferred PBMC. The antitumor effect was most likely due to NK cells, because it was conferred by unprimed PBMC and CD16+, CD56+ cells, which predominated in the tumor.

As previously mentioned, the inhibitory effect of the K562DR1 transfectant on NK-lysis appeared to be mediated by endogenous peptides presented by the HLA-DR1 molecule: protection from lysis occurred equally with NK cells matched or mismatched with HLA-DR1 and was abrogated by brefeldin (an inhibitor of endogenous antigen processing) [93]. It is possible that the same peptides stimulated the proliferative CD4+ response, since both HLA-DR1 matched and mismatched T cells responded equally to the transfected cell line. Thus the presentation of antigen through HLA-DR1 appeared to be the central factor governing tumor susceptibility to NK cells and the alteration in the effector cell response.

The development of in vivo models of allogeneic antileukemia responses may shed light on some of the mechanisms of GVL in clinical BMT. The variation of the strength of GVL in different type of leukemias and different stages of the same disease is not well understood. Many early leukemia progenitor cells express both MHC class I and II molecules and therefore represent good targets for T-cell attack, if appropriate allo-antigens are presented. In solid tumors, the down-regulation in surface expression of MHC class I and II is a frequent occurrence which may render the tumor resistant to T-cell attack. Such MHC deficient cells should however become targets for NK cell attack [211]. Similar changes occur in leukemia relapsing after BMT [212]. Since many myeloid leukemias are MHC class II positive [189], it is interesting to speculate whether differences in class II expression might explain different susceptibilities of leukemia to the GVL effect. During myeloid differentiation CD33+ cells down regulate HLA class II. Such cells should therefore be more susceptible to NK cell–mediated killing. The stronger GVL reaction seen in CML when compared with AML [3] could be related to the preponderance of DR negative, CD33+, NK sensitive cells in CML in chronic phase. However other key surface molecules such as B7.1 costimulatory molecules [190] and fas antigen [140,191] may have equal or greater significance in determining immunogenicity and susceptibility to killing of leukemia cells. The relative importance of these molecules in determining alloimmune responses to leukemia could be studied further using the approaches described here.

VI. FUTURE DIRECTIONS

Since our understanding of the GVL effect has much improved during the last decade and in practice, we have advanced from the stage of trying to prove the existence of a GVL effect to applying it more efficiently. There remain many challenging issues related to the GVL effector cells to be studied. Examples of approachable questions are as follows:

1. What is the role of monocyte/macrophages in GVL? Monocyte/macrophage is the most important effector in innate immunity and at the first line of immune responses. Its role in regulating GVL and GVHD should be deemed to be more important than what we currently understand. For example, the low incidence of GVHD with G-CSF mobilized stem-cell transplantation has been attributed to the higher numbers of CD14+ presented in the graft [213]. The mechanisms by which CD14+ monocytes regulate GVHD or GVL is not understood.
2. Since CD34+ progenitor cells can be induced to develop into NK cells [214] or T cells, is it possible, in vitro, to study the selection mechanisms by which immune cells can be educated to mediate GVL not GVHD?
3. Is there any specific T-cell suppression to its antileukemia immune responses?
4. What are the factors that result in variable strength of GVL effect observed in different leukemias?
5. Can effector cells be more specifically defined so that GVL and GVHD can be separated on the base of T-cell functions rather than phenotypes?

REFERENCES

1. Goldman JM. Allogeneic bone marrow transplantation for chronic myeloid leukemia:experimental hematology today. In: Baum SJ, Santos GW, and Takaku F, eds. Recent Advances and Future Directions in Bone Marrow Transplantation. New York: Springer Verlag, 1987.
2. Talpaz M, Kantarjian M, Kurzrock R, Gutterman J. Update on therapeutic options for chronic myelogenous leukemia. Semin Hematol 1990; 27 (suppl 4):31–36.
3. Horowitz MM, Gale RP, Sondel PM, Goldman JM, Kersey J, Kolb H-J, Rimm AA, Ringden O, Rozman C, Speck B, Truitt RL, Zwaan FE, Bortin MM. Graft-versus-leukemia reactions after bone marrow transplantation. Blood 1990; 75:555–562.
4. Weiden PL, Flournoy N, Thomas ED, Prentice R, Fefer A, Buckner CD, Storb R. Antileukemia effect of graft-versus-host disease in human recipients of allogeneic marrow graft. N Engl J Med 1979; 300:1068–1073.
5. Collins RH, Rogers ZR, Bennett M, Kumar V, Niekein A, Fay JW. Hematologic relapse of chronic myelogenous leukemia following allogeneic bone marrow transplantation: apparent graft-versus-leukemia effect following abrupt discontinuation of immunosuppression. Bone Marrow Transplant 1992; 10:391–395.
6. Goldman JM, Gale RP, Horowitz MM, Biggs JC, Champlin RE, Gluckman E, Hoffmann RG, Jacobsen SJ, Marmont AM, McGlave PB, Messner HA, Rimm A, Rozman C, Speck B, Tura S, Weiner R, Bortin MM. Bone marrow transplantation for

chronic myelogenous leukemia in chronic phase: increased risk of relapse associated with T cell depletion. Ann Intern Med 1988; 108:806–814.

7. Martin P, Hansen JA, Buckner CD, Sanders JE, Deeg J, Stewart P, Appelbaum FR, Clift R, Fefer A, Witherspoon RP, Kennedy MS, Sullivan KM, Flournoy N, Storb R, Thomas ED. Effects of in vitro depletion of T cells in HLA identical allogeneic marrow grafts. Blood 1985; 66:664–672.
8. Apperley JF, Jones L, Hale G, Goldman JM. Bone marrow transplantation for patients with chronic myeloid leukemia: T cell depletion with Campath-1 reduces the incidence of GVHD but may increase the risk of leukemia relapse. Bone Marrow Transplant 1986; 1:53–68.
9. van Rhee F, Kolb HJ. Donor leukocyte transfusions for leukemic relapse. Curr Opin Hematol 1995; 2:423–430.
10. Cullis JO, Jiang YZ, Schwarer AP, Hughes TP, Barrett AJ, Goldman JM. Donor leukocyte infusion in the treatment of chronic myeloid leukaemia in relapse following allogenic bone marrow transplantation. Blood 1992; 79:1379–1381.
11. Jiang YZ, Cullis JO, Kanfer EJ, Goldman JM, Barrett AJ. T cell and NK cell mediated graft versus leukemia reactivity following donor buffy coat transfusion to treat relapse after marrow transplantation for chronic myeloid leukemia. Bone Marrow Transplant 1993; 11:133–138.
12. Papadopoulos E, Ladanyi M, Emanuel D, Mackinnon S, Boulad F, Carabasi M, Castro-Malaspina H, Childs BH, Gillio AP, Small TN, Young JW, Kernan NA, O'Reilly RJ. Infusion of donor leukocytes to treat EBV associated lymphoproliferative disorders after allogeneic bone marrow transplantation. N Engl J Med 1994; 330:1185–1191.
13. Tricot G, Vesole D, Jagannath S, Hilton J, Munshi N, Barlogie B. Graft-versus-myeloma effect: proof of principle. Blood 1996; 87:1196–1198.
14. Verdonck LF, Lokhorst HM, Dekker AW, Nieuwenhuis HK, Petersen EJ. Graft-versus-myeloma effect in two cases. Lancet 1996; 347:800–801.
15. Eibl B, Schwaighofer H, Nachbaur D, Marth C, Gachter A, Knapp R, Bock G, Gassner C, Schiller L, Petersen F, Niederwieser D. Evidence of a graft-versus tumor effect in a patient treated with marrow ablative chemotherapy and allogeneic bone marrow transplantation for breast cancer. Blood 1996; 88:1501–1508.
16. Nimer SD, Giorgi J, Gajewski JL, Ku N, Schiller GJ, Lee K, Territo M, Ho W, Feig S, Selch M, Isacescu V, Reichert TA, Champlin RE. Selective depletion of CD8+ cells for prevention of graft-versus-host disease after bone marrow transplantation. Transplantation 1994; 57:82–87.
17. Giralt S, Hester J, Huh Y, Hirsch-Ginsberg C, Rondn G, Seong D, Lee M, Gajewski J, Van Besien K, Khouri I, Mehra R, Przepiorka D, Kirbling M, Talpaz M, Kantarjian H, Fischer H, Deisseroth A, Champlin R. CD8-depleted donor lymphocyte infusion as treatment for relapsed chronic myelogenous leukemia after allogeneic bone marrow transplantation. Blood 1995; 86:4337–4343.
18. Palathumpat V, Dejbakhsh-Jones S, Strober S. The role of purified CD8+ T cells in graft-versus-leukemia activity and engraftment after allogeneic bone marrow transplantation. Transplantation 1995; 60:355–361.
19. Herrera C, Martin C, Garcia-Castellano JM, Roman J, Alvarez MA, Flores R, Garcia MJ, de la Torre MJ, Sanchez J, Martines F, Gomez P, Torres A. Prevention of

GVHD by selective CD4+ T cell depletion plus adjustment of the CD8+ cell content in donor bone marrow (abstr). Blood 1995; 86 (suppl 1):571a.

20. Jiang YZ, Barrett AJ, Goldman JM and Mavroudis DA. Association of natural killer cell immune recovery with a graft-vs-leukemia effect independent of graft vs host disease after allogeneic bone marrow transplantation. Ann Hematol 1996; 74:1–6.
21. Glass B, Uharek L, Zeis M, Loeffler H, Mueller-Ruchholtz W, Gassmann W. Graft-versus-leukaemia activity can be predicted by natural cytotoxicity against leukaemia cells. Br J Haematol 1996; 93:412–420.
22. Glass B, Uharek L, Gassmann W, Focks B, Bolouri H, Loeffler H, Mueller-Ruchholtz W. Graft-versus-leukemia activity after bone marrow transplantation does not require graft-versus-host disease. Ann Hematol 1992; 64:255–259.
23. Haynes B. The human thymic microenvironment. Adv Immunol 1984; 36:87–142.
24. Tjonnfjord GE, Veiby OP, Steen R, Egeland T. T lymphocyte differentiation in vitro from adult human prethymic CD34+ bone marrow cells. J Exp Med 1993; 177:1531–1539.
25. Murray L, Chen B, Galy S, Tushinski R, Uchida N, Negrin R, Tricot G, Jagannath S, Vesole D, Narlogie B, Hoffman R, Tsukamoto A. Enrichment of human hematopoietic stem cell activity in the CD34+Thy1+Lin-subpopulation from mobilized peripheral blood. Blood 1995; 85:368–378.
26. DiGiusto D, Chen S, Combs J, Webb S, Namikawa R, Tsukamoto A, Chen BP, Galy AHM. Human fetal bone marrow early progenitors for T, B and myeloid cells are found exclusively in the population expressing high levels of CD34. Blood 1994; 84:421–432.
27. Freedman AR, Zhu H, Levine JD, Kalams S, Scadden DT. Generation of human T lymphocytes from bone marrow CD34+ cells in vitro. Nature Med 1996; 2:46–51.
28. Ardavin C, Wu L, Shortman K. Thymic dendritic cells and T cells develop simultaneously in the thymus from a common precursor population. Nature 1993; 362: 761–763.
29. Spits H, Lanier LL, Phillips JH. Development of human T and natural killer cells. Blood 1995; 85:2654–2670.
30. Mombaerts P, Clarke AR, Rudnicki MA, Iacomini J, Itohara S, Lafaille JJ, Wang L, Ichikawa Y, Jaenisch R, Hooper MI, Tonegawa S. Mutations in T cell receptor gene a and b block thymocyte development at different stages. Nature 1992; 360: 225–231.
31. Raulet DH, Garman RD, Saito H, Tonegawa S. Developmental regulation of T cell receptor gene expression. Nature 1985; 314:103–107.
32. Hori T, Spits H. Clonal analysis of human CD4-CD8-CD3-thymocytes purified from postnatal thymus. J Immunol 1991; 146:2116.
33. Ernst BB, Surh CD, Sprent J. Bone marrow derived cells fail to induce positive selection in thymus reaggregation cultures. J Exp Med 1996; 183:1235–1240.
34. Testi R, Phillips JH, Lanier LL: Constitutive expression of a phosphorylated activated antigen (Leu 23) by CD3bright human thymocytes. J Immunol 1988; 141: 2557–2563.

35. Vanderkerckhove BAE, Barcena A, Schols D, Mohan-Peterson S, Spits H, Roncarolo MG. In vivo cytokine expression in the thymus: CD3high human thymocytes are activated and already functionally differentiated in helper and cytotoxic cells. J Immunol 1994; 152:1738.
36. Lanier LL, Allison JP, Phillips JH. Correlation of cell surface antigen exprcssion on human thymocytes by multi-color flow cytometric analysis: implications for differentiation. J Immunol 1986; 137:2501–2507.
37. Robey E, Chang D, Itano A, Cado D, Alexander H, Lans D, Weinmaster G, Salmon P. An activated form of Notch influences the choice between CD4 and CD8 T cell lineages. Cell 1996; 87:483–492.
38. Constant SL, Bottomly K: Induction of Th1 and Th2 CD4+ T cell responses: the alternative approaches. Annu Rev Immunol 1997; 15:297–322.
39. Rolink A, ten Boekel E, Melchers F, Fearon DT, Krop I, Andersson J. A subpopulation of B220+ cells in murine bone marrow does not express CD19 and contains natural killer cell progenitors. J Exp Med 1996; 183:187–194.
40. Phillips JH, Lanier LL. Acquisition of non-MHC restricted cytotoxic function by IL2 activated thymocytes with an immature antigenic phenotype. J Immunol 1987; 139:683–687.
41. Sanchez MJ, Muench MO, Roncarolo MG, Lanier L, Phillips JH. Identification of a common T/NK cell progenitor in human fetal thymus. J Exp Med 1994; 180: 569.
42. Lotzova E, Savary CA, Gray KN, Raulston GL, Jardine JH. Natural killer cell profile of two random-bred strains of athymic rats. Exp Hematol 1984; 12:633–640.
43. Sirianni MC, Businco L, Seminara R, Aiuti F. Severe combined immunodeficiency primary T cell defects and digeorge syndrome in human: characterization by monoclonal antibodies and natural killer cell activity. Clin Immunol Immunopathol 1983; 28:361–370.
44. Raulet DH, Held W. Natural killer cell receptors: the offs and ons of NK cell recognition. Cell 1995; 82:697–700.
45. Davis SJ, van der Merwe PA: The structure and ligand interactions of CD2: implications for T-cell function. Immunol Today 1996; 17:177–186.
46. Springer TK, Martin SD. The LFA-1, CD2 and LFA3 molecules: cell adhesion receptors of the immune system. Annu Rev Immunol 1987; 5:223–252.
47. Bierer BE, Sleckman BP, Rotnofsky SE, Burakoff SJ. The biological roles of CD2, CD4, and CD8 in T-cell activation. Annu Rev Immunol 1989; 7:579–600.
48. McCloskey MA, Poo MM. Contact-induced redistribution of specific membrane components: local accumulation and development of adhesion. J Cell Biol 1986; 102:2185–2196.
49. Dustin ML, Springer TA. T-cell receptor cross-linking transiently stimulates adhesiveness through LFA-1. Nature 1989; 341:619–624.
50. van Gool S, Vandenberghe P, de Boer M, Ceuppens JL. CD80, CD86 and CD40 provide accessory signals in a multiple-step T-cell activation model. Immunol Rev 1996; 153:47–82.
51. Falk K, Rotzschke O, Deres K, Metzger J, Jung G, Rammensee HG. Identification of naturally processed viral nonapeptides allows their quantification in infected cells

and suggests an allele-specific T cell epitope forecast. J Exp Med 1991; 174:425–434.

52. Cantrell D. T cell antigen receptor signal transduction pathways. Annu Rev Immunol 1996; 14:259–274.
53. Ward SG, June CH, Olive D. PI 3-kinase: a pivotal pathway in T cell activation? Immunol Today 1996; 17:187–197.
54. Alberola-Ila J, Takaki S, Kerner JD, Perlmutter RM. Differential signaling by lymphocyte antigen receptors. Annu Rev Immunol 1997; 15:125–154.
55. Gauen LKT, Zhu YX, Letourneur F, Hu Q, Bolen JB, Matis LA, Klausner RD, Shaw AS. Interactions of p59fyn and ZAP70 with TCR activation motifs: defining the nature of a signaling motif. Mol Cell Biol 1994; 14:3729–3741.
56. Rudd CE, Trevillyan JM, Dasgupta JD, Wong LL, Schlossman SF. The CD4 receptor is complexed in detergent lysates to a protein-tyrosine kinase (pp58) from human T lymphocytes. Proc Natl Acad Sci USA 1988; 85:5190.
57. Goldman F, Crabtree J, Hollenback C, Koretzky G. Sequestration of p56lck by gp120, a model for TCR desensitization. J Immunol 1997; 158:2017–2024.
58. Mescher MF. Molecular interactions in the activation of effector and precursor cytotoxic T lymphocytes. Immunol Rev 1995; 146:177–210.
59. Burridge K, and Connell LJ. A new protein of adhesion plaques and ruffling membranes. J Cell Biol 1983; 97:359–367.
60. Kupfer A, Singer SJ. The specific interaction of helper T cells and antigen-presenting B cells: IV. Membrane and cytoskeletal reorganizations in the bound T cell as a function of antigen dose. J Exp Med 1989; 170:1697–1713.
61. Waters JB, Oldstone MBA, Hahn KM. Changes in the cytoplasmic structure of CTLs during target cell recognition and killing. J Immunol 1996; 157:3396–3403.
62. Kupfer A, Singer SJ. Cell biology of cytotoxic and helper T cell functions: immunoflurescence microscopic studies of single cells and cell couples. Annu Rev Immunol 1989; 7:309–337.
63. Yannelli JR, Sullivan JA, Mandell GL, Engelhard VH. Reorientation and fusion of cytotoxic T lymphocyte granules after interaction with target cells as determined by high resolution micrography. J Immunol 1986; 136:377–382.
64. Hamblin AS. Lymphokines. Oxford: IRL Press, 1988.
65. Suda T, Takahashi T, Golstein P, Nagata S. Molecular cloning and expression of the Fas ligand, a novel member of the tumor necrosis factor family. Cell 1993; 75: 1169–1178.
66. Amlot PL, Tahami F, Chinn D, Rawlings E. Activation antigen expression on human T cells: analysis by two-colour flow cytometry of umbilical cord blood, adult blood and lymphoid tissue. Clin Exp Immunol 1996; 105:176–182.
67. Podack ER, Kupfer A. T-cell effector functions: mechanisms for delivery of cytotoxicity and help. Annu Rev Cell Biol 1991; 7:479–504.
68. Herberman RB, Reynolds CW, Taldo JR. Mechanism of cytotoxicity by natural killer cells. Annu Rev Immunol 1986; 4:651–680.
69. Sanchez MJ, Gutierrez-Ramos JC, Fernandez E, Leonardo E, Lozano J, Martinez C, Toribio ML. Putative prethymic T-cell precursors within the early human embryonic liver: a molecular and functional analysis. J Exp Med 1993; 177:19.
70. Moretta A, Vitale M, Bottino L, Orengo AM, Morelli L, Angugliaro R, Barbaresi

M, Ciccone E, Moretta L. P58 molecules as putative receptors for major histocompatibility complex (MHC) class I molecules in human NK cells: anti-p58 antibodies reconstitute lysis of MHC class I-protected cells in NK clones displaying different specificities. J Exp Med 1993; 178:597–604.

71. Litwin V, Gumperz J, Parham P, Phillips JH, Lanier LL. NKB1: a natural killer cell receptor involved in the recognition of polymorphic HLA-B molecules. J Exp Med 1994; 180:537–543.
72. D'Andrea A, Chang C, Franz-Bacon K, McClanahan T, Phillips JH, Lanier LL. Molecular cloning of NKB1: a natural killer cell receptor for HLA-B allotypes. J Immunol 1995; 155:2306–2310.
73. Gumperz JE, Litwin V, Phillips JH, Lanier LL, Parham P. The Bw4 public epitope of HLA-B molecules confers reactivity with natural killer cell clones that express NKB1, a putative HLA receptor. J Exp Med 1995; 181:1133–1144.
74. Dohring C, Scheidegger D, Samaridis J, Cella M, Colonna M. A human killer inhibitory receptor specific for HLA-A. J Immunol 1996; 156:3098–3101.
75. Peruzzi M, Wagtmann N, Long EO. A p70 killer cell inhibitory receptor specific for several HLA-B allotypes discriminated among peptides bound to HLA-B*2705. J Exp Med 1996; 184:1585–1590.
76. Phillips JH, Chang CW, Mattson J, Gumperz JE, Parham P, Lanier LL. CD94 and a novel associated protein (94AP) form a NK cell receptor involved in the recognition of HLA-A, B and C allotypes. Immunity 1996; 5:163–172.
77. Brumbaugh KM, Perez-Villar JJ, Dick CJ, Schoon RA, Lopez-Botet M, Leibson PJ. Clonotypic differences in signaling from CD94 (kp43) on NK cells lead to divergent cellular responses. J Immunol 1996; 157:2804–2812.
78. Wagtman N, Biassoni R, Cantoni C, Verdiani S, Malnati MS, Vitale M, Bottino C, Moretta L, Moretta A, Long EO. Molecular cloning of the p58 NK cell receptor reveal immunoglobulin related molecules with diversity in both the extra- and intracellular domains. Immunity 1995; 2:439–449.
79. Colonna M, Samaridis J. Cloning of immunoglobulin superfamily members associated with HLA-C and HLA-B recognition by human natural killer cells. Science 1995; 268:405–408.
80. Vitale M, Sivori S, Pende D, Moretta L, Moretta A. The coexpression of two functionally independent p58 inhibitory receptors in human NK cell clones results in the inability to kill all normal allogeneic target cells. Proc Natl Acad Sci USA 1995; 92:3536–3540.
81. Lanier LL, Gumperz JE, Parham P, Melero I, Botet ML, Phillips JH. The NKB1 and HP-3E4 NK cell receptors are structurally distinct glycoproteins and independently recognize polymorphic HLA-B and HLA-C molecules. J Immunol 1995; 154: 3320–3327.
82. Lanier LL, Phillips JH. Inhibitory MHC class I receptors on NK and T cells. Immunol Today 1996; 17:86–91.
83. Ciccone E, Grossi CE, Velardi A. Opposing functions of activatory TCR and inhibitory NK cell receptors on CTLs. Immunol Today 1996; 17:450–452.
84. Moretta A, Bottino C, Vitale M, Pende D, Biassoni R, Mingari MC, Moretta L. Receptors for HLA class I molecules in human natural killer cells. Annu Rev Immunol 1996; 14:619–648.

85. Long EO, Burshtyn DN, Clark WP, Peruzzi M, Rajagopalan S, Rojo S, Wagtmann N, Winter CC. Killer cell inhibitory receptors: diversity, specificity, and function. Immunol Rev 1997; 155:135–144.
86. Renard V, Cambiaggi A, Vely F, Blery M, Olcese L, Olivero S, Bouchet M, Vivier E. Transduction of cytotoxic signals in natural killer cells: a general model of fine tuning between activatory pathways in lymphocytes. Immunol Rev 1997; 155:205–221.
87. Rammensee HG, Falk K, Rotzschke O. Peptides naturally presented by MHC class I molecules. Annu Rev Immunol 1993; 11:213–244.
88. Malnati MS, Peruzzi M., Parker KC, Biddison WE, Ciccone E. Moretta A, Long EO. Peptide specificity in the recognition of MHC class I by natural killer cell clones. Science 1995; 267:1016.
89. Rajagopalan S, Long EO. The direct binding of a p58 killer cell inhibitory receptor to human histocompatibility leukocyte antigen (HLA)-Cw4 exhibits peptide selectivity. J Exp Med 1997; 185:1523–1528.
90. Nakajima H, Takiguchi M. Regulaton of CTL recognition by receptors for HLA-DR molecules. J Immunol 1996; 157:2239–2242.
91. Lobo PI, Pencer CE. Use of anti-HLA antibodies to mask major histocompatibility complex gene products on tumour cells can enhance susceptibility of these cells to lysis by natural killer cells. J Clin Invest 1989; 83:278–287.
92. Lobo PI, Patel HC. A novel role for MHC class II antigens: evidence implicating a protective effect on tumour cells against cytotoxicity by NK and LAK cells. Immunology 1994; 83:240.
93. Jiang YZ, Couriel D, Mavroudis D, Lewalle P, Malkovska V, Hensel N, Dermime S, Molldrem J, Barrett AJ. Interaction of NK cells with MHC class II: reversal of HLA-DR1 mediated protection of K562 transfectant from NK cell mediated cytolysis by Brefeldin-A. Immunology 1996; 87:481–486.
94. Kurago ZB, Smith KD, Charles TL. NK cell recognition of MHC class I: NK cells are sensitive to peptide-binding groove and surface α-helical mutations that affect T cells. J Immunol 1995; 154:2631–2641.
95. Kaufman DS, Schoon RA, Leibson PJ. Role for major histocompatibility complex class I in regulating natural killer cell–mediated killing of virus-infected cells. Proc Natl Acad Sci USA 1992; 89:8337.
96. Pinet V, Malnati MS, Long EO. Two processing pathways for the MHC class II restricted presentation of exogenous influenza virus antigen. J Immunol 1994; 152: 4852.
97. Nuchtern JG, Biddison WE, Klausner RD. Class II MHC molecules can use the endogenous pathway of antigen presentation. Nature 1990; 343:74–76.
98. Rudensky AY, Preston-Hurlburt P, Hong S-C, Barlow A, Janeway CA. Sequence analysis of peptides bound to MHC class II molecules. Nature 1991; 353:622–627.
99. Ciccone E, Pende D, Viale O, Di Donato C, Tripodi G, Orengo AM, Uardiola J, Moretta A, Moretta L. Evidence of a NK cell repertoire for (allo) antigen recognition: definition of five distinct NK-determined allospecificities in humans. J Exp Med 1992; 175:709–718.
100. Kung SK, Miller RG. Mouse natural killer subsets defined by their target specificity

and their ability to be separately rendered unresponsive in vivo. J Immunol 1997; 158:2616–2626.

101. Biassoni R, Falco M, Cambiaggi A, Costa P, Verdiani S, Pende D, Conte R, di Donato C, Parham P, Moretta L. Amino acid substitutions can influence the NK-mediated recognition of HLA-C molecules. Role of serine-77 and lysine-80 in the target cell protection from lysis mediated by group 2 or group 1 NK clones. J Exp Med 1995; 182:605–609.

102. Storkus WJ, Salter RD, Alexander J. Class I induced NK resistance in human B cell targets: identification of non-permissive residues in HLA-A2. Proc Natl Acad Sci USA 1991; 88:5989–5993.

103. Schulz RJ, Parkes A, Mizoguchi E, Bhan A, Koyasu S. Development of CD4-CD8-abTCR+NK1.1+T lymphocytes: thymic selection by self antigen. J Immunol 1996; 157:4379–4389.

104. Vivier E, Rocher N, Kovhan J-P, Presky DH, Schlossman SF, Anderson P. Structure similarities between Fc receptors and TCR: expression of the g subuint of FceRI in human T cells, NK cells, and thymocytes. J Immunol 1991; 147:4263–4270.

105. Wirthmueller U, Kurosaki T, Murakami MS, Ravetch JV. Signal transduction by FcgRIII (CD16) is mediated through the γ chain. J Exp Med 1992; 175:1381–1390.

106. Salcedo TW, Kurosaki T, Kanakaraj P, Ravetch J, Perussia B. Physical and functional association of p56lck with FcgRIIIa (CD16) in natural killer cells. J Exp Med 1993; 177:1475–1480.

107. Anegon I, Cuturi MC, Trinchieri G, Perussia B. Interaction of Fc receptor (CD16) ligands induces transcription of interleukin 2 receptor (CD25) and lymphokine genes and expression of their products in human natural killer cells. J Exp Med 1988; 167:452–471.

108. Ryan JC, Niemi EC, Nakamura MC, Seaman WE. NKR-P1 A is a target specific receptor that activates natural killer cell cytotoxicity. J Exp Med 1995; 181:1911–1915.

109. Ryan JC, Niemi EC, Doldfien RD, Hiserodt JC, Seaman WE. NKR-p1, an activating molecule on rat natural killer cells, stimulates phospho-inositide turnover and a rise in intracellular calcium. J Immunol 1991; 147:3244–3250.

110. Yokoyama WM, Seaman WE. The LY49 and NKR-P1 gene families encoding lectin-like receptors on natural killer cells: the NK gene complex. Annu Rev Immunol 1993; 11:613–635.

111. Santis AG, Lopez-Cabrera M, Hamann J, Strauss M, Sanchez-Madrid F. Structure of the gene coding for the human early lymphocytes activation antigen CD69: a C-type lectin receptor evolutionarily related with the gene families of natural killer cell specific receptors. Eur J Immunol 1994; 24:1692–1697.

112. Triebel F, Jitsukawa S, Baxeras E, Roman-Roman S, Genevee C, Viegas-pequignot E, Hercend T. Lag-3, a novel lymphocyte activation gene closely related to CD4. J Exp Med 1990; 171:1393–1405.

113. Moretta A, Ciccone E, Pantaleo G, Tambussi G, Bottino C, Melioli G, Migari MC, Moretta L. Surface molecules involved in the activation and regulation of T or natural killer lymphocytes in human. Immunol Rev 1989; 111:145–175.

114. Grogg D, Hahn S, Erb P. CD4+ T-cell-mediated killing of major histocompatibility

complex class-II-positive antigen-presenting cells:III. CD4+ cytotoxic T-cells induce apoptosis of APC. Eur J Immunol 1992; 22:267.

115. Ju ST, Ruddle NH, Strack P, Dorf ME, DeKruyff RH. Expression of two distinct cytolytic mechanisms among murine CD4 subsets. J Immunol 1990; 144:23–31.
116. Stadler T. Fas antigen is the major target molecule for CD4+ mediated cytotoxicity. J Immunol 1994; 152:1127–1134.
117. Suda T, Nagata S. Purification and characterization of the Fas-ligand that induces apoptosis. J Exp Med 1994; 179:873.
118. Peitsch MC, Tschopp J, Comparative molecular modelling of the fas-ligand and other members of the TNF family. Mol Immunol 1995; 32:761.
119. Smith CA, Farrah T, Goodwin RG. The TNF receptor superfamily of cellular and viral proteins: activation, costimulation, and death. Cell 1994; 76:959.
120. Wanatanabe-Fukunaga R, Brannan CI, Copeland NG, Jenkins NA, Nagata S. Lymphoproliferation disorder in mice explained by defects in Fas antigen that mediates apoptosis. Nature 1992; 356:314–317.
121. Miyawaki T, Uehara T, Nibu R, Tsuji T, Yachie A, Yonehara S, Taniguchi N. Differential expression of apoptosis-related Fas antigen on lymphocyte subpopulations in human peripheral blood. J Immunol 1992; 149:3753–3758.
122. Itoh N, Yonehara S, Ishii A, Yonehara M, Mizushima S, Sameshima M, Hase A, Set V, Nagata S. The polypeptide encoded by the cDNA for human cell surface antigen Fas can mediate apoptosis. Cell 1991; 66:233–243.
123. Nagata S. Apoptosis: telling cells their time is up. Curr Biol 1996; 6:1241–1243.
124. Kagi D, Vignaux F, Ledermenn B, Burki K, Depraetere V, Nagata S, Hengartner H, Golstein P. Fas and perforin pathways as major mechanisms of T cell-mediated cytotoxicity. Science 1994; 265:528–530.
125. Brossart P, Bevan MJ. Selective activation of Fas/Fas ligand-mediated cytotoxicity by a self peptide. J Exp Med 1996; 183:2449–2458.
126. Berke G. Review: the fas-based mechanism of lymphocytotoxicity. Human Immunol 1997; 54:1–7.
127. Kagi D, Ledermann B, Burki K, Seiler P, Odermatt B, Olsen KJ, Posack ER, Zinkernagel RM, Hengartner H. Cytotoxicity mediated by T cells and NK cells is greatly impaired in perforin deficient mice. Nature 1994; 369:31–37.
128. Hahn S, Gehri R, Erb P. Mechanism and biological significance of CD4-mediated cytotoxicity. Immunol Rev 1995; 146:57–79.
129. Velotti F, MacDonald HR, Nabholz M. Granzyme A secretion by normal activated Lyt-2+ and L3T4+ T cells in response to antigenic stimulation. Eur J Immunol 1987; 17:1095–1090.
130. Williams NS, Engelhard VH. Identification of a population of CD4+CTL that utilizes a perforin-rather than a Fas ligand-dependent cytotoxic mechanism. J Immunol 1996; 156:153–159.
131. Liu CC, Persechini PM, and Young JDE. Perforin and lymphocyte-mediated cytolysis. Immunol Rev 1995; 146:145–175.
132. Susskind B, Shornick MD, Iannotti MR, Duffy B, Mehrotra nee Tanden P, Siegel JP, Mohanakumar T. Cytolytic effector mechanisms of human CD4+ cytotoxic T lymphocytes. Hum Immunol 1996; 45:64.
133. Welsh RM, Selin LK, and Razvi ES. Role of apoptosis in the regulation of virus-

induced T cell response, immune suppression and memory. J Cell Biochem 1995; 59:135–142.
134. Akbar AN, Salmon M. Cellular environments and apoptosis: tissue microenvironment control activated T-cell death. Immunol Today 1997; 18:72–76.
135. Alderson MR, Armitage RJ, Maraskovsky E, Tough TW, Roux E, Schools V, Ramsdell F, Lynch DH. Fas transduces activation signals in normal human T lymphocytes. J Exp Med 1993; 178:2231–2235.
136. Clark WR, Walsh CM, Glass AA, Hayashi F, Matloubian M, Ahmed R. Molecular pathways of CTL-mediated cytotoxicity. Immunol Rev 1995; 146:33–43.
137. Trenn G, Takayama H, Sitkovsky MV. Exocytosis of cytolytic granules may not be required for target cell lysis by CTL. Nature 1987; 330:72–74.
138. Kagi D, Ledermann B, Burki K, Zinkernagel RM, Hengartner H. Lymphocyte-mediated cytotoxicity in vitro and in vivo: mechanisms and significance. Immunol Rev 1996; 146:95–115.
139. Ogasawara J, Watanabe-Fukunaga R, Adachi M, Matsuzawa A, Kasugai T, Kitamura Y, Itoh N, Suda T, Nagata S. Lethal effect of the anti-fas antibody in mice. Nature 1993; 364:806–809.
140. Yagita H, Hanabuchi S, Asano Y, Tamura T, Nariuchi H, Okumura K. Fas-mediated cytotoxicity—a new immunoregulatory and pathogenic function of Th1 CD4+ T cells. Immunol Rev 1995; 146:223–239.
141. Young JD, Cohn ZA, Podack ER. The 9th component of complement and the pore-forming protein (perforin 1) from cytotoxsic T cells: structural, immunological, and functional similarities. Science 1986; 233:184–190.
142. Nakajima H, Henkart PA. Cytoxic lymphocyte granzymes trigger a target cell internal disintegration pathway leading to cytolysis and DNA breakdown. J Immunol 1994; 152:1057–1063.
143. Shinkai Y, Takio K, Okumura K. Homology of perforin to the ninth component of complement (c9). Nature 1988; 334:525–527.
144. Yagita H, Nakata M, Kawasaki A, Shinkai Y, Okumura K. Role of perforin in lymphocyte-mediated cytolysis. Adv Immunol 1992; 51:215–242.
145. Young JDE, Hengartner H, Podack ER, Cohn ZA. Purification and characterization of a cytolytic pore forming protein from granules of cloned lymphocytes with natural killer activity. Cell 1986; 44:849.
146. Jenne DE, Tschopp J. Granzymes, a family of serine proteases released from granules of cytotoxic T lymphocytes upon T cell receptor stimulation. Immunol Rev 1988; 103:53–71.
147. Jenne DE, Masson D, Zimmer M, Haefliger JA, Li WH, Tschopp J. Isolation and complete structure of the lymphocyte serine protease granzyme G: a novel member of the granzyme multigene family in murine cytolytic T lymphocytes: evolutionary origin of lymphocyte proteases. Biochemistry 1989; 28:7953–7961.
148. Peters PJ, Borst J, Oorschot V, Fukuda M, Krahenbuhl O, Tschopp J, Slot JW, Geuze HJ. Cytotoxic T lymphocyte granules are secretory lysosomes, containing both perforin and granzymes. J Exp Med 1991; 173:1099–1109.
149. Heusel JW, Wesselschmidt RL, Hresta S, Russel JH, and Ley TJ. Cytotoxic lymphocytes require granzyme B for the rapid induction of DNA fragmentation and apoptosis in allogeneic target cells. Cell 1994; 76:977–987.

150. Nakajima H, Park HL, Henkart PA. Synergistic roles of granzymes A and B in mediating target cell death by rat basophilic leukemia mast cell tumors also expressing cytolysin/perforin. J Exp Med 1995; 181:1037–1046.
151. Shresta A, Heusel JW, Macivor DM, Wesselschmidt RL, Russel JH, Ley T. Granzyme B plays a critical role in cytotoxic lymphocyte-induced apoptosis. Immunol Rev 1995; 146:211–221.
152. Ojcius DM, Zheng LM, Spicas EC, Zychlinsky A, and Young JDE. Subcellular localization of perforin and serine esterase in lymphokine activated killer cells and cytotoxic T cells by immunogold labeling. J Immunol 1991; 146:4427–4432.
153. Tsutsui H, Nakanishi K, Matsui K, Higashino K, Okamura H, Miyazawa Y, and Kaneda K. IFN-r inducing factor up-regulates Fas ligand-mediated cytotoxic activity of murine NK clones. J Immunol 1996; 157:3967–3973.
154. Tanaka M, Suda T, Takahashi T, Nagata S. Expression of the functional soluble form of human Fas ligand in activated lymphocytes. EBMO J 1995; 14:1129.
155. Tanaka M, Suda T, Haze K, Nakamura N, Sato K, Kimura F, Motoyoshi K, Mizuki M, Tagawa S, Ohga S, Hatake K, Drummond AH, Nagata S. Fas ligand in human serum. Nature Med 1996; 2:317.
156. Kolb H, Schattenberg A, Goldman JM, Hertenstein B, Jacobsen N, Arcese W, Ljungman P, Ferrant A, Verdonck L, Niederwieser D, van Rhee F, Mittermueller J, de Witte T, Holler E, Ansari H. Graft vs leukemia effect of donor lymphocyte transfusions in marrow grafted patients. Blood 1995; 86:2041–2050.
157. Soiffer RJ, Murray C, Gonin R, Ritz J. Effect of low dose IL2 on disease relapse after T cell depleted allogeneic bone marrow transplantation. Blood 1994; 84:964–971.
158. Blaise D, Olive D, Michallet M, Marit G, Leblond V, Maraninchi D. Impairment of leukemia free survival by addition of interleukin-2 receptor antibody to standard graft-vs-host prophylaxis. Lancet 1995; 345:1144–1146.
159. Hebart H, Ehninger G, Schmidt H, Berner B, Reuss-Borst M, Waller HD, Muller HD, and Einsele H. Treatment of steroid-resistant graft versus host disease after allogeneic bone marrow transplantation with anti- CD3/TCR monoclonal antibodies. Bone Marrow Transplant 1995; 15:891–894.
160. Blazar BR, Sharpe AH, Taylor PA, Mortari AP, Gray GS, Korngold R, Vallera DA. Infusion of anti-B7.1 (CD80) and anti-B7.2 (CD86) monoclonal antibodies inhibits murine graft-vs-host disease lethality in part via direct effects on CD4+ and CD8+ T cells. J Immunol 1996; 157:3250–3259.
161. Higano CS, Brixey M, Bryant EM, Durnam DM, Doney K, Sullivan KM, Singer JW. Durable complete remission of acute non-lymphoblastic leukemia associated with discontinuation of immunosuppression following relapse after allogeneic bone marrow transplantation—a case report of a probable GVL effect. Transplantation 1990; 50:175–177.
162. Falkenburg F, Goselink H, van der Harst D, van Lyxemburg-Heijs AA, Kooy-Winkelaar YM, Faber M, de Kroon J, Brand A, Fibbe WE, Willemze R. Growth inhibition of clonogenic leukemic precursor ells by minor histocompatibility antigen specific cytotoxic T lymphocytes. J Exp Med 1991; 174:27–33.
163. Hoffmann T, Theobald M, Bunkes D, Weiss M, Heimpel H, Heit W. Frequency

of bone marrow T cells responding to HLA-identical nonleukemic and leukemic stimulator cells. Bone Marrow Transplant 1993; 12:1–8.
164. Jiang YZ, Kanfer E, MacDonald M, Cullis JO, Goldman JM, Barrett AJ. Graft versus leukemia effect following allogeneic bone marrow transplantation: emergence of cytotoxic T lymphocytes to host leukemia cells. Bone Marrow Transplant 1991; 8:253–258.
165. Bunjes D, Theobald M, Hertenstein B, Wiesneth M, Novotny J, Arnold R, Heimpel H. Successful therapy with donor buffy coat transfusions in patients with relapsed chronic myeloid leukemia after bone marrow transplantation is associated with high frequencies of host reactive interleukin-2 secreting T helper cells. Bone Marrow Transplant 1995; 15:713–719.
166. Townsend RM, Paterson A, Hsieh MH, Korngold R. Studies of the graft-versus-myeloid leukemia responses following murine bone marrow transplantation. (abstr). Blood 1996; 88(suppl 1):244.
167. Korngold R, Sprent J. T cell subsets and graft versus host disease. Transplantation 1987; 44:335–339.
168. O'Kunewick J, Kociban D, Machen L, Buffo M. Effect of selective donor T-cell depletion on the graft-versus-leukemia reaction in allogeneic marrow transplantation. Transplant Proc 1992; 24:2998–2999.
169. Truitt RL, Atasoylu AA: Contribution of CD4+ and CD8+ T cells to graft-versus-host disease and graft-versus-leukemia reactivity after transplantation of MHC-compatible bone marrow. Bone Marrow Transplant 1991; 8:51–58.
170. Jiang YZ, Barrett AJ. Cellular and cytokine mediated effects of CD4+ lymphocyte lines generated in vitro against chronic myelogenous leukemia. Exp Hematol 1995; 23:1167–1172.
171. Oettel KR, Wesly OH, Albertini MR, Hank JA, Iliopolis O, Sosman JA, Voelkerding K, Wu S, Clark SS, Sondel PM. Allogeneic T-cell clones able to selectively destroy Philadelphia chromosome-bearing (Ph1+) human leukemia lines can also recognize Ph1- cells from the same patient. Blood 1994; 83:3390–3402.
172. Mackinnon S, Papadopoulos EB, Carabsi M, Reich L, Collins NH, Boulad F, Castro-Malaspina H, Childs BH, Gillio AP, Kernan NA, Small TN, Young JW, O'Reilly RJ. Adoptive immunotherapy evaluating escalating doses of donor leukocytes for relapse of CML after bone marrow transplantation: separation of graft versus leukemia responses from graft versus host disease. Blood 1995; 86:1261–1270.
173. Moss PAH, Bell JI. The human T cell receptor repertoire. In: Bell JI, Owen MJ, Simpson E, eds. T Cell Receptors. Oxford:Oxford University Press, 1995.
174. Pinet V, Malnati MS, Long EO. Two processing pathways for the MHC class II restricted presentation of exogenous influenza virus antigen. J Immunol 1994; 152: 4852–4860.
175. Gale RP. Graft versus host disease. Immunol Rev 1985; 88:19–212.
176. Naume B, Gately M, Espevik T. A comparative study of IL12, IL2 and IL7 induced effectors on immunomagnetically purified CD56 NK cells. J Immunol 1992; 148: 2429–2436.
177. Lamont AG, Adorini L. IL-12: a key cytokine in immune regulation. Immunol Today 1996; 17:214–217.

178. Niederwieser D, Aubock J, Troppmair J, Herold M, Schuler G, Boeck G, Lotz J, Fritsch P, Huber C. IFN-mediated induction of MHC antigen expression on human keratinocytes and its influence on in vitro alloimmune responses. J Immunol 1988; 140:2556–2564.
179. Vanky F, Hising C, Sjowalk K, Larsson B, Rodriguez L, Orre L, Klein E. Immunogenicity and immunosensitivity of ex vivo human carcinomas: interferon-r and tumor necrosis factor-a treatment of tumor cells potentiates their interaction with autologous blood lymphocytes. Cancer Immunol Immunother 1995; 41:217–226.
180. Oyaizu N, McCloskey TW, Than S, Hu R, Kalyanaraman VS, Pahwa S. Cross-linking of CD4 molecules up-regulates Fas antigen expression in lymphocytes by inducing interferon-gamma and tumor necrosis factor-alpha secretion. Blood 1994; 84:2622–2631.
181. Cohen JJ. Apoptosis. Immunol Today 1993; 14:126–130.
182. Trinchieri G: Biology of natural killer cells. Adv Immunol 1989; 47:187–376.
183. Hercend T, Takvorian T, Nowill A, Tantravahi R, Moingeon P, Anderson KC, Murray C, Bohuon C, Ythier A, Ritz J. Characterization of natural killer cells with anti-leukemia activity following allogeneic bone marrow transplantation. Blood 1986; 76:722–728.
184. Keevr CA, Klein J, Leong N, Copelan EA, Avalos BR, Kapoor N, Cunningham I, Tutschka PJ. Effect of GVHD on the recovery of NK cell activity and LAK precursors following BMT. Bone Marrow Transplant 1993; 12:289–295.
185. Silla LMR, Pincus SM, Locker JD, Glover J, Elder EM, Donnenberg AD, Nardi NB, Bryant J, Ball ED, Whiteside TL. Generation of activated natural killer cells in patients with chronic myelogenous leukemia and their role in the in vitro disappearance of BCR/abl-positive targets. Br J Hematol 1996; 93:375–385.
186. Zeis M, Uharck L, Glass B, Steinmann J, Dreger P, Gassmann W, Schmitz N. Allogeneic MHC-mismatched activated natural killer cells administered after bone marrow transplantation provide a strong graft-vs-leukemia effect in mice. Br J Hematol 1997; 96:757–761.
187. Tajima F, Kawatani T, Endo A, Kawasaki H. Natural killer cell activity and cytokine production as prognostic factors in adult acute leukemia. Leukemia 1996; 10: 478–482.
188. Niederwieser D, Gastl G, Rumpold H, Marth Ch, Kraft D, Huber H. Rapid reappearance of large granular lymphocytes with concomitant reconstitution of natural killer activity after human bone marrow transplantation. Br J Hematol 1987; 65: 301–305.
189. Delain M, Tiberghien P, Racadot E, Billot M, Pariset J, Chabod J, Cahn JY, Herve P. Variability of the alloreactivity T-cell response to human leukemia blasts. Leukemia 1994; 8:642–647.
190. Matulonis UA, Dosiou C, Lamont C, Freeman GJ, Mauch P, Nadler LM, Griffin JD. Role of B7-1 in mediating an immune response to myeloid leukemia cells. Blood 1995;85:2507–2515.
191. Munker R, Lubbert M, Yonehara S, Tuhnitz A, Mertelsmann R, Wilmanns W. Expression of the fas antigen on primary human leukemia cells. Ann Hematol 1995; 70:15–22.

192. Antin JH, Ferrara JLM. Cytokine dysregulation and acute graft-versus-host disease. Blood 1992; 80:2964–2970.
193. Johnson BD, Truitt RI. A decrease in graft-vs-host disease without loss of graft-vs-leukemia reactivity after MHC-matched bone marrow transplantation by selective depletion of donor NK cells in vivo. Transplantation 1992; 54:104.
194. Borland A, Mowat AM, Parrott DM: Augmentation of intestinal and peripheral natural killer cell activity during the graft-vs-host reaction in mice. Transplantation 1983; 36:513.
195. Rhoades JL, Cibull ML, Thompson JS, Henslee-Downey PJ, Jennings CD, Sinn HP, Brown SA, Eichhorn TR, Cave ML, Jezek DA. Role of natural killer cells in the pathogenesis of human acute graft vs host disease. Transplantation 1993; 56: 113–120.
196. Laughlin MJ, Kurtzberg J, Weinhold K, Ferrari G, Pilgrim A, Gelber C, Nair S, Gilboa E, Smith CA, Martinek L, DeOliveria D, Lyerly HK. Generation of T lymphocyte clones specific for acute lymphoblastic leukemia (ALL) via dendritic cell (abstr). Blood 1996; 88(suppl 1): 375.
197. Falkenburg JHF, van Bergen CAM, Smit WM, Willemze R. Induction of apoptic death of CD34+ chronic myeloid leukemia precursor cells by CD4+ T cells (abstr). Blood 1996; 88(suppl 1):243.
198. Jiang YZ, Mavroudis DA, Dermime S, Hensel NF, Couriel D, Molldrem J, Barrett AJ. Alloreactive CD4+ T lymphocytes can exert cytotoxicity to CML cells processing and presenting exogenous antigen. Br J Hematol 1996; 93:606–612.
199. Mizoguchi H, O'Shea J, Longo D, Loeffler C, McVicar D, Ochoa A. Alterations in signal transduction molecules in T lymphocytes from tumor-bearing mice. Science 1992; 258:1795–1798.
200. Nakagomi H, Pisa P, Pisa EK, Yamamoto Y, Halapi E, Backlin K, Juhlin C, Kiessling R. Lack of interleukin-2 expression and selective expression of IL-10 mRNA in human renal cell carcinoma. Int J Cancer 1995; 63:366–371.
201. Finke J, Zea A, Stanley J, Longo DL, Mizoguchi H, Tubbs RR, Wiltraut RH, O'Shea JJ, Kudoh S, Klein E, Bukowski RM, Ochoa A. Loss of T cell receptor zeta chain and p561ck in T cells infiltrating human renal cell carcinoma. Cancer Res 1993; 53:5613–5616.
202. Matsuda N, Petersson M, Lenkei R, Tampin J, Magnusson I, Mellstedt H, Anderson P, Kiessling R. Alterations in the signal transducing molecules of T cell and NK cells in colorectal tumor infiltrating, GUT mucosal and peripheral lymphocytes: correlation with stage of the disease. Int J Cancer 1995; 61:765–772.
203. Zea A, Curti B, Longo D, Alvord WG, Strobl SL, Mizoguchi H, Creekmore SP, O'Shea JJ, Powes GC, Urba WJ, Ochoa AC. Alterations in T cell receptor and signal transduction molecules in melanoma patients. Clin Can Res 1995; 1:1327–1335.
204. Wang Q, Stanley J, Kudoh S, Myles J, Kolenko V, Yi T, Tubbs R, Bukowski R, Finke J: T cells infiltrating non-Hodgkin's B cell lymphoma show altered tyrosine phosphorylation pattern even though T cell receptor/CD3 associated kinase are present. J Immunol 1995; 155:1382–1392.
205. Lewalle P, Hensel NF, Guimaraes A, Couriel D, Jiang YZ, Mavroudis D, Barrett

AJ. Helper and cytotoxic lymphocyte responses to CML: implications for adoptive immunotherapy with T cells. Br J Hematol 1996; 92:587–594.

206. Gale RP, Horowitz MM, Ash R, Champlin RE, Goldman JM, Rimm AA, Ringden O, Stone JA, Bortin MM. Identical twin bone marrow transplants for leukemia. Ann Intern Med 1994; 120:646–652.

207. Faber L, van Luxemberg-Heijs S, Veenhof W, Willemze R, Falkenburg JHF. Generation of CD4+ cytotoxic T-lymphocyte clones from a patient with severe graft versus host disease after allogeneic bone marrow transplantation: implications for graft versos leukemia reactivity. Blood 1995; 86:2821–2828.

208. Munker R, Koeffler P. In vitro action of tumor necrosis factor on myeloid leukemia cells. Blood 1987; 69:1102–1108.

209. Backx B, Broeders L, Bot FJ, Lowenberg B. Positive and negative effects of tumor necrosis factor on colony growth from highly purified normal marrow progenitors. Leukemia 1991; 5:66–70.

210. Weichold F, Jiang YZ, Dunn DE, Bloom M, Malkovska V, Hensel NF, Barrett AJ. Regulation of a graft vs leukemia effect by major histocompatibility complex class II molecules on leukemia cells: HLA-DR1 expression renders K562 cell tumors resistant to adoptively transferred lymphocytes in severe combined immunodeficiency/nonobese diabetic mice. Blood 1997; 90:4553–4558.

211. Garrido F, Ruiz-Cabello F, Cabrera T, Perez-Villar JJ, Lopez-Botet M, Duggan-Keen M, Stern PL. Implications for immunosurveillance of altered HLA class I phenotypes in human tumors. Immunol Today 1997; 18:89–95.

212. Dermime S, Mavroudis D, Jiang YZ, Hensel N, Couriel D, Molldrem J, Barrett AJ. Mechanism of leukemia escape from graft-vs-leukemia effect: down-regulation of surface molecules and impairment of immune effector activity. Bone Marrow Transplant 1997; 19:989–999.

213. Mielcarek M, Martin P, Torok-Storb B. Suppression of alloantigen-induced T cell proliferation by large numbers of CD14+ cells in G-CSF mobilized peripheral blood mononuclear cells. (abstr). Blood 1996; 88(suppl 1):249.

214. Takenaka K, Mizuno S, Harada M, Nagafuji K, Miyamoto T, Iwasaki H, Fujisaki T, Kubota A, Ohno Y, Arima F, Shigenatsu H, Gondo H, Okamura T, Okamura S, Inaba S, and Niho Y. Generation of human natural killer cells from peripheral blood CD34+ cells mobilized by granulocyte colony-stimulating factor. Br J Hematol 1997; 92:788–794.

5
Minor Histocompatibility Antigens in GVL

Tuna Mutis and Els Goulmy
Leiden University Medical Center
Leiden, The Netherlands

I. INTRODUCTION

In syngeneic bone marrow transplantation (BMT) and in recipients of autologous BMT, relapse rates are high. No MHC or minor histocompatibility antigen (mHag) disparities exist and thus no alloreactivities can be induced. This is clearly different in allogeneic BMT, where the relapse rates are significantly lower and a relationship is seen between the graft versus leukemia (GVL) effect and acute and chronic graft-versus-host disease (GVHD). Likewise, donor lymphocyte infusion (DLI) therapy, inducing remission in relapsed chronic myeloid leukemia (CML) after allogeneic BMT, is frequently accompanied by GVHD. Thus, one may conclude that alloreactive donor T cells are involved in antileukemia reactivities. Human mHag are polymorphic antigens that are independent from HLA, expressed on leukemic cells, and recognized by alloreactive immune bone marrow donor T cells. It is therefore likely that in the HLA-identical situation, mHag participate in GVL reactivities. This review does not cover the information regarding the GVL effect of murine mHag. These and other experimental animal studies are described in Chapter 3. Here we summarize current knowledge of the putative impact of human mHag on the GVL effect in BMT and discusses the possible clinical application of mHag for immunotherapy of leukemia.

II. HUMAN mHag: CELLULAR IDENTIFICATION AND CHARACTERISTICS

mHag have been defined by MHC-restricted T cells obtained from individuals primed in vivo. In humans mHag studies have predominantly been performed in the HLA-identical BMT setting. mHag-specific T cells can be isolated in vitro from a patient's peripheral blood lymphocytes (PBL) after HLA-identical BMT. The concept of generating antihost CTL and T helper (Th) cells with specific activity for mHag is based on the following assumption: the patient's posttransplant (i.e., donor) cells, when sensitized against the patient's own pretransplant cells, are directed against patient-specific target structures, such as mHag, which are absent from the donor cells and present on the patient's pretransplant cells. In this way, a series of mHag-specific CTL and Th cells have been described. With these T cells, information on human mHag—such as genetics, tissue distribution, and clinical relevance—has been gathered [1]. Recent technical advances have resulted in the identification of the chemical nature of the first series of human mHag [2–5]. It is now clear that mHag are peptides, derived from polymorphic self proteins, that can associate with MHC molecules.

The major characteristics of human mHag recognized by MHC-restricted T cells are (1) variable phenotype frequencies with low polymorphism; (2) Mendelian segregation that is independent from HLA, and (3) restricted or broad tissue distribution. Translating these characteristics into a GVH/GVL effect after HLA-identical but mHag-mismatched BMT, one could postulate that BM donor T cells would mount an immune response against patient's mHag, which are expressed on patient's hematopoietic cells, including leukemic cells, and—depending on the individual mHag—also on nonhematopoietic cells and tissues [6].

III. mHag: IN VIVO GVL RESPONSES IN CLINICAL STUDIES

Already in the early years of BMT, it was observed that allogeneic BMT not only restores patient's hematopoiesis but also possesses a curative graft-versus-leukemia (GVL) effect. Since then, several clinical studies have indicated that the eradication of leukemia could be related to the presence of alloreactive T cells in the grafted bone marrow. The involvement of donor-derived alloreactive T cells in the GVL effect is clearly demonstrated in an analysis by the International Bone Marrow Transplant Registry of 2254 leukemia patients receiving HLA-identical sibling bone marrow [7]. In relation to our working hypothesis, we focus on two aspects of these results. First, the GVL effect after allogeneic BMT is mediated to a great extent by donor-derived T cells. The probability of relapse in patients who received T cell–depleted BMT was 41%, which is significantly higher than the non-T cell–depleted BMT group, which varied between 7 and 25% (Table 1). Second, minor histocompatibility disparities between donor and patient may play an important role in the GVL effect. The lowest GVL effect was observed in BMT from identical twins (syngeneic BMT), with a relapse rate of 46%. The supposition that (1) donor T cells are involved in the GVL effect and (2) mHag disparities facilitate this effect is plausible, since the GVL-associated alloimmune response is often not restricted to the leukemia cells. Patients receiving non-T cell–depleted BMT demonstrated a probability of relapse that was inversely correlated with the development of GVHD (Table 1): relapse rates of 25% were seen in patients who did not develop GVHD compared with 7% in patients who developed both acute and chronic GVHD. A more recent analysis comprising 1294 patients transplanted for CML (in the first chronic phase) confirmed these results [8]. Moreover, the relapse rates were inversely correlated with the severity of acute GVHD (aGVHD). Nevertheless, aGVHD grade 1 was most favorable for leukemia-free survival, since higher grades of GVHD were associated with transplant-related mortality (Figure 1).

Another indication of the involvement of donor-derived allogeneic T cells in the GVL effect is the successful use of donor lymphocyte infusions (DLI) as adoptive immunotherapy for CML relapsing after BMT [9]. Clinical response rates exceeding 80% had been achieved in several studies. CML patients are the best responders to DLI; response rates of ALL and AML patients are substantially lower [10,11]. Although the reason for this discrepancy is not known, the clinical data clearly demonstrate that the outcome of the DLI treatment is strongly associated with the development of GVHD, regardless of the type of malignancy. This is illustrated in Table 2 showing the published data of DLI performed between HLA-identical donor-patient sibling pairs [9,12–24]. Both in the high-responder CML group and in the low-responder AML/ALL/MDS group, the GVL effect (i.e., complete remission, molecular or cytogenetic remission) is strongly corre-

Table 1 Correlation Between the GVL Effect and Alloimmune Donor T Cells

Allogeneic non-T-cell-depleted BMT	Number of Patients	% Probability of Relapse
No GVHD	433	25
Acute GVHD	738	22
Chronic GVHD	127	10
Acute and chronic GVHD	485	7
Allogeneic T-cell-depleted BMT	401	41
Syngeneic BMT	70	46

Source: From Ref. 7.

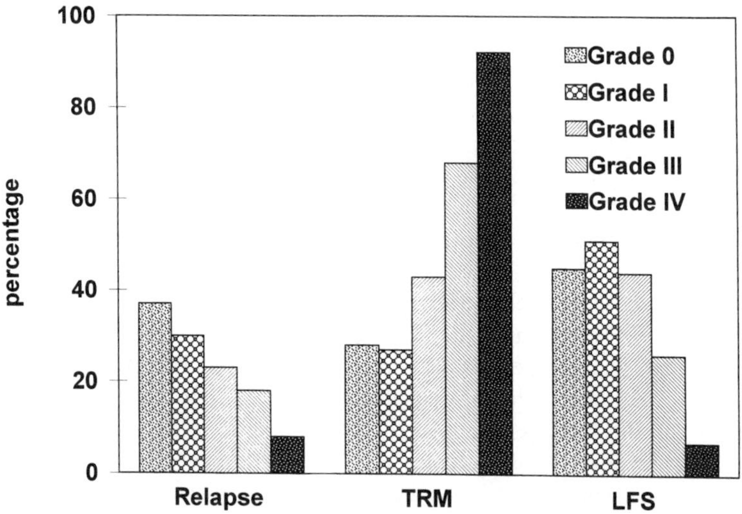

Figure 1 Inverse correlation between the acute GVHD grade and relapses in CML patients after BMT. TRM, Transplantation-related mortality; LFS, Leukemia free survival. (From Ref. 8.)

lated with the development of GVHD. Thus, the therapeutic effect of DLI is mediated to a large extent by alloreactive T cells recognizing patient-specific mHag on different tissues and cells, including the patient's leukemic cells. The occurrence of GVL without any sign of GVHD in some CML patients indicates that, clinically, GVHD can be separable from GVL. In those cases, the effector mechanisms may involve leukemia-specific T cells, NK cells, or T cells recognizing mHag that show restricted tissue distribution. The latter possibility is dis-

Table 2 Correlation of GVL with GVHD in Leukemia Patients Receiving DLI from HLA-Identical Sibling Donors

	CML Patients[a]		AML/ALL/MDS Patients[b]	
	GVL	No GVL	GVL	No GVL
GVHD	46	5	13	5
No GVHD	7	9	1	12

[a] Data are pooled from Refs. 9, 12–19, 23, and 24.
[b] Data are pooled from Refs. 15, 16, and 19–22.

cussed below. For the involvement of NK cells in GVL, the reader is referred to Ref. 25.

IV. mHag: IN VITRO STUDIES OF IN VIVO GVL RESPONSES

In line with the results of the clinical studies, a close relationship between GVL responses and the presence of donor-derived host-reactive T cells has been shown in vitro. Changes in the host-reactive T-cell precursor frequencies after BMT or DLI were correlated with the GVL effect of these treatments. In an in vitro analysis of 18 CML patients (11 receiving marrow grafts from HLA-identical sibling donors), Jiang et al. have demonstrated that leukemia-reactive CTL precursor frequencies (Lk-CTLp) increase after BMT [26]. High Lk-CTLp frequencies correlated with both GVHD and the leukemia-free survival. Lk-CTLp frequencies higher than 1:400,000 were associated with severe GVHD, whereas Lk-CTLp frequencies lower than 1:400,000 were observed in patients with leukemic relapse.

Similarly, Bunjes et al. have demonstrated high frequencies of host-reactive IL-2 secreting T-helper precursor (Th-p) in all patients who entered molecular remission after receiving DLI for relapsed CML [13]. In four of five responding patients, the presence of Th-p was associated with symptoms of GVHD, suggesting T-cell reactivity against mHag expressed on both leukemic cells and host tissues. No host-reactive Th-p were detectable in one patient who did not respond to DLI treatment. In this study, antihost CTLp were detected in only three responder patients.

Previously, we studied both antihost CTL and Th-cell activities at different times after HLA genotypically identical BMT [27,28]. In Table 3, the analysis

Table 3 Effects of mHag-Specific CTL/Th Cells on GVHD and GVL in HLA Genotypically Identical Patient-Donor Pairs

Number of Patients	Antihost T-Cell Activities		Status
	CTL	Th	GVHD/Relapse
3	None	None	No/relapse
2	Yes	None	No
2	Yes	Yes	No
1	None	Yes	Acute > II
2	Yes	None	Acute > II
5	Yes	Yes	Acute > II
5	Yes	Yes	Acute and chronic

of either CTL- and Th-cell responses in each individual patient is scored. We observed both absence and presence of antihost CTL- and Th-cell activities in patients without any clinical signs of GVHD (Table 3). It was notable that in all three cases without antihost T-cell activities, leukemia relapse was manifest. On the other hand, the presence of either anti-host CTL or Th cells in the absence of GVHD and relapse (n = 4) argues for the possible role of these T cells in the antileukemic activity. Subsequently, some post-BMT antihost T cell responses were analyzed in vitro for their putative antileukemic activity [29]. Figure 2 shows the antihost CTL activities we observed. CTL lines were generated using posttransplant lymphocytes from an HLA-identical sibling, which lysed both the patient's normal (i.e., PHA blast and EBV-LCLs) and leukemic cells at different times after BMT. Subsequent cloning of these CTL lines yielded CTL clones with ''GVHD''- and ''GVL''-related activities. The latter type of CTL clones recognized the patient's neoplastic cells only. The former type of CTL clones were reactive with ligands, presumed to be mHag shared by host PHA blasts and leukemic cells (Table 4).

An elegant in vitro study was performed in a patient who had been treated with BMT as a therapy for breast cancer [30]. Resolution of liver metastases was observed simultaneously with clinical GVHD in the first weeks after transplant.

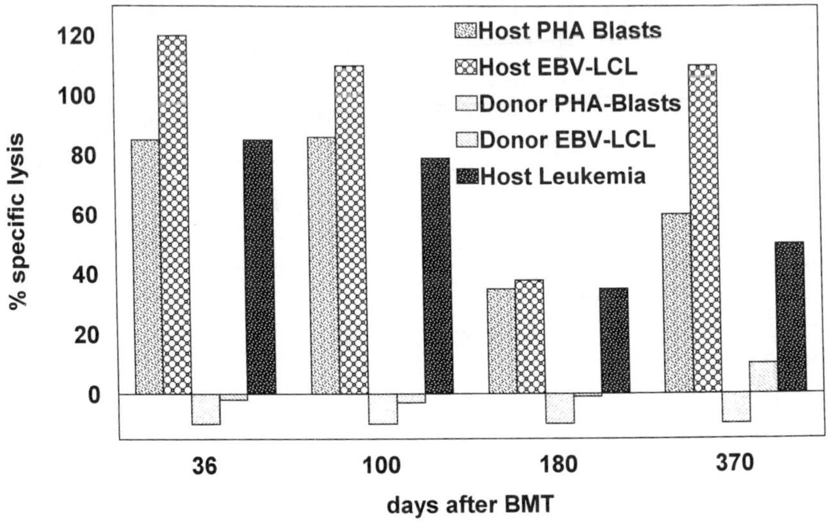

Figure 2 Close association between antihost (GVH) and antileukemia (GVL) CTL reactivities in leukemia patients after BMT.

Table 4 Antihost GVH and GVL T-cell reactivities After HLA Genotypically Identical BMT

Number of Clones	Reactivity at PHA Blasts	Reactivity at Leukemic Cells	Putative Specificity
7	Yes	Yes	T and leukemic cells
4	Yes	No	T cells
4	No	Yes	Leukemic cells

Coincidentally, mHag-specific CTL recognizing breast carcinoma target cells were isolated from the blood of the patient. A clear example of antihost mHag-specific CTL responses that show leukemia-associated recognition was recently reported by Dolstra et al. [31]. Isolated CTL, after HLA-identical BMT, recognized a mHag expressed solely on B-acute lymphoblastic leukemla (B-ALL) cells and EBV-LCL.

Not only donor-derived CD8 CTL but also CD4 mHag-specific CTL clones generated postallogeneic BMT are implicated in the GVL effect [32] (see also Chapter 18).

V. mHag: PRIMARY IN VITRO ANTILEUKEMIA RESPONSES

In the previous section, we discussed GVL reactivities conferred by T cells primed by BMT. Here we give some examples of primary in vitro responses against leukemic cells. These studies also indicate an association between host-reactive T cells and GVL reactivities. For instance, to determine whether donor-derived host-specific T-helper cell precursor (Th-p) frequencies are associated with GVHD and/or relapse, Lachance et al. measured pretransplant host-specific Th-p frequencies in donors of 32 HLA-identical marrow graft recipients [33]. The Th-p frequencies were significantly higher in patients who developed aGVHD grade II or more as compared with patients without GVHD. In 88% of the patients who relapsed, host-reactive Th-p frequencies were significantly lower ($\leq$1:200,000) than in those who did not relapse. Similarly, Datta et al. have found that in HLA-identical sibling donors of CML patients, higher responses to CML cells correlated with GVHD grade $\geq$2 [34]. In the latter study, some degree of CML-selective reactivity could be achieved after depletion of the proliferative response to nonleukemic T-cell blasts, suggesting that CML cells may express specific antigens that are recognized by T cells. This issue was also addressed by Hoffmann et al., who studied CTLp/Th-p in the HLA-identical donors of leukemic patients. Upon stimulation with nonleukemic cells (T-cell blasts) 90% of the clones reacted only with nonleukemic cells, whereas upon stimulation with leukemic cells, 75% of the generated clones were exclusively reactive with leukemic cells [35]. Whether this leukemia cell selectivity is due to tissue-restricted mHag remains to be investigated. Another point of consideration in these in vitro studies is that the selective leukemia reactivity observed in the primary limiting dilution analyses may be transient or not representative of a genuine leukemia specificity. In several studies, T cells initially thought to selectively recognize leukemic cells appeared also to recognize normal target cells. For example Oettel et al. generated T-cell lines and clones that initially lysed only bcr/abl-positive but not bcr/abl-negative target cells. Upon prolonged culture, bcr/abl-negative target cells were recognized as well [36]. Several CD4- or CD8-positive T cells generated from HLA-identical sibling donors using leukemic cells as stimulator cells appear to recognize mHag with either restricted or broad tissue specificity [37,38]. Using in vitro primary stimulation protocols, Falkenburg et al. recently successfully transferred leukemia-reactive CTL to treat refractory leukemia [39]. This issue is covered in more detail in Chapter 18. We have generated leukemia-reactive CD4-positive T-cell lines and clones from the HLA-identical sibling donor of an AML patient using CD80 transfected leukemic cells as stimulator cells. While some T cells preferentially recognized leukemic cells, the majority of the leukemia-reactive T-cell lines and clones did not discriminate between leukemic and nonleukemic cells, indicating that the target antigens are patient-specific mHag present on both leukemic and nonleukemic cells [40].

VI. mHag: IN VITRO TISSUE DISTRIBUTION STUDIES RELEVANT FOR GVL RESPONSES

The previous sections discussed both in vivo and in vitro GVL responses of patients with limited or extended GVHD. The former could be the result of alloimmune responses mainly directed against mHag, with limited tissue distribution. The extended GVH forms can be explained by T-cell reactivities against ubiquitously expressed mHag. Our tissue distribution studies of five mHag underline this notion [41]. Our analysis of the membrane expression of a limited number of mHag, by means of functional assays, revealed differential expression: mHag (i.e., H-Y, HA-3, and HA-4) are expressed on hematopoletic as well as on nonhematopoietic cells, while the expression of other mHag (HA-1 and HA-2) is limited to cells of the hematopoietic lineage only. Thus, we observed either broad or restricted mHag expression, as summarized in Table 5. It should be stressed that all mHag are present on clonogenic leukemic precursor cells [42,44]

Table 5 mHag Tissue Distribution Studies

Restricted Expression	Broad Expression
Hematopoietic progenitor cells	Fibroblasts
Hematopoietic cells	Keratinocytes
Leukemic progenitors (lymphoid and myeloid)	Melanocytes
Leukemic cells (lymphoid and myeloid)	Endothelial cells
	Epithelial cells
	Corneal tissue
	Liver cells

as well as on circulating leukemic cells of lymphocytic and myeloid origin [44,45].

VII. mHag: APPLICATION FOR IMMUNOTHERAPY OF LEUKEMIA

The recent insights into the chemical nature of mHag not only reveal their physiological function but, more importantly, provide the basic ingredients for the use of CTL specific for mHag peptides for the treatment of refractory, residual, or relapsed leukemia. This proposal is in principle similar to the adoptive immunotherapy of donor buffy coat cells, which can successfully induce remission in CML patients relapsing after allogeneic BMT. Success of DLI therapy is, however, limited by significant GVHD. Furthermore, DLI for relapsed ALL and AML patients is far less effective.

The usage of mHag-specific CTL as adoptive immunotherapy for leukemia is based on their restricted and specific target cell damage. We will take advantage of three of the known characteristics of human mHag: (1) MHC-restricted recognition by T cells; (2) variable phenotype frequencies, (i.e., mHag polymorphism); and (3) restricted tissue distribution. Moreover, since mHag are clearly expressed on circulating leukemic cells and clonogenic leukemic precursor cells of both myeloid and lymphoid origin, both types of leukemias can be targeted. Clearly, the mHag with ''restricted'' tissue distribution (Table 5) are candidates for adoptive immunotherapy of leukemia. Currently, suitable candidates meeting the above criteria are mHag HA-1 and HA-2, whose amino acid sequence is known. Their characteristics are summarized in Table 6.

As exemplified in Figure 3, we will generate mHag peptide CTL ex vivo from mHag-negative BM donors for mHag-positive patients with high risk of relapse. Upon transfusion (either pre-BMT as part of the conditioning regimen

Table 6 Characteristics of mHag to Be Used for Adoptive Immunotherapy of Leukemia[a]

mHag	Restriction Molecule	Peptide Sequence	Population Frequency	Tissue Distribution
HA-1	HLA-A*0201	VLHDDLLEA	69%	restricted
HA-2	HLA-A*0201	YIGEVLVSV	95%	restricted

[a] As of December 1997.
Sources: Refs. 2 and 3.

or post-BMT as adjuvant therapy), the mHag peptide-specific CTL will eliminate the mHag-positive patient's hematopoietic cells, including the patient's leukemic cells. Since the mHag have restricted expression on the hematopoietic cell lineage, the nonhematopoietic cells will be spared. If necessary, the patient's hematopoietic system could be reconstituted with mHag-negative marrow from the original BM donor. We have already succeeded in inducing, ex vivo, mHag peptide-specific CTL showing specific cytotoxic activity in vitro against hematopoetic cells, including leukemic cells expressing the relevant mHag ligand [46]. A universal option would be to generate ''off the shelf'' mHag peptide-specific CTL using mHag-negative healthy blood donors with frequent HLA-homozygous haplotypes. Patients positive for certain mHag matching the HLA typing of the CTL donor could be treated with such allogeneic mHag peptide-specific CTL.

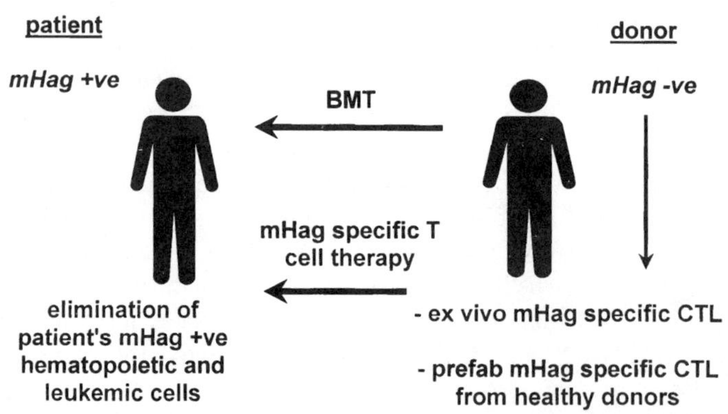

Figure 3 Flowchart of mHag-specific adoptive immunotherapy in HLA-identical, mHag-mismatched BMT.

Transduction of CTL with a suicide gene could also be performed to make possible the elimination of the CTL in case adverse effects occur.

ACKNOWLEDGMENTS

We are grateful to Machteld Oudshoorn and Jon van Rood for their critical reading and Leny de Vries for typing the manuscript. This work was supported in part by grants from the Dutch Organization for Scientific Research (NWO), the Dutch Cancer Foundation, the J.A. Cohen Institute for Radiopathology and Radiation Protection (IRS), the Macropa Foundation, and the Leukemia Society of America.

REFERENCES

1. Goulmy E. Human minor histocompatibility antigens. Curr Opin Immunol 1996; 8: 75–81.
2. den Haan JM, Sherman NE, Blokland E, Huczko E, Koning F, Drijfhout JW, Skipper J, Shabanowitz J, Hunt DF, Engelhard VH, Goulmy E. Identification of a graft versus host disease–associated human minor histocompatibility antigen. Science 1995; 268: 1476–1480.
3. den Haan JM, Meadows LM, Wang W, Pool J, Blokland E, Bischop TL, Reinhardus C, Shabanowitz J, Offringa R, Hunt DF, Engelhard VH, Goulmy E. The minor histocompatibility antigen HA-1: a diallelic gene with a single aminoacid polymorphism. Science. 1998; 279:1054–1057.
4. Wang W, Meadows LR, den Haan JM, Sherman NE, Chen Y, Blokland E, Shabanowitz J, Agulnik AI, Hendrickson RC, Bishop CE, Hunt DF, Goulmy E, Engelhard VH. Human H-Y: a male-specific histocompatibility antigen derived from the SMCY protein. Science 1995; 269:1588–1590.
5. Meadows L, Wang W, den Haan JM, Blokland E, Reinhardus C, Drijfhout JW, Shabanowitz J, Pierce R, Agulnik AI, Bishop CE, Hunt DF, Goulmy E, Engelhard VH. The HLA-A*0201-restricted H-Y antigen contains a posttranslationally modified cysteine that significantly affects T cell recognition. Immunity 1997; 6:273–281.
6. Goulmy E. Human minor histocompatibility antigens: new concepts for marrow transplantation and adoptive immunotherapy. Immunol Rev 1997; 157:125–140.
7. Horowitz MM, Gale RP, Sondel PM, Goldman JM, Kersey J, Kolb HJ, Rimm AA, Ringden O, Rozman C, Speck B, Truitt RL, Zwaan FE, Bortin MM. Graft-versus-leukemia reactions after bone marrow transplantation. Blood 1990; 75:555–562.
8. Gratwohl A, Hermans J, Apperley JF, Arcese W, Bacigalupo A, Bandini G, di-Bartolomeo P, Boogaerts M, Bosi A, Carreras E, Devergie A, Ferrant A, Fibbe WE, Frassoni F, Gahrton G, Goldman JM, Iriondo A, Jacobsen N, Kolb HJ, Link H, Michallet M, Prentice HG, Reiffers J, van Rhee F, Ruutu T, Schwaighofer H, Ver-

nant JP, de Witte T, Niederwieser D. Acute graft-versus-host disease: grade and outcome in patients with chronic myelogenous leukemia: Working Party Chronic Leukemia of the European Group for Blood and Marrow Transplantation. Blood 1995; 86:813–818.

9. Kolb HJ, Mittermuller J, Clemm C, Holler E, Ledderose G, Brehm G, Heim M, Wilmanns W. Donor leukocyte transfusions for treatment of recurrent chronic myelogenous leukemia in marrow transplant patients. Blood 1990; 76:2462–2465.
10. Kolb HJ, Schattenberg A, Goldman JM, Hertenstein B, Jacobsen N, Arcese W, Ljungman P, Ferrant A, Verdonck L, Niederwieser D, van Rhee F, Mittermuller J, de Witte T, Holler E, Ansari H. Graft-versus-leukemia effect of donor lymphocyte transfusions in marrow grafted patients: European Group for Blood and Marrow Transplantation Working Party Chronic Leukemia. Blood 1995; 86:2041–2050.
11. Porter DL, Roth MS, Lee SJ, McGarigle C, Ferrara JL, Antin JH. Adoptive immunotherapy with donor mononuclear cell infusions to treat relapse of acute leukemia or myelodysplasia after allogeneic bone marrrow transplantation. Bone Marrow Transplant 1996; 18:975–980.
12. Bär BM, Schattenberg A, Mensink EJ, Geurts Van Kessel A, Smetsers TF, Knops GH, Linders EH, De Witte T. Donor leukocyte infusions for chronic myelold leukemia relapsed after allogeneic bone marrow transplantation. J Clin Oncol 1993, 11: 513–519.
13. Bunjes D, Theobald M, Hertenstein B, Wiesneth M, Novotny J, Arnold R, Heimpel H. Successful therapy with donor buffy coat transfusions in patients with relapsed chronic myeloid leukemia after bone marrow transplantation is associated with high frequencies of host-reactive interleukin 2–secreting T helper cells. Bone Marrow Transplant 1995; 15:713–719.
14. Cullis JO, Jiang YZ Schwarer AP, Hughes TP, Barrett AJ, Goldman JM. Donor leukocyte infusions for chronic myelold leukemia in relapse after allogeneic bone marrow transplantation (letter). Blood 1995; 79:1379–1381.
15. Kell F, Hass OA, Fritsch G, Kalhs P, Lechner K, Mannhalter C, Reiter E, Niederwieser D, Hoecker P, Greinix HT. Donor leukocyte infusions for leukemic relapse after allogeneic marrow transplantation: lack of residual donor hematopoiesis predicts aplasia. Blood 1997; 89:3113–3117.
16. Slavin S, Naparstek E, Nagler A, Ackerstein A, Samuel S, Kapelushnik J, Brautbar C, Or R. Allogeneic cell therapy with donor peripheral blood cells and recombinant human interleukin-2 to treat leukemia relapse after allogeneic bone marrow transplantation. Blood 1996; 87:2195–2204.
17. Drobyski WR, Keever CA, Roth MS, Koethe S, Hanson G, McFadden P, Gottschall JL, Ash RC, van Tuinen P, Horowitz MM, Flomenberg N. Salvage immunotherapy using donor leukocyte infusions as treatment for relapsed chronic myelogenous leukemia after allogeneic bone marrow transplantation: efficacy and toxicity of a defined T-cell dose. Blood 1993; 82:2310–2318.
18. Porter DL, Roth MS, McGarigle C, Ferrara JL, Antin JH. Induction of graft-versus-host disease as immunotherapy for relapsed chronic myeloid leukemia. N Engl J Med 1994; 330:100–106.
19. Russell LA, Jacobsen N, Heilmann C, Simonsen AC, Christensen LD, Vlndelov LL.

Treatment of relapse after allogeneic BMT with donor leukocyte infusions in 16 patients. Bone Marrow Transplant 1996; 18:411–414.

20. Szer J, Grigg AP, Phillips GL, Sheridan WP. Donor leucocyte infusions after chemotherapy for patients relapsing with acute leukaemia following allogeneic BMT. Bone Marrow Transplant 1993; 11:109–111.
21. Tzeng CH, Lin JS, Lee JC, Yung CH, Hu HY, Chen PM. Transfusion of donor peripheral blood buffy coat cells as effective treatment for relapsed acute leukemia after transplantation of allogeneic bone marrow or peripheral blood stem cells from the same donor. Transfusion 1996; 36:685–690.
22. Fores R, Diez-Martin JL, Briz M, Cabrera JR, Sanjuan I, Regidor C, Garcia-Talavera J, Fernandez MN. Donor leukocyte infusions for treatment of relapsed acute myeloid leukemia after allogeneic bone marrow transplantation. Bone Marrow Transplant 1996; 17:439–441.
23. Hertenstein B, Wiesneth M, Novotny J, Bunjes D, Stefanic M, Heinze B, Hubner G, Heimpel H, Arnold R. Interferon-alpha and donor buffy coat transfusions for treatment of relapsed chronic myeloid leukemia after allogenic bone marrow transplantation. Transplantation 1993; 56:1114–1118.
24. Helg C, Roux E, Beris P, Cabrol C, Wacker P, Darbellay R, Wyss M, Jeannet M, Chapuis B, Roosnek E. Adoptive immunotherapy for recurrent CML after BMT. Bone Marrow Transplant 1993; 12:125–129.
25. Murphy WJ, Longo DL. The potential role of NK cells in the separation of graft-versus-tumor effects from graft-versus-host disease after allogeneic bone marrow transplantation. Immunol Rev 1997; 157:167–176.
26. Jiang YZ, Kanfer EJ, Macdonald D, Cullis JO, Goldman JM, Barrett AJ. Graft-versus-leukaemia following allogeneic bone marrow transplantation: emergence of cytotoxic T lymphocytes reacting to host leukaemia cells. Bone Marrow Transplant 1991; 8:253–258.
27. van Els CA, Bakker A, Zwinderman AH, Zwaan FE, van Rood JJ, Goulmy E. Effector mechanisms in graft-versus-host disease in response to minor histocompatibility antigens: I. Absence of correlation with cytotoxic effector cells. Transplantation 1990; 50:62–66.
28. van Els CA, Bakker A, Zwinderman AH, Zwaan FE, van Rood JJ, Goulmy E. Effector mechanisms in graft-versus-host disease in response to minor histocompatibility antigens: II. Evidence of a possible involvement of proliferative T cells. Transplantation 1990; 50:67–71.
29. van Lochem E, de Gast B, Goulmy E. In vitro separation of host specific graft-versus-host and graft-versus- leukemia cytotoxic T cell activities. Bone Marrow Transplant 1992; 10:181–183.
30. Eibl B, Schwaighofer H, Nachbaur D, Marth C, Gachter A, Knapp R, Bock G, Gassner C, Schiller L, Petersen F, Niederwieser D. Evidence for a graft-versus-tumor effect in a patient treated with marrow ablative chemotherapy and allogeneic bone marrow transplantation for breast cancer. Blood 1996; 88:1501–1508.
31. Dolstra H, Fredrix H, Preijers F, Goulmy E, Figdor CG, de Witte TM, van de Wiel-van Kemenade E. Recognition of a B cell leukemia–associated minor histocompatibility antigen by CTL. J Immunol 1997; 158:560–565.

32. Faber LM, van Luxemburg-Heijs SA, Veenhof WF, Willemze R, Falkenburg JHF. Generation of CD4+ cytotoxic T-lymphocyte clones from a patient with severe graft-versus-host disease after allogenic bone marrow transplantation: implications for graft-versus-leukemia reactivity. Blood 1995; 86:2821–2828.
33. Lachance S, Le Gouvello S, Roudot F, Kuentz M, Bernaudin F, Beaujean F, Bierling P, Cordonnier C, Farcet JP, Vernant JP. Predictive value of host-specific donor helper T-cell precursor frequency for acute graft-versus-host disease and relapse in HLA-identical siblings receiving allogeneic bone marrow transplantation for hematological malignancies. Transplantation 1997; 64:1147–1152.
34. Datta AR, Barrett AJ, Jiang YZ, Guimaraes A, Mavroudis DA, van Rhee F, Gordon AA, Madrigal A. Distinct T cell populations distinguish chronic myeloid leukaemia cells from lymphocytes in the same individual: a model for separating GVHD from GVL reactions. Bone Marrow Transplant 1994; 14:517–524.
35. Hoffmann T, Theobald M, Bunjes D, Weiss M, Heimpel H, Heit W. Frequency of bone marrow T cells responding to HLA-identical non-leukemic and leukemic stimulator cells. Bone Marrow Transplant 1993; 12:1–8.
36. Oettel KR, Wesly OH, Albertinl MR, Hank JA, Illopolis O, Sosman JA, Voelkerding K, Wu SQ, Clark SS, Sondel PM. Allogeneic T-cell clones able to selectively destroy Philadelphia chromosome-bearing (Ph1+) human leukemia lines can also recognize Ph1- cells from the same patient. Blood 1994; 83:3390–3402.
37. Faber LM, van Luxemburg-Heijs SA, Willemze R, Falkenburg JHF. Generation of leukemia-reactive cytotoxic T lymphocyte clones from the HLA-identical bone marrow donor of a patient with leukemia. J Exp Med 1992; 176:1283–1289.
38. Falkenburg JHF, Faber LM, van den Elshout M, van Luxemburg-Heijs SA, Hooftman-den Otter A, Smit WM, Voogt PJ, Willemze R. Generation of donor-derived antileukemic cytotoxic T-lymphocyte responses for treatment of relapsed leukemia after allogeneic HLA identical bone marrow transplantation. J Immunother 1993; 14:305–309.
39. Falkenburg JHF, Wafelman AR, van Bergen CAM, Bongaerts R, Lurvink EGA, Posthuma EFM, Smit WM, Joosten P, Landegent JE, Kluin-Nelemans JC, Fibbe WE, Willemze R. Leukemia-reactive cytotoxic T lymphocytes (CTL) induce complete remission in a patients with refractory accelerated chronic myeloid leukemia (CML) (abstr). 1997; 90(suppl 1):589.
40. Mutis T, Schrama E, Melief CJM, Goulmy E. CD80 transfected acute myeloid leukemia cells induce primary T cell responses directed at patient specific minor histocompatibility antigens and leukemia associated antigens. Blood 1998; 92:1677–1684.
41. de Bueger M, Bakker A, van Rood JJ, Van der Woude F, Goulmy E. Tissue distribution of human minor histocompatibility antigens: ubiquitous versus restricted tissue distribution indicates heterogeneity among human cytotoxic T lymphocyte-defined non-MHC antigens. J Immunol 1992; 149:1788–1794.
42. Falkenburg JHF, Goselink HM, van der Harst D, van Luxemburg-Heijs SA, Kooy-Winkelaar YM, Faber LM, de Kroon J, Brand A, Flbbe WE, Willemze R, Goulmy E. Growth inhibition of clonogenic leukemic precursor cells by minor histocompatibility antigen-specific cytotoxic T lymphocytes. J Exp Med 1991; 174:27–33.
43. Faber LM, van der Hoeven J, Goulmy E, Hooftman-den Otter AL, van Luxemburg-Heijs SA, Willemze R, Falkenburg JHF. Recognition of clonogenic leukemic cells,

remission bone marrow and HLA-identical donor bone marrow by CD8+ or CD4+ minor histocompatibility antigen-specific cytotoxic T lymphocytes. J Clin Invest 1995; 96:877–883.

44. Niederwieser D, Grassegger A, Aubock J, Herold M, Nachbaur D, Rosenmayr A, Gachter A, Nussbaumer W, Gaggl S, Ritter M, Huber C. Correlation of minor histocompatibility antigen-specific cytotoxic T lymphocytes with graft-versus-host disease status and analyses of tissue distribution of their target antigens. Blood 1993; 81:2200–2208.
45. van der Harst D, Goulmy E, Falkenburg JHF, Kooij-Winkelaar YM, van Luxemburg-Heijs SA, Goselink HM, Brand A. Recognition of minor histocompatibility antigens on lymphocytic and myeloid leukemic cells by cytotoxic T-cell clones. Blood 1994; 83:1060–1066.
46. Mutis T, Verdijk R, Schrama E, Esendam B, Brand A, Goulmy E. Feasibility of immunotherapy of relapsed leukemia with ex vivo-generated cytotoxic T lymphocytes specific for hematopoietic system-restricted minor histocompatibility antigens. Blood 1999; 93:2336–2341.

6
Tissue-Specific Antigens in GVL

Jeffrey J. Molldrem
M. D. Anderson Cancer Center
Houston, Texas

I. INTRODUCTION

Immunity directed against leukemia in the setting of allogeneic bone marrow transplant, which has been termed GVL, is often accompanied by unwanted GVHD. Much clinical and laboratory evidence now exists showing that both reactions are mediated by T cells contained in the graft [1–3] as detailed in other chapters. Methods to reduce GVHD have included infusions of marrow or peripheral blood following depletion of T cells by either ''nonselective'' (anti-CD3) or ''semiselective'' (anti-CD8, -T10B9, or -Campath) means. Although GVHD is sometimes diminished by these maneuvers, none result in the infusion of only leukemia-specific T cells. If marrow or peripheral blood grafts could be enriched for such leukemia-specific T cells, GVHD might be significantly reduced or even eliminated.

Attempts to select and expand leukemia-reactive lymphocytes ex vivo have shown us that such lymphocytes, when infused into the patient, can induce remission [4]. This demonstrates an important ''proof of principle'': namely, that T cells selected for leukemia reactivity can be used to produce GVL in the absence of GVHD. However, not until we are able to identify the target antigens of the GVL-producing T cells will we be able to harness the full therapeutic benefit of this immune response. Once such target molecules are identified, they could be used in the development of both active and passive immunotherapeutic strategies.

Several methods to identify specific leukemia-associated antigens (LAA) have been used, within both the autologous and allogeneic settings. While strategies using allogeneic T lymphocytes are certain to uncover LAA, which are distinct for some donor-recipient pairs, there may also be many LAA derived from self-proteins that can be recognized by T cells from both donor and recipient. These common LAA may not be immunodominant, however, which might explain why the host does not rid itself of the leukemia cells. Recently, work on other tumors has shown us that many tumor-associated antigens (TAA) recognized by T cells are epitopes derived from self proteins and that previous host tolerance to such TAA can be overcome. These TAA can then be used to focus the immune response preferentially against the tumor. In this chapter, hematopoietic tissue-restricted proteins are highlighted as a potential source of LAA for targeting the GVL response.

II. HISTORICAL BACKGROUND

Harnessing the immune system to treat malignancy is an old concept, and recent attempts at clinical development of antitumor immunotherapy have taken two parallel paths. The subject of this chapter, how tissue-specific antigens might be used to focus the antitumor immune response associated with bone marrow transplantation (BMT), lies at the crossroads of these two approaches. The approach taken by marrow transplanters began following the observations first made by Barnes and colleagues in 1956 using inbred mouse models of BMT to treat recipient mice with leukemia [5]. They observed that an allogeneic reaction of the graft against the recipient's leukemia might be necessary to cure the leukemia. However, not until 1958 were leukocyte antigens first described [6], and BMT performed with the knowledge of these antigens did not occur until 1968 [7]. In the years following, the problems of engraftment and GVHD prevention remained the primary preoccupation for BMT immunologists. More recently, attention has shifted to separating the specific elements of the donor antitumor response so that it can be selectively exploited.

Even before the turn of this century, however, physicians were using immunity to treat human tumors. Based upon the observation that patients with malignancies who developed severe infections would occasionally experience regression of their tumors, physicians in Europe were inducing bacterial infections in cancer patients [8]. When the tumor showed signs of regression, the patient would be treated for the infection. Dr. William B. Coley, a New York physician, documented many anecdotal cases of such treatments using bacterial extracts instead of bacteria, which subsequently became known as "Coley's toxins." The active component of Coley's toxin was later identified as lipopolysaccharide (LPS), and it was ultimately found that the observed antitumor phenomenon was an indirect effect of LPS on host macrophages, causing them to become activated and develop antitumor cell activity.

The intentional use of cellular immunity to treat tumors followed observations made during the 1940s, using inbred mouse models of transplanted tumors. It was found that when chemically induced sarcoma cells were used to elicit immunity in one animal, the resulting sarcoma-specific T lymphocytes could be adoptively transferred to syngeneic naïve recipient animals and that this would protect against secondary tumor challenges [9,10]. The use of allogeneic tumor–sensitized lymphocytes in humans was first reported in 1966 and did not involve BMT [11]. Tumors from one patient were subcutaneously implanted into the thigh of another patient, and 2 weeks later 500 mL of blood containing leukocytes from the recipient were transfused back into the original tumor donor daily for 3 weeks. Even though no attempts were made to immunosuppress the leukocyte recipients to prevent leukocyte rejection and HLA-matching was not performed, some minor responses were reported, although they could not be reproduced.

These early attempts with unmodified leukocytes were repeated by others, but this eventually gave way to the use of recombinant cytokines (such as interleukin-2, or IL-2) to generate autologous lymphocytes with antitumor activity. Such lymphokine activated killer (LAK) cells were first defined in 1980; since then, LAK cells with or without IL-2 have been used to treat patients with many different tumor types [12–14]. Currently, IL-2 with or without LAK cells is used to treat patients with renal cell cancer and melanoma, with response rates seen in 15–30% of patients [15].

Beginning in 1988, so-called tumor infiltrating lymphocytes (TIL), derived from autologous lymphocytes collected from human melanoma lesions and expanded ex vivo with IL-2, were used to successfully induce both complete and partial regressions [16]. Interestingly, there was no significant relationship between response rate and the number of infused TIL, although there was a highly significant association of tumor response with the ability of TIL to lyse autologous tumor targets in vitro [17]. In addition, prior administration of cyclophosphamide was significantly associated with the ability of TIL to localize to tumor, and localization to tumor correlated with clinical response [18].

TIL taken either directly from the tumors or from the peripheral blood of these patients exhibit cross-reactivity with autologous and allogeneic tumors in a MHC-restricted manner. These observations led to the first successful characterization of a human tumor antigen in 1991, called MAGE-1, which was isolated following the stable transfection of a genomic DNA library into a melanoma antigen-loss variant and then using T lymphocyte clones specific for the melanoma to screen the transfected cells [19]. The phenomenon of MHC-restricted tumor-cell specificity has now also been observed in patients with breast cancer, renal cell cancer, ovarian cancer, cervical cancer, and squamous cell carcinoma of the lung; many other TAA have since been isolated [20,21].

III. IMPORTANT CONCEPTS IN TUMOR IMMUNITY

It is now well established that CD8+ and CD4+ T cells recognize peptide antigens in the context of either MHC I or MHC II, respectively. After ligation of the T cell receptor (TCR) by the peptide, β_2-microglobulin, and MHC complex, the T cell may receive a second costimulatory signal via B7.1 or B7.2 expressed on the antigen-presenting cell (APC) or tumor cell and become activated. A cascade of events then takes place, including autologous IL-2 secretion, subsequent proliferation, and activation of various effector functions of the cell. Adhesion molecules such as ICAM-1 (CD54) help to stabilize the interaction between the T cell and the target cell, which facilitates the antigen recognition process. As shown in Figure 1, it is in the context of a heightened expression of the MHC, costimulatory, and adhesion molecules that an immune response is made against the antigen.

The known tumor antigens can be categorized as shown in Figure 2. They are derived from proteins that may be normal self proteins, oncogenes altered as a result of mutation or translocation events, or foreign proteins such as viral gene products expressed only in the tumor. The majority of identified tumor antigens are derived from the first group: self proteins that are either overexpressed or aberrantly expressed in the tumor [22]. Since these self antigens are also expressed in normal tissues, it is likely that T lymphocytes can distinguish the different level of expression in the tumor and therefore preferentially attack the tumor cells over normal cells. This may be due to a critical threshold level of expression of self peptide plus MHC that must be present to trigger T-cell recognition, which is related to the level of expression of the parent protein. This overlap between autoimmunity and tumor immunity blurs the distinction between self antigens and tumor antigens.

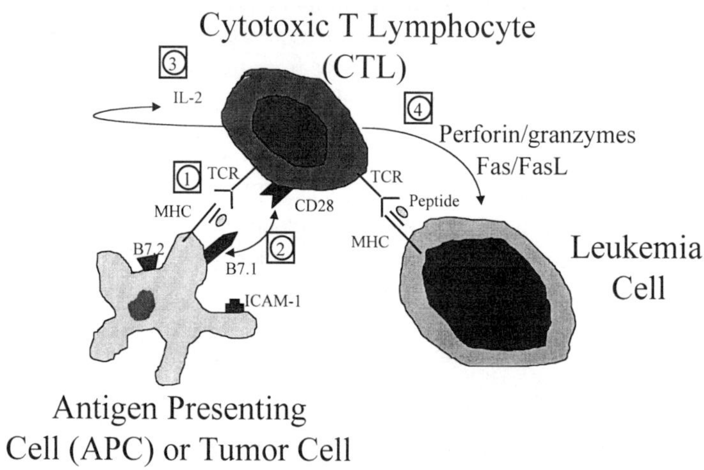

Figure 1 Lymphocyte activation.

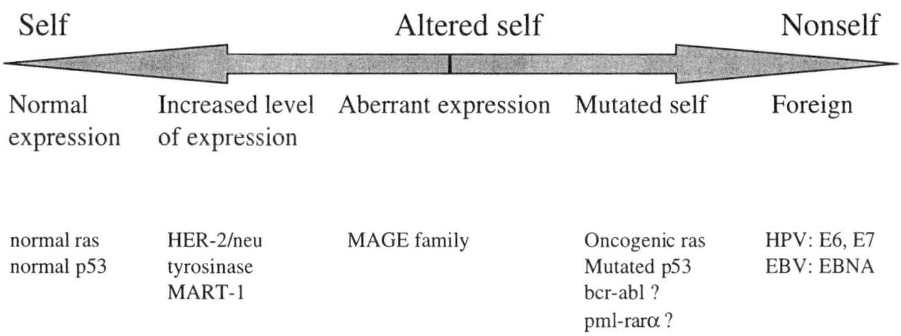

Figure 2 Spectrum of tumor antigens.

Several examples of self antigens that are also TAA are the melanoma antigens MAGE-1 and MAGE-3, expressed in testes, and MART-1 and gp100, expressed in the retina and in normal melanocytes [23]. Another example is HER-2/neu, a growth-factor receptor homologous to epidermal growth factor receptor, which is also expressed in most normal tissues [24,25]. This self protein is over-expressed in 25–30% of patients with breast cancer and ovarian cancer and is present at a 40- to 50-fold higher level of expression in malignant cells than in normal tissues [26].

Since the immune system responds against self proteins expressed in tumor cells as well as normal cells, preferential tumor recognition may be due to the different level of self-antigen expression in each cell type [26]. In support of this explanation, when mice were recently immunized with a self antigen, CTL with low antigen avidity were elicited; these rejected tumors that expressed high levels of the target self antigen but left normal cells that expressed low antigen levels alone. This shows how immunizing with self antigens can recruit CTL into responding against tumor cells while also remaining tolerant to normal cells [27].

It has been shown that several patients with breast and ovarian cancer have existent immune recognition of HER-2/neu, including T-cell recognition of specific HER-2/neu–derived peptides [28]. The following question then naturally arises: Why do patients have cancer despite an immune recognition of the tumor antigens? There are probably many reasons for this. For instance, in tumors, there is heterogeneity in the level of expression of MHC, B7.1, and ICAM-1 on individual tumor cells [29]. The cells with a low level of expression of these molecules may escape immune recognition and may come to predominate in the tumor. In experiments where previously underexpressed costimulatory molecules were either increased on leukemia cells or added by addition of bystander cells with highly expressed costimulatory molecules, autologous leukemia-specific T-cell responses could be elicited in vitro.

Another reason the immune system may not respond to the self tumor antigens is because of quantitative differences in antigen processing and presentation in the tumor cells. For example, fibroblasts infected with virus elicit CTL with lytic responses only against the subdominant epitopes, whereas dendritic cells (DC) infected with virus elicit lytic responses against the dominant epitopes [30]. However, when sensitized to peptide antigens presented by either cell type, T cells retain the ability to recognize both the dominant and subdominant epitopes. These different cell types were found to process and present the same set of virus proteins in quantitatively different ways to T cells.

Tumor cells, like the virus-infected fibroblasts, may not process and present the tumor antigens to elicit a response against the dominant epitopes. However, lytic responses directed against subdominant epitopes might be uncovered if the immune response could be heightened to be directed against these epitopes. This might result in preferential targeting of the tumor cells over normal cells owing to aberrant expression of the subdominant self-antigens in the tumor cells.

This concept may be important in the search for tumor antigens among self antigens in many tumors such as leukemia. For instance, T-cell recognition of self proteins expressed in hematopoietic tissues might be preserved against many subdominant epitopes because the T cells that recognize them have escaped negative selection and may be tolerant to such epitopes. Furthermore, tolerance to these self-antigens may be quantitative rather than absolute. In animal models, vaccination with such self-antigens can activate specific T cells that are able to reject tumor cells expressing high levels of the self antigen. If we could determine what might be the subdominant epitopes selectively expressed in hematopoietic tissues, they might provide a reservoir of leukemia-specific targets. Cytotoxic T lymphocytes (CTL) might then be coaxed into recognizing these target antigens in order to selectively destroy leukemic cells.

IV. METHODS TO IDENTIFY TUMOR ANTIGENS

Tumor antigens recognized by CTLs consist of peptides derived from endogenous proteins and presented by MHC molecules. Three methods have been used to identify the peptides presented to tumor-specific T cells. The first is a genetic approach using the transfection of recombinant DNA libraries made from tumor cells into cell lines co-transfected with the presenting MHC molecule in order to isolate the gene encoding the antigen. Tumor-specific CTL clones are used to screen the library of transfected cells for the antigen-encoding cell. Once the gene is isolated, the antigenic peptide is deduced from the sequence of the putative protein. The first melanoma antigen, MAGE-1, was found using this method [19].

The second method is biochemical and involves acid-eluting the peptides bound to MHC molecules expressed by the tumor cells. The eluted peptides are then separated into fractions by high-pressure liquid chromatography (HPLC). Each peptide fraction is tested using tumor-specific CTL to screen for the peptide's ability to reconstitute the antigen when pulsed onto MHC-matched APC. The peptide sequence is then deduced using Edman degradation (if there is sufficient peptide present) or mass spectrometry.

The third, or immunological, method is the reverse of the first two. Rather than starting with a tumor-specific CTL, the starting point is the sequence of a putative tumor antigen. The target antigen might be selected based on the general paradigm of many known tumor antigens, as highlighted in the previous section. Peptides of 9 to 11 amino acids in length, selected from the putative tumor antigen for their high-affinity binding to a given MHC class I molecule, are loaded on APC in order to stimulate lymphocytes in vitro. Peptide-specific CTL are readily obtainable by this procedure, but a number of them do not recognize HLA-matched tumor cells expressing protein endogenously.

The melanoma antigen MAGE-3 is an example of a TAA that was found using two of the methods described above. HLA-A1 and -A2 present melanoma peptide antigens derived from MAGE-3 proteins to melanoma-specific CTL. This protein belongs to a family of proteins expressed in melanoma cells and in normal testis, and a MAGE-3–derived peptide was determined by separate groups, one using the immunological method and the other a genetic method (using tumor antigen-deficient mutants), to be antigenic for CTL [31,32]. What may be critical for tumor-specific destruction by CTL is the density of the overexpressed peptide-MHC complexes, the tumor cell type's ability to process and present the proper epitopes, and the expression of costimulatory signals that influence activation of the otherwise silent tumor-specific T-cell repertoire.

V. TISSUE ANTIGENS AS TARGETS FOR GVL

A. Self Proteins Can Be Tissue Antigens for GVL

In order to find LAA, we have studied aberrantly expressed myeloid-restricted proteins based on the paradigm that such self proteins can also be TAA. Myeloid leukemias express a number of differentiation antigens associated with granule formation as shown in Figure 3. One of those, proteinase 3 (diagrammed in Figure 4), is a 26,000-Da neutral serine protease that is stored in primary azurophil granules and maximally expressed at the promyelocyte stage of differentiation [33,34]. The human gene contains five exons, is localized on chromosome 19p, and has recently been cloned [35]. Proteinase 3 (P3) is overexpressed in a variety of myeloid leukemia cells, including 75% of those of CML patients, approximately 50% of those of acute myeloid leukemia patients, and approximately 30% of those of myelodsyplastic syndrome patients [36].

P3 may also be centrally involved either in the process of leukemic transfor-

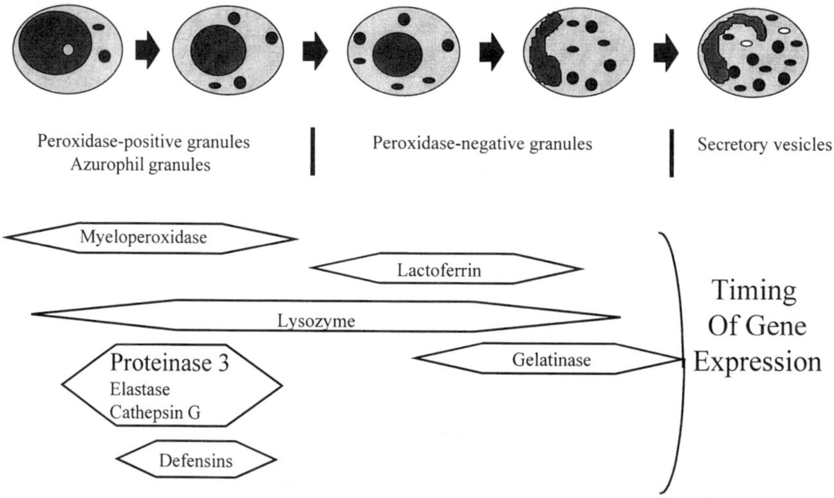

Figure 3 Normal myeloid development.

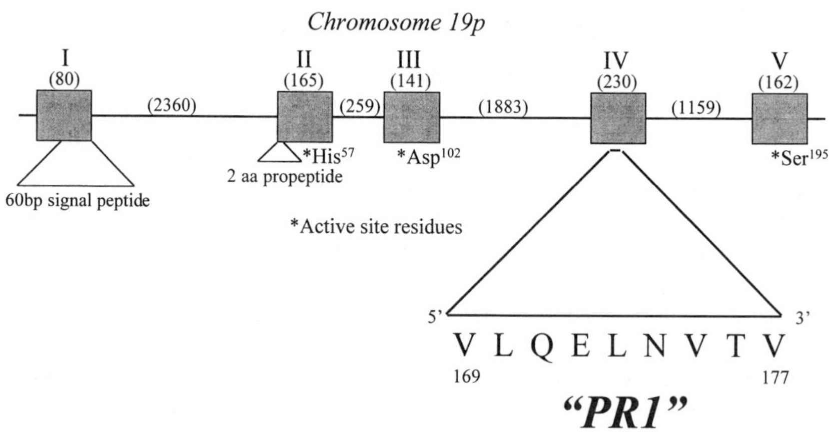

Figure 4 Structure of human proteinase 3 gene.

mation or the maintenance of the leukemia phenotype, since inhibition of P3 expression by antisense oligodeoxynucleotides inhibits cell proliferation and induces differentiation in the HL60 human leukemia cell line [37]. Although leukemia cells with mutant forms of the P3 protein might escape immune recognition, they might also lose their ability to maintain the leukemic phenotype if the mutation involved an essential portion of the molecule.

The P3 protein is also a target of autoimmune attack in Wegener's granulomatosis (WG) [38,39]. This chronic disease is associated with the production of IgG antineutrophil cytoplasmic antibodies (ANCA) with specificity for P3, which suggests that T-cell help is required for P3 antigen recognition. Acute flareups of WG and other autoimmune disorders associated with ANCA are strongly associated with an increase in the ANCA titer [39,40]. P3 may also be present in endothelial cells, and the level of expression can be increased after exposure to TNF-α [41]. Although ANCA have been shown to bind P3 on human umbilical vein endothelial cells in vitro [42], biopsy material from active sites of disease in WG patients failed to demonstrate the presence of ANCA on endothelial cells [43,44], raising the question of the immunopathological relevance of these findings [45].

T cells taken from peripheral blood or biopsy of active sites of disease in individuals with WG proliferate in response to crude extracts from azurophilic granules and to the purified P3 protein [46–48]. These findings suggest that T-cell responses to P3 exist in patients with WG and that therefore peptides from P3 should be contained in the T-cell repertoire. This also suggested that CTL responses to peptides derived from P3, as opposed to other myeloid proteins, might be easier to elicit. Furthermore, if such peptides could be found, this strategy might be useful when other tissue-restricted protein targets were being considered.

It was found that PR1 (aa sequence VLQELNVTV), a 9 aa peptide derived from P3 (aa 169–177) that binds to HLA-A*0201, can be used to elicit CTL from HLA-A*0201 normal donors in vitro, which demonstrate preferential cytotoxicity toward allogeneic HLA-A*0201 myeloid leukemia cells [49]. The sequence of PR1 is compared with other TAA and to two recently discovered minor antigens (Figure 5), PR1-specific CTL also inhibit granulocyte-macrophage colony-forming units (GM-CFU) from the marrow of CML patients, but not GM-CFU from normal HLA-matched donors [50]. P3 is highly expressed in CD34+ CML blasts in some patients (unpublished observations), which indicates that leukemia progenitor cells contain the aberrantly expressed parent protein. Both the lysis of fresh leukemia cells and the inhibition of leukemia progenitors was highly correlated with the amount of P3 expression in the target cells [49,50]. The region coding for the PR1 peptide has been sequenced in a number of CTL and leukemia cells from these experiments, and no polymorphisms have been found, which eliminates the possibility that PR1 is a minor antigen [50].

	Position								
	1	2	3	4	5	6	7	8	9
Anchor residues		L M				V			V L
PR-1	**V**	**L**	**Q**	**E**	**L**	**N**	**V**	**T**	**V**
Tyrosinase	M	L	L	A	L	L	Y	C	L
MART-1	A	A	G	I	G	I	L	T	V
HA-1	V	L	H	D	D	L	L	E	A
HA-2	Y	I	G	E	V	L	V	S	V

Figure 5 HLA-A*0201 binding motif.

PR1 is therefore the first self-peptide antigen that can elicit specific CTL lysis of fresh human myeloid leukemia cells. Based on preclinical studies, a phase I/II clinical trial will investigate the toxicity and efficacy of a PR1 peptide vaccine administered with incomplete Freund's adjuvant to patients with refractory or relapsed myeloid leukemias. Clinical studies using PR1-specific adoptive cellular therapies may hold promise as well, since normal allogeneic cells used as effector cells would circumvent potential TCR signalling defects that have been described in autologous T cells [51].

Other peptides from P3 are predicted to bind to HLA-A2.1, but not all of these have been tested for their potential to elicit CTL immunity. In addition, P3 was recently found to contain a polymorphism outside of the region coding for PR1, and two synthetic peptides inclusive of this polymorphism have been shown to bind to HLA-A*0201 [52]. Should CTL responses be found in individuals with peptide discordance, these peptides might be useful as minor antigens for targeted allogeneic adoptive immunotherapy of myeloid leukemias.

In support of the concept that self antigens can be presented as targets by leukemia cells, Papadopoulos et al. recently identified naturally processed peptides bound to HLA class I and II molecules on CML blasts [53]. Following elution from MHC molecules with weak acetic acid, peptides were separated by reverse-phase HPLC and single fractions were sequenced. The sequences of the MHC-bound peptides were then compared with known protein sequences. They found a high copy number of self peptides bound to HLA-A, HLA-B, and HLA-DR molecules. Specifically, they found a peptide derived from P3 bound to an HLA-B allele, which provides confirmatory evidence that P3 is naturally processed and presented with MHC molecules in CML.

It is uncertain whether PR1 might also be a CTL target in WG patients. In one study of five WG patients, T-cell lines established from tissue biopsies of active sites of disease proliferated in response to purified P3 [47]. However, when various peptides from P3 that bound to HLA-A*0201 were investigated, these same T cells demonstrated no cytotoxicity against PR1-loaded T2 target cells. In addition, these investigators could not generate PR1-specific CTL in culture from T cells taken from biopsy sites in these WG patients. The concentration of peptide is critical to elicit specific CTL responses, however, and these investigators used concentrations different from those used to elicit PR1-specific CTL from normal individuals. In addition, the source of the T cells was a biopsy site instead of peripheral blood, and T cells at those sites are likely to be highly selected T cells that might not recognize the PR1 peptide.

The PR1 aa sequence is also found in another serine protease restricted to myeloid cells, neutrophil elastase (NE), at aa 168–176. The genes for both NE and P3 are localized to a 50-kb segment near the telomere of chromosome 19p. Expression of both genes appears to be coordinately regulated, since transcripts for both NE and P3 are first detected in myeloblasts and are maximal at the promyelocyte stage [54]. This redundancy may be beneficial if PR1 can elicit an immune response in leukemia patients, since mutations in PR1 that might allow immune escape are less likely to occur simultaneously in both genes.

There is additional evidence to support the theory that such developmentally regulated hematopoietic proteins are targets of GVL. Mutis et al. have isolated a CD4+ T-cell clone from a normal individual that lysed leukemia cells from an HLA-DR mismatched unrelated AML patient [55]. The clone was derived by stimulating responder lymphocytes with HLA-DR mismatched leukemic cells. This lytic CD4+ clone could lyse leukemia cells from other AML patients in an HLA-DR-restricted fashion as well as CD34+ normal cells, but not CD34− cells or more differentiated marrow precursors. The target antigen for this CD4+ T-cell clone was therefore thought to be a developmentally regulated hematopoietic tissue–restricted protein. Serody et al. have shown similar data with CD4+ lymphocytes derived from five normal donors [56].

Recent evidence suggests that alloreactive T cells recognize unique peptide-MHC complexes and not a common peptide dependent conformation of the MHC molecule, where multiple peptides could provide the conformation necessary for T-cell recognition [57]. Consequently, even though alloreactive CD4+ T cells recognized target antigen in the context of mismatched allogeneic HLA-DR in the study by Mutis et al., it is possible that the peptide antigen is common to all early hematopoietic precursors and is therefore either a unique self protein or a minor antigen (mH). Figure 6 highlights the various immune reactions that are possible when allogeneic lymphocytes are transfused to illustrate this point.

Based on the common observation of aberrant expression in leukemia cells and autoimmune diseases associated with many granule proteins, one would predict that other epitopes might be found within this group of proteins as shown in Table 1. The fact that two of these granule proteins, P3 and cathepsin G, are naturally processed and presented on CML cells supports future efforts to uncover such epitopes.

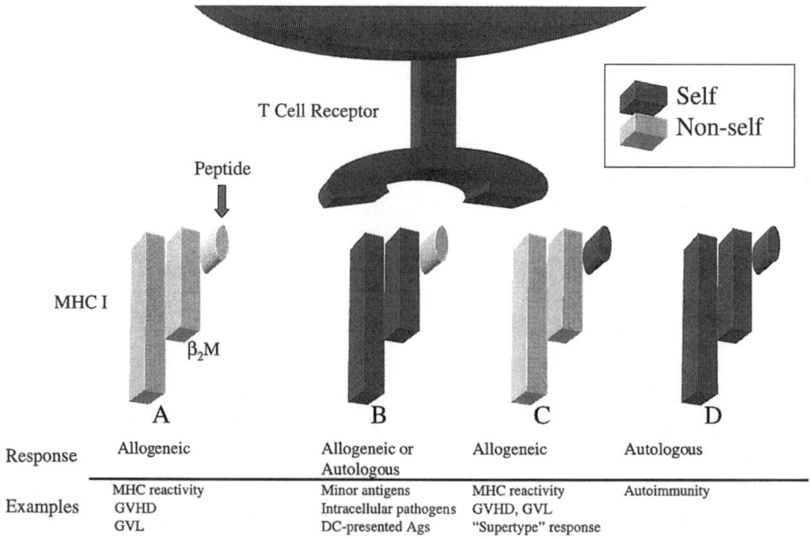

Figure 6 Possible immune reactions with transfused allogeneic lymphocytes.

Table 1 Myeloid Proteins as Leukemia Antigens

		mRNA		
Protein	Chromosome	Normal CD34+	Leukemic CD34+	Autoimmune Syndrome
Proteinase 3[a]	19p	−/+	+	Wegener's
Neutrophil elastase	19p	−	+	Wegener's and vasculitis
Myelo-peroxidase	17q22	+	++	Vasculitis
Cathepsin G[a]	14q11.2	−	+	Sclerosing cholangitis

[a]Naturally processed and presented by CML blasts

VI. MINOR ANTIGENS CAN BE TISSUE ANTIGENS FOR GVL

Some of the methods used to separate GVL from GVHD have demonstrated that T lymphocytes that recognize target antigens with clear tissue-specific distribution can be generated in the laboratory. In particular, CTL clones elicited from patients after HLA-matched BMT were used to define several mH. Four of these—HA-1, HA-2, HA-5, and HB-1—are selectively expressed in hematopoietic tissues [58–61]. A recent analysis showed a significant correlation between severe GVHD and HA-1 mismatching [62]. This suggests that HA-1 is not a good candidate antigen for selective GVL reactivity. However, neither HA-2 nor HA-5 disparity predicted severe GVHD, which may reflect a lack of immunodominance, or they may reflect another type of immune reactivity, such as GVL.

Warren, et al., in Seattle, have found 17 other CTL-defined mH in a study involving 10 allogeneic BMT donor/recipient pairs [63]. Of these, the majority (12) were expressed in hematopoietic cells but not in skin fibroblasts from the recipients. In two out of four donor/recipient pairs from whom CTL clones with hematopoietic tissue reactivity were isolated, clinical GVHD did not develop, suggesting that hematopoietic mH-specific CTL might be safely used in adoptive immunotherapy. They also found many of the mH to have sufficiently high phenotype frequencies, which would be necessary if targeting of such mH in discordant donor-recipient pairs were to be clinically useful.

If more of the genes encoding these mH could be identified, then a more accurate assessment of the tissue distribution could be made. Until then, it remains uncertain whether these mH are limited to hematopoietic tissues. Efforts using both the genetic and biochemical approaches discussed above are currently under way to determine the genes for these mH.

VII. OTHER METHODS TO SELECT TISSUE ANTIGENS FOR GVL

Recently, the HLA alleles have been grouped into four so-called supertypes, as shown in Table 2 [64]. Peptides that bind to one HLA allele within a supertype may be able to bind to other alleles and be presented to T cells, a process referred to as promiscuous or degenerative recognition, which provides for broader recognition of these peptide antigens.

This has important implications for the use of peptides derived from tumor antigens in immunotherapy strategies. First, if a single peptide can bind to many HLA types, it would hold greater potential as a useful peptide antigen for immunotherapy, since a greater number of patients with diverse HLA types might recognize the peptide. Second, nearly all peptide epitopes that bind to the HLA

Table 2 HLA Super Motifs

- A2-like
  —A∗0201, A∗0202, A∗0203, A∗0204, A∗0205, A∗0206, A∗6802, A∗6901
- A3-like
  —A∗0301, A∗1101, A∗3101, A∗3301, A∗6801
- B7-like
  —B∗0702-5, B∗3501-3, B∗5101-5, B∗5301, B∗5401, B∗5501-2, B∗5601, B∗6701, B∗7801
- B44-like
  —Acidic residue at 2; hydrophobic/aromatic C-terminus

supertypes have been found to be immunogenic [64]. If this concept were applied to the paradigm of self antigens also as tumor antigens, it might facilitate the selection of more relevant CTL target peptides.

There is recent evidence that such supertype recognition is important in antitumor immunity. An antigenic peptide derived from a melanoma antigen that could bind to multiple HLA alleles of the HLA-A3 supertype was also recognized as a TAA by CTL from patients of diverse HLA class I alleles [65]. This might mean that the immune response is focused on only a few select epitopes—an observation that could be applied to the design of peptide-based immunotherapy strategies.

REFERENCES

1. Drobyski WR, Ash RC, Casper JT, McAuliffe T, Horowitz MM, Lawton C, Keever C, Baxter-Lowe LA, Camitta B, Garbrecht F. Effect of T-cell depletion as graft-versus-host disease prophylaxis on engraftment, relapse, and disease-free survival in unrelated marrow transplantation for chronic myelogenous leukemia. Blood 1994; 83:1980–1987.
2. Kolb HJ, Schattenberg A, Goldman JM, Hertenstein B, Jacobsen N, Arcese W, Ljungman P, Ferrant A, Verdonck L, Niederwieser D. Graft-versus-leukemia effect of donor lymphocyte transfusions in marrow grafted patients: European Group for Blood and Marrow Transplantation Working Party Chronic Leukemia. Blood 1995; 86:2041–2050.
3. Kolb HJ, Holler E. Adoptive immunotherapy with donor lymphocyte transfusions. Curr Opin Oncol 1997; 9:139–145.
4. Falkenburg JHF, Wafelman AR, van Bergen CAM, Bongaerts R, Lurvink EGA, Smit WM, Joosten P, Landegent JE, Kluen-Nelemans JC, Fibbe WE, Willemze P. Leukemia-reactive cytotoxic T lymphocytes induce complete remission in a patient

with refractory accelerated phase chronic myeloid leukemia. Blood 1997; 10(suppl 1):2619.
5. Barnes DWH, Corp MJ, Loutit JF, Neal FE. Treatment of murine leukemia with x-rays and homologous bone marrow: preliminary communication. Br Med 1956; 2: 626–627.
6. Dausset J. Iso-leuco-anticorps. Acta Haematol 1958; 20:156–166.
7. Gatti RA, Meuwissen HJ, Allen HD, Hong R, Good RA. Immunological reconstitution of sex-linked lymphopenic immunological deficiency. Lancet 1968; 2:1366–1369.
8. Didot A. Essai sur la prophylaxie du cancer. Bull Acad R Sol Belge 1851; 11:100–172.
9. Gross L. Intradermal immunization of C3H mice against a sarcoma that originated in an animal of the same line. Cancer Res 1943; 3:326–330.
10. Foley EJ. Antigenic properties of methylcholanthrene-induced tumors in mice of the strain of origin. Cancer Res 1953; 13:835–844.
11. Nadler SH, Moore GE. Clinical immunologic study of malignant disease: response to tumor transplants and transfer of leukocytes. Ann Surg 1966; pp. 482–490.
12. Lotze MT, Line BR, Mathisen DJ. The in vivo distribution of autologous human and murine lymphoid cells grown in T cell growth factor (TCGF): implications for the adoptive immunotherapy of tumors. J Immunol 1980; 125:1487–1493.
13. Mazumder A, Eberlein TJ, Grimm EA. Phase I study of the adoptive immunotherapy of human cancer with lectin activated autologous mononuclear cells. Cancer 1984; 53:896–905.
14. Rosenberg SA. Immunotherapy of cancer by the systemic administration of lymphoid cells plus interleukin-2. J Biol Resp Mod 1984; 3:501–511.
15. Rosenberg SA. Cell Transfer Therapy: Clinical Applications, 2d ed. Philadelphia: Lippincott, 1995.
16. Rosenberg SA, Packard BS, Aebersold PM. Use of tumor-infiltrating lymphocytes and interleukin-2 in the immunotherapy of patients with metastatic melanoma, special report. N Engl J Med 1988; 319:1676–1680.
17. Schwartzentruber DJ, Hom SS, Dadmarz R, White DE, Yannelli JR, Steinberg SM, Rosenberg SA, Topalian SI. In vitro predictors of therapeutic response in melanoma patients receiving tumor-infiltrating lymphocytes and interleukin-2. J Clin Oncol 1994; 12:1475–1483.
18. Pockaj BA, Sherry R, Wei J, Yannelli JR, Carter CS, Leitman SF, Carrasquillo JR, White DE, Steinberg S, Rosenberg SA, Yang JD. Localization of Indium-111-labelled tumor infiltrating lymphocytes to tumor in patients receiving adoptive immunotherapy: augmentation with cyclophosphamide in association with response. Cancer 1994; 73:1731–1737.
19. van der Bruggen P, Traversari C, Chomez P, Lurquin C, De Plaen E, Van den Eynde B, Knuth A, Boon T. A gene encoding an antigen recognized by cytolytic T lymphocytes on a human melanoma. Science 1991; 254:1643–1646.
20. Robbins PF, Kawakami Y. Human tumor antigens recognized by T cells. Curr Opin Immunol 1996; 8:628–636.
21. Boon T, Coulie PG, Van den Eynde B. Tumor antigens recognized by T cells. Immunol Today 1997; 18:267–268.

22. Nanda NK, Sercarz EE: Induction of anti-self-immunity to cure cancer. Cell 1995; 82:13–17.
23. Marincola FM, Hijazi YM, Fetsch P. Salgaller ML, Rivoltini L, Cormier J, Simonis TB, Duray PH, Herlyn M, Kawakami Y, Rosenberg SA. Analysis of expression of the melanoma-associated antigens MART-1 and gp100 in metastatic melanoma cell lines and in situ lesions. J Immunother Emphasis Tumor Immunol 1996; 19:192–205.
24. Peoples GE, Smith RC, Linehan DC, Yoshino I, Goedegebuure PS, Eberlein TJ. Shared T cell epitopes in epithelial tumors. Cell Immunol 1995; 164:279–286.
25. Linehan DC, Goedegebuure PS, Peoples GE, Rogers SO, Eberlein TJ. Tumor-specific and HLA-A2-restricted cytolysis by tumor-associated lymphocytes in human metastatic breast cancer. J Immunol 1995; 155:4486–4491.
26. Yoshino I, Peoples GE, Goedegebuure PS, Maziarz R, Eberlein TJ. Association of HER2/neu expression with sensitivity to tumor-specific CTL in human ovarian cancer. J Immunol 1994; 152:2393–2400.
27. Morgan DJ, Kreuwel HTC, Fleck S, Levitsky HI, Pardoll DM, Sherman LA. Activation of low avidity CTL specific for a self epitope results in tumor rejection but not autoimmunity. J Immunol 1998; 160:643–651.
28. Disis ML, Cheever MA. HER-2/neu protein: a target for antigen-specific immunotherapy of human cancer. Adv Cancer Res 1997; 71:343–371.
29. Dermime S, Mavroudis D, Jiang YZ, Hensel N, Molldrem J, Barrett AJ. Immune escape from a graft-versus-leukemia effect may play a role in the relapse of myeloid leukemias following allogeneic bone marrow transplantation. Bone Marrow Transplant 1997; 19:989–999.
30. Butz EA, Bevan MJ. Differential presentation of the same MHC class I epitopes by fibroblasts and dendritic cells. J Immunol 1998; 160:2139–2144.
31. Celis E, Tsai V, Crimi C. DeMars R, Wentworth PA, Chesnut RW, Grey HM, Sette A, Serra HM. Induction of anti-tumor cytotoxic T lymphocytes in normal humans using primary cultures and synthetic peptide epitopes. Proc Natl Acad Sci USA 1994; 91:2105–2109.
32. Gaugler B, Van den Eynde B, Van der Bruggen P, Romero P, Gaforio JJ, De Plaen E, Lethe B, Brasseur F, Boon T. Human gene MAGE-3 codes for an antigen recognized on a melanoma by autologous cytolytic T lymphocytes. J Exp Med 1994; 179: 921–930.
33. Rao NV, Wehner NG, Marshall BC, Gray WR, Gray BH, Hoidal JR. Characterization of proteinase-3 (PR-3), a neutrophil serine proteinase. J Biol Chem 1991; 266: 9540.
34. Muller-Berat N, Minowada J, Tsuji-Takayama K, Drexler H, Lanotte M, Wieslander J, Wiik A. The phylogeny of proteinase 3/myeloblastin, the autoantigen in Wegener's granulomatosis, and myeloperoxidase as shown by immunohistochemical studies on human leukemic cell lines. Clin Immunol Immunopathol 1994; 70:51–59.
35. Sturrock AB, Franklin KF, Rao G, Marshall BC, Rebentisch MB, Lemons RS, Hoidal JR. Structure, chromosomal assignment, and expression of the gene for proteinase 3. J Biol Chem 1992; 267:21193.
36. Dengler R, Munstermann U, al-Batran S, Hausner I, Faderl S, Nerl C, Emmerich

B. Immunocytochemical and flow cytometric detection of proteinase 3 (myeloblastin) in normal and leukaemic myeloid cells. Br J Haematol 1995; 89:250–257.
37. Bories D, Raynal MC, Solomon DH, Darzynkiewicz Z, Cayre YE. Down-regulation of a serine protease, myeloblastin, causes gwoth arrest and differentiation of promyelocytic leukemia cells. Cell 1989; 59:959.
38. Spronk PE, Bootsma H, Horst G, Huitema MG, Limburg PC, Cohen Tervaert JW, Kallenberg CG. Antineutrophil cytoplasmic antibodies in systemic lupus erythematosus. Br J Rheumatol 1996; 35:625–631.
39. Stegeman CA, Cohen Tervaert JW, Kallenberg CG, Kallenberg CG, Brouwer E, Mulder AH, Stegeman CA. Anti-neutrophil cytoplasmic antibodies: tools for diagnosis and follow-up in systemic vasculitis ANCA—pathophysiology revisited. Ann Med Interne 1994; 145:523–532.
40. Tervaert JW, Stegeman CA, Huitema MG, Kallenberg CG. Anti-neutrophil cytoplasmic antibodies (ANCA) in sera from patients with inflammatory bowel disease (IBD): relation to disease pattern and disease activity. Arthritis Rheum 1994; 37: 596–597.
41. Sibelius U, Hattar K, Schenkel A, Noll T, Scernok E, Gross W, Werner-Johannes M, Hans-Michael P, Seeger W, Grimminger F. Wegener's granulomatosis: anti-proteinase 3 antibodies are potent inductors of human endothelial cell signalling and leakage response. J Exp Med 1998; 187:497–503.
42. Mayet WJ, Csernok E, Szymkowiak C, Gross WL, Meyer ZUM, Buschenfelde KH. Human endothelial cells express proteinase 3, the target antigen of anticytoplasmic antibodies in Wegener's granulomatosis. Blood 1993; 82:1221–1229.
43. Brouwer E, Huitema MG, Mulder AH, Heeringa P, van Goor H, Tervaert JW, Weening JJ, Kallenberg CG. Neutrophil activation in vitro and in vivo in Wegener's granulomatosis. Kidney Int 1994; 45:1120–1131.
44. Mrowka C, Csernok E, Gross WL, Feucht HE, Bechtel U, Thoenes GH. Distribution of the granulocyte serine proteinases proteinase 3 and elastase in human glomerulonephritis. Am J Kidney Dis 1995; 25:253–261.
45. Gross WL, Scernok E. Immunodiagnostic and pathophysiologic aspects of antineutrophil cytoplasmic antibodies in vasculitis. Curr Opin Rheumatol 1995; 7:11–19.
46. Brouwer E, Stegeman CA, Huitema MG, Limburg PC, Kallenberg CG. T cell reactivity to proteinase 3 and myeloperoxidase in patients with Wegener's granulomatosis (WG). Clin Exp Immunol 1994; 98:448–453.
47. Ballieux BE, van der Burg SH, Hagen EC, van der Woude FJ, Melief CJ, Daha MR. Cell-mediated autoimmunity in patients with Wegener's granulomatosis (WG). Clin Exp Immunol 1995; 100:186–193.
48. Griffith ME, Coulthart A, Pusey CD. T cell responses to myeloperoxidase (MPO) and proteinase 3 (PR3) in patients with systemic vasculitis. Clin Exp Immunol 1996; 103:253–258.
49. Molldrem J, Dermime S, Parker K, Jiang YZ, Mavroudis D, Hensel N, Fukushima P, Barrett AJ. Targeted T-cell therapy for human leukemia: cytotoxic T lymphocytes specific for a peptide derived from proteinase 3 preferentially lyse human myeloid leukemia cells. Blood 1996; 88:2450–2457.
50. Molldrem JJ, Clave E, Jiang YZ, Mavroudis D, Raptis A, Hensel N, Agarwala V,

Barrett AJ. Cytotoxic T lymphocytes specific for a nonpolymorphic proteinase 3 peptide preferentially inhibit chronic myeloid leukemia colony-forming units. Blood 1997; 90:2529–2534.

51. Boussiotis VA, Barber DL, Nakarai T, Freeman GJ, Gribben JG, Bernstein GM, D'Andrea AD, Ritz J, Nadler LM. Prevention of T cell anergy by signaling through the gamma c chain of the IL-2 receptor. Science 1994; 266:1039–1042.
52. Clave E, Molldrem J, Hensel N, Raptis A, Barrett AJ. Donor-recipient polymorphism of the proteinase 3 gene: a potential target for T cell alloresponses to myeloid leukemia. J Immunother 1999; 22(1):1–6.
53. Papadopoulos K, Suciu-Foca N, Hesdorffer C, Tugulea S, Maffei A, Harris P. Naturally processed tissue- and differentiation stage-specific autologous peptides bound by HLA class I and II molecules of chronic myeloid leukemia blasts. Blood 1997; 90:4938–4946.
54. Fouret P, DuBois RM, Bernaudin J-F, Takahashi H, Ferrans VJ, Crystal RG. Expression of the neutrophil elastase gene during human bone marrow cell differentiation. J Exp Med 1989; 169:833–845.
55. Mutis T, Schrama E, van Luxemburg-Heijs SA, Falkenburg JH, Melief CJ, Goulmy E. HLA class II restricted T-cell reactivity to a developmentally regulated antigen shared by leukemic cells and CD34+ early progenitor cells. Blood 1997; 90:1083–1090.
56. Serody JS, Brecher ME, Dent G, Bentley SA, Frelinger JA, Shea TC. A method for the production of CD4+ chronic myelogenous leukemia-specific allogeneic T lymphocytes. Cancer Res 1997; 57:1547–1553.
57. Wang W, Man S, Gulden PH, Hunt DF, Engelhard VH. Class I-restricted alloreactive cytotoxic T lymphocytes recognize a complex array of specific MHC-associated peptides. J Immunol 1998; 160:1091–1097.
58. van der Harst D, Goulmy E, Falkenburg JH, Kooij-Winkelaar YM, van Luxemburg-Heijs SA, Goselink HM, Brand A. Recognition of minor histocompatibility antigens on lymphocytic and myeloid leukemic cells by cytotoxic T-cell clones. Blood 1994; 83:1060–1066.
59. Marijt WA, Veenhof WF, Goulmy E, Willemze R, van Rood JJ, Falkenburg JH. Minor histocompatibility antigens HA-1, -2, and -4, and HY-specific cytotoxic T-cell clones inhibit human hematopoietic progenitor cell growth by a mechanism that is dependent on direct cell-cell contact. Blood 1995; 82:3778–3785.
60. de Bueger M, Bakker A, Van Rood JJ, Van der Woulde F, Goulmy E. Tissue distribution of human minor histocompatibility antigens: ubiquitous versus restricted tissue distribution indicates heterogeneity among human cytotoxic T lymphocyte-defined non-MHC antigens. J Immunol 1992; 149:1788–1798.
61. Dolstra H, Fredrix H, Preijers F, Goulmy E, Figdor CG, de Witte TM, van de Wiel-van Kemenade E. Recognition of a B cell leukemia-associated minor histocompatibility antigen by CTL. J Immunol 1997; 158:560–565.
62. Goulmy E, Schipper R, Pool J, Blokland E, Falkenburg JH, Vossen J, Grathwohl A, Vogelsang GB, van Houwelingen HC, van Rood JJ. Mismatches of minor histocompatibility antigens between HLA-identical donors and recipients and the development of graft-versus-host disease after bone marrow transplantation. N Engl J Med 1996; 334:281–285.

63. Warren EH, Greenberg PD, Riddell SR. Cytotoxic T-lymphocyte-defined human minor histocompatibility antigens with a restricted tissue distribution. Blood 1998; 91:2197–2207.
64. Sidney J, Grey HM, Kubo RT, Sette A. Practical, biochemical and evolutionary implications of the discovery of HLA class I supermotifs. Immunol Today 1996; 17:261–266.
65. Wang R-F, Johnston SL, Southwood S, Sette A, Rosenberg SA. Recognition of an antigenic peptide derived from tyrosinase-related protein-2 by CTL in the context of HLA-A31 and -A33. J Immunol 1998; 160:890–897.

7

Oncoproteins as Tumor-Specific Antigens

Carlo Gambacorti-Passerini
National Cancer Institute
Milan, Italy

I. INTRODUCTION

In this chapter the biological relevance of T cell–mediated recognition of human oncogenic proteins expressed in malignant cells is discussed and the potential and limitations of oncogene-based immunotherapy are addressed.

The transformation of normal cells into neoplastic ones is a multistep process in which several genetic lesions accumulate to produce the transformed phenotype. Much knowledge of the genes involved in malignant transformation has been accumulated since the seminal discovery of *ras* mutations in human cancer in 1980 [1]. Nearly all the genes so far discovered are implicated either in the transmission of a proliferative signal from the cytoplasm to the nucleus, the regulation of DNA repair, cellular adhesion, differentiation, or apoptosis. They are collectively and somewhat loosely designated as *oncogenes*.

Oncogenic proteins represent modifications of normal proteins derived from their normal proto-oncogene counterparts. Three main molecular pathways lead to the generation of oncoproteins (Figure 1): (1) The normal protein becomes overexpressed or inappropriately expressed—i.e., in a cell lineage in which the gene is normally silent—as a result of translocations in which the entire open reading frame goes under the control of a new promotor or enhancer—e.g., *myc* in Burkitt's lymphoma, and *bcl*-2 in follicular lymphomas [2,3]; (2) Mutations can change the conformation of the molecule, locking the oncoprotein into a permanently ''on'' state in which a proliferative signal is continuously transmitted in the absence of a physiological external stimulus.—e.g., ras genes [1]. (3)

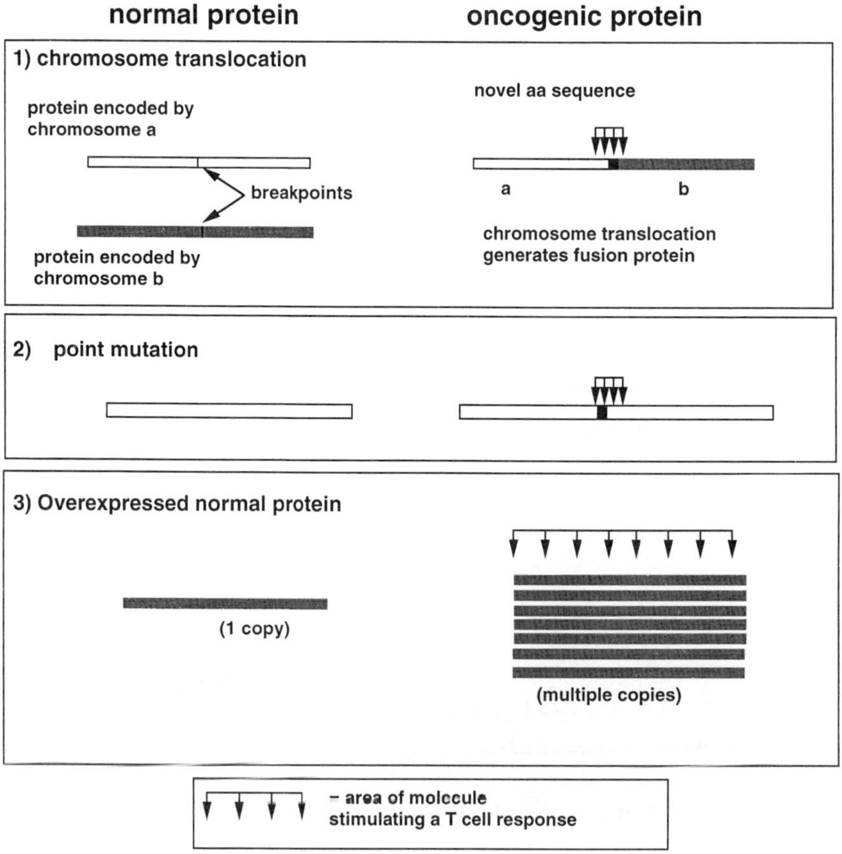

Figure 1 Mechanisms of formation of oncogenic proteins.

Chromosomal translocations cause the fusion of exons from different genes to produce oncogenic fusion proteins (OFP)—e.g., many hematological malignancies—BCR/ABL, PML/RARα, AML1/ETO, in humans and NPM/ALK in mice [4,7]. Sometimes more than one mechanism operates to produce the malignant phenotype: The NPM/ALK murine lymphoid malignancy is characterized by the overexpression of the NPM/ALK fusion protein [7]. In all these examples a causal relationship between the molecular abnormality and the neoplastic phenotype has been established using transgenic or "knock-in" animal models [4–7]. Their causative role in the generation of a particular type of malignancy is therefore well accepted. There exist, however, many situations where the relationship between a genetic alteration and cell transformation is likely but not formally proven—for example, the overexpression of the Her-2-neu gene [8–10]. Her-2/neu is overexpressed in approximately 30% of ovarian and breast cancers and other epithelial cancers. Its causative role is, however, far from established in all these cases, and the overexpression could represent the consequence and not the cause of the activation state of the transformed cells [11]. Since malignant transformation is a multistep process with progressive DNA alteration and damage, genetic alterations developing as a consequence, not a cause, of a malignant process probably represent the commonest form of genetic alteration [12]. Substances affecting DNA, such as radiation and alkylating agents, do so randomly, generating numerous nontransforming mutations throughout the genome, which differ from cell to cell. Malignant transformation in an oncogene represents a relatively rare initiating event. The central difference between these transformational and nontransformational genetic changes is that only the transforming genes and their products are present throughout the malignant cell population, since there is a strong selection pressure for cells containing the genes responsible for the malignant phenotype [12].

In recent years the focus of antitumor immunotherapy has moved from generally unsuccessful approaches to nonspecifically activate the immune system—as with IL-2 [13,14]—to targeting tumor cells specifically. The specific tumor-restricted recognition of neoplastic cells by the immune system represents a central requirement for this approach. As immunological targets, the products of transforming genes are obviously of more interest than the heterogeneously expressed proteins generated by random DNA damage. Two categories of oncogene products could be targets of immunotherapy: those where a new protein polypeptide sequence is generated and those where a normal protein is overexpressed. T cell–mediated immunity, unlike humoral immunity, is not restricted to the recognition of membrane-bound molecules, being theoretically able to recognize peptides originating from any cell-derived protein [15]. The search for tumor-specific antigens remained elusive until recently, when investigators identified several proteins recognized by the lymphocytes of cancer patients [16,17]. Tumor antigen targets should not only be tumor-specific but also closely related to the malignant process in order to avoid failure of immunotherapy by the selection of viable antigen-negative tumor cells in the malignant population [18].

Discussed below are specific examples of known immune interactions with oncogene products. The current status of research and the potentials and limitations of these tumor targets for T cell–mediated immunotherapy is outlined.

II. ONCOGENIC FUSION PROTEINS (OFPs)

OFPs represent a major category of tumor-specific transformation-related (TSTR) antigens. Many examples of OFPs occur in myeloid and lymphoid malignancies in humans as well as a growing number of solid tumors, such as Ewing's sarcoma and papillary thyroid carcinoma [19,20] (Table 1). OFPs have not so far been found in the more common solid tumors, but improved techniques of cytogenetic analysis in these tumors may in future reveal small and currently hidden translocations. Genes involved in OFPs include tyrosine kinases or transcription factors. Tumor specificity in OFPs is linked to the junctional region of the hybrid protein; therefore tumor-specific peptides span the fusion region. Most work with OFPs has been directed to the BCR/ABL fusion proteins in Ph+ chronic myelogenous leukemia and the PML/RARa fusion proteins characteristic of promyelocytic leukemia.

A. PML RARα

Acute promyelocytic leukemia (APL) is characterized by a 15;17 chromosome translocation that blocks the normal retinoic acid–induced differentiation of promyelocytes, which are the predominant cell in APL. PML/RARα represents the first OFP in which a human T cell–mediated response was documented [21]. CD4+ lymphocytes obtained from healthy HLA DR11–positive donors recognize a 19-mer peptide spanning the fusion region of PML/RARα. The peptide elicited both proliferative and cytotoxic T-cell responses. T-cell clones specific for the fusion protein also recognized autologous cells transfected with the PML/RARα gene and expressing the associated polypeptide. The ability to induce cytotoxic lymphocytes specific for the naturally processed and presented fusion peptide looked promising for possible clinical application. Unfortunately, the translation of these data into therapeutic strategies has been limited by the lack of HLA class II expression on the APL cell and the absence of detectable MHC class I–restricted T-cell responses [22]. The main reason for the absent class I expression appeared to be the lack of HLA class I binding motifs at the junctional region of PML/RARα [23]. In the case of OFP, a tumor-specific response can develop only against junctional peptides; therefore the number of tumor-specific peptidase that can be generated is limited. The constraints imposed by the single area of variability at the fusion junction may be a general limiting factor to developing a tumor immune response targeting fusion proteins. It remains puzzling, however, that an immune response can be demonstrated against OFP, only in the context of a restriction element (HLA DR) that is not expressed by the leukemic cells. It may represent an elegant mechanism for tumor escape from an immune response. It is possible that the immune response against junctional-region peptides play a role in selecting OFPs destined to give rise to clinical disease. A second limitation resides in the frequently impaired immune function found after chemotherapy in many patients with leukemia and solid tumors, this can persist for years after treatment without concomitant leukemic relapse [23]. In fact, al-

Table 1 Oncogenic Translocations and Fusion Genes in Hematological and Nonhematological Malignancies

Disease and Subtype	Chromosome Translocation	Fusion Gene
Myeloid leukemias	t(821)	AML1-ETO
Acute myelomonocytic leukemia (AML M4 Eo)	inv16	CBFb-MYH11
AML M2 inv16	t(15;17)	PML-RARa
Acute promyelocytic leukemia (AML M3)	t(3;v)	EV11
AML/AUL	t(3;5)	NPM-MLF1
	t(6;9)	DEK-CAN
	t(16;21)	FUS-ERG
	t(7;11)	NUP98-HOXA9
	t(9;11)	MLL-AF9
Chronic myeloid leukemia	t(9;22)	BCR-ABL (b2a2/b3a2)
Myelodysplastic syndrome	t(3;21)	AML1-EAP
Lymphoid malignancies		
High-risk B-ALL	t(1;19)	E2A-PBX
	t(12;21)	TEL-AML1
	t(1;11) t(4;11) t(11;19)	MLL fusions
	t(9;22)	BCR-ABL (e1a2)
	t(1;19)	E2A-PBX1
	t(17;19)	E2A-HLF
ALL, B lymphomas, chronic lymphocytic leukemia (CLL)	t(8;14), t(2;8), t(8;22)	MYC fusions
T-cell leukemias	14/TCRaδ or 7/TCR β	HOX11,LMO1/2-LYL1,TAL1/2,MYC
Solid tumors		
Ewing's sarcoma	t(11;22)	FLI1-EWS
	t(21;22)	ERG-EWS
Papillary thyroid carcinoma	inv 10	RET-D10S170
Melanoma of soft parts	t(12;22)	ATF1-EWS
Liposarcoma	t(12;16)	CHOP-FUS
Rhabdomyosarcoma	t(2;13)	PAX3-FKHR
Synovial sarcoma	t(X;18)	SYT-SSX

though anti-PML/RARα CD4+ cells could be found in healthy donors they were not detected in APL patients.

B. BCR/ABL

The Philadelphia chromosome (9;22) occurs in most patients with chronic myeloid leukemia (CML), some patients with acute lymphoblastic leukemia (ALL) and occasional patients with acute myelomonocytic leukemia (AML). The product of the 9;22 Philadelphia chromosome translocation was the first to be cloned in 1982 [24,25]. Both the b2a2 and the b3a2 fusions (the dominant types in CML) have several binding motifs for common HLA specificities [26,27]. The classic strategy for inducing peptide-specific T cells is illustrated in Figure 2. Bocchia et al [27] showed that A3-restricted CD8-specific lymphocytes could be elicited against several b3a2 junctional peptides with the induction of specific cytotoxicity. Both Bocchia and ten Bosch et al. [27,28] also analyzed the proliferative response of CD4+ cells to longer peptides and identified specific responses using b3a2 peptides in DR11 and DR0401 individuals [29]. While the Leiden group could elegantly demonstrate the recognition of blast-crisis leukemic cells and transfected LCL by peptide-specific lymphocytes, Bocchia did not show cross-reactivity. Therefore it is not clear whether class I–restricted anti-BCR/ABL–specific T cells actually recognize leukemic cells. Another limitation of these data resides in the fact that only healthy donors were used and not patients. Using the b3a2 DR0401–restricted fusion peptide used by the Leiden group, our group tested the ability of two immunocompetent b3a2-positive DR 0401-positive individuals with CML to generate peptide-specific T cells. Although these patients could mount normal proliferative responses to common antigens, no peptide-specific immune recognition was detected (manuscript in preparation). Currently, therefore, while several groups have been successful in generating b3a2-specific T cells, the demonstration that such effectors exist in patients is still lacking. The apparent recognition of blast-crisis CML cells and not of chronic-phase cells [30] is also noteworthy, since it is known that in blast crisis CML cells express higher amounts of BCR/ABL protein than in chronic phase. In fact, a relationship between the level of expression of a particular protein and its immunogenicity is now established [31]. As a consequence, immunogenic proteins are often expressed at high levels, while most OFPs are not.

C. Reactivity Against Other OFPs

Several groups have raised specific T cells recognizing peptides derived from the fusion region of different OFPs, including the DEK/AN, DRB4 0103-restricted fusion protein [32], and the Tel/AML1, HLA A0201-restricted fusion peptide [33]. In all of these cases the lymphocytes were usually obtained from

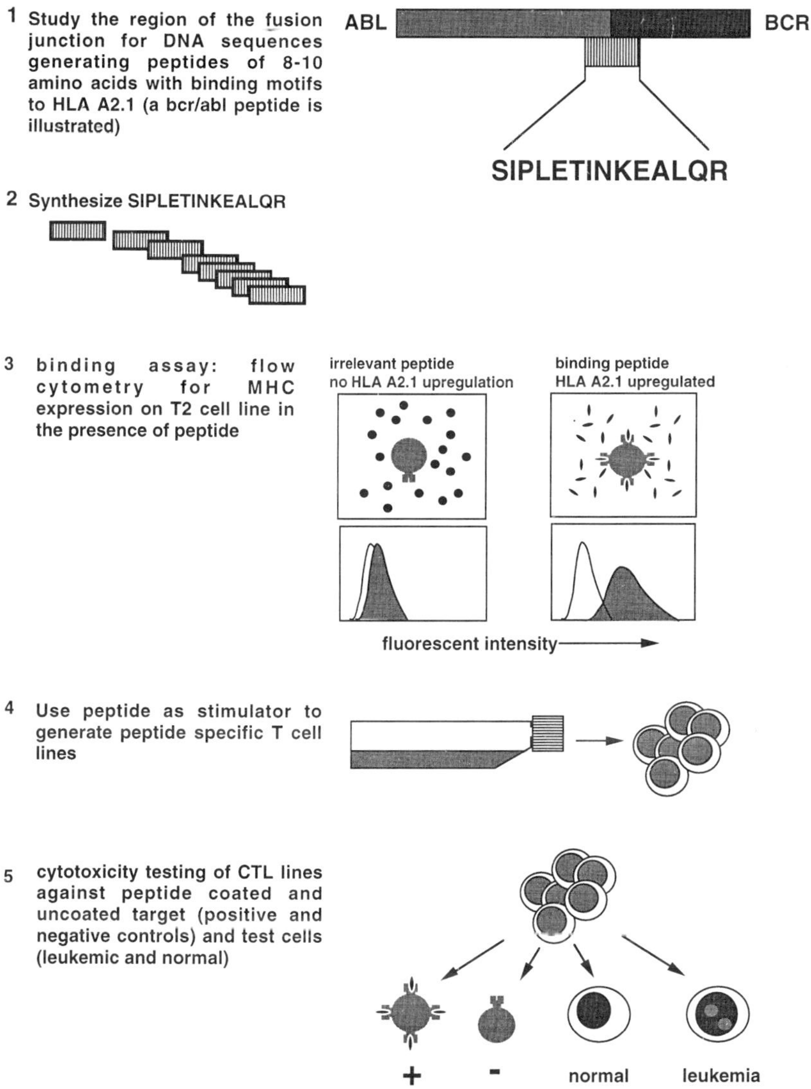

Figure 2 Strategy for generating fusion peptide–Specific cytotoxic T cells.

the donors and cross-reactivity with leukemic cells was not unequivocally demonstrated.

In conclusion, the immunogenicity of OFPs is a fascinating issue. It may well be possible that the immune response against junctional peptides can play a role in selecting OFPs causing clinically evident disease. In fact, peptides obtained from the fusion region of OFPs bind to HLA molecules significantly less efficiently than batches of random peptides containing the same binding motifs [23]. In other words, junctional peptides derived from OFPs seem to derive from larger pools of fusion peptides by a negative immune selection that eliminates cells presenting most immunogenic peptides. In addition, as recently described [34], some HLA specificities could be protective for the development of certain leukemias. On the other hand, some OFPs are definitely immunogenic and some leukemia cells can be recognized by peptide-specific clones; however, the complexity of the system (having to match different subtypes of OFP with different HLA specificities), the frequent inability of patients to mount an effective immune response to OFPs, the normally low level of expression of OFPs, and the lack of expression of the relevant HLA class in some leukemias renders the use of anti-OFP–specific lymphocytes as therapeutic effectors still premature and in need of further study.

III. Her-2/Neu

This protein is a member of the family of epidermal growth factor receptors and is considered to function as a potential growth factor receptor. Her-2/Neu is membrane-bound, with a cytoplasmic domain with tyrosine-kinase activity and an extracellular (ligand-binding) domain. Her-2/Neu represents the prototype of an overexpressed tumor-specific protein. It is expressed during development and at very low levels in epithelial cells thereafter. In several different neoplastic tissues—mostly adenocarcinomas and approximately 30% of breast and ovarian cancer—it becomes overexpressed through gene amplification and increased transcription [35]. The her-2/neu gene encodes for a tyrosine kinase that imparts a strong proliferative signal to cells expressing it. This ability of the molecule to regulate the cell cycle makes it a strong candidate for an oncogene. Transgenic animals expressing Her-2/Neu under the control of a mammary-specific promotor develop breast tumors [36], although additional alterations are clearly necessary for transformation [36,37]. The casual role of Her-2/Neu in cancers other than breast cancers is less secure.

Numerous publications from several groups demonstrate the specific recognition of different Her-2/Neu epitopes by lymphocytes from breast, ovarian, and pancreatic cancer patients. Both tumor-associated/infiltrating lymphocytes and peripheral blood lymphocytes were used. At least three different groups have shown the presence of CD8+ lymphocytes able to recognize Her-2/Neu peptides. These effectors recognized peptide-pulsed cells, transfected lymphoblastoid cell lines (ALL), and neoplastic cells overexpressing Her-2/Neu [38–41]. Different peptides can be recognized by these HLA class I–restricted cytotoxic T lymphocytes (CTL) with at least two dominant epitopes (E78, aa 369-377; C85 aa971–979). In addition, antibodies to Her-2/Neu are present in up to 40% of Her-2/Neu positive breast cancer patients. The correlation of these antibodies with prognosis is complex, depending on the stage of the tumor and the presence or absence of a lymphocyte infiltrate [44]. Predictably, when CD8+ responses and Her-2/Neu antibodies occur, a helper T-cell response has also been detected. Disis et al. [42] found proliferative CD4+ cell responses to several Her-2/Neu peptides in breast cancer patients. Taken together, these data indicate the presence of a response to Her-2/Neu in cancer patients. It might therefore be possible to modulate such a response for therapeutic advantage. These positive findings suggest the conditions that may be favorable for developing an immune response to a tumor: overexpression of the target protein, availability of multiple epitopes, and the presence of tumor cells bearing the appropriate restriction element. On a cautionary note, however: it is important not to lose sight of the fact that the immune responses are detected in patients with progressive malignancies. Clearly, the immune response was not adequate to eliminate the cancer. Furthermore, one report [41] indicates that the selection of tumor variants resistant to specific CTLs is a relatively frequent occurrence. In the three resistant variants examined, no down-regulation of the target Her-2/Neu antigen was observed, as can be predicted for transformation-related molecules. Instead, two of the three variants showed reduced expression of the relevant MHC molecule, thus preventing Her-2/Neu presentation and permitting immune escape by the tumor. Thus, the tumor continues to produce the protein essential for its malignant phenotype but prevents a T-cell response to the protein by masking the surface expression of its associated peptides. This situation is in contrast to the tumor escape behavior of nontransforming lineage-specific antigens in melanoma, where loss of antigen has been described [18].

IV. Ras PROTEINS

The Ras proteins are well-characterized examples of oncogenic proteins resulting from a single somatic mutation. The three *ras* proto-oncogenes identified (H-*ras*, K-*ras*, and N-*ras*) encode a highly conserved family of 21-kDa proteins called p21-Ras (2). Mutations of the *ras* proto-oncogene are among the most frequent alterations found in human tumors and are predominantly at a limited number of residues: 12,3 or 61. *ras* gene mutations can be found in 20–30% of all human malignancies, in particular in about 90% of pancreatic adenocarcinomas. In this tumor, all mutations are located at codon 12 [44,45]. The commonest mutations result in the substitution of Gly with Asp (39%) or Val (33%) at position 12. Other mutations involve Arg, Cys, and Ala [46]. The activating mutations impair the intrinsic GTPase activity of the protein, locking it into a constitutively activated form. The presence of a mutation inside the oncogenic protein indicates that immunogenic peptides could be generated. In fact the Ras peptides contain binding motifs and have been shown to bind to several HLA specificities, including A0201 and A0301. In vitro, Ras peptides have been shown to generate both CD4+ and CD8+ T-cell responses. In both normal individuals and patients, tumor cells and the full-length protein were also recognized in some but not all studies [47–51]. These results indicate that mutated Ras proteins have the potential to serve as targets of immunotherapy with T cells [50]. However, a review of the data (which includes analyses of antibody specificities to the Ras protein) indicates that the response is directed against normal portions of the protein [52]. The major immune response to Ras is probably, therefore, not tumor-specific. Since RAS is not overexpressed in malignant cells and is present in normal cells an immune response to Ras would not show selectively against tumor. The relevance of immunity to Ras protein in human malignancy thus remains unsettled.

V. p53 PROTEIN

Overexpression of p53, a cell-cycle controller and apoptosis inducer, is observed in up to 40% of all cancers [53]. Increased levels of p53 frequently result from mutations that prolong the protein half-life by decreasing its catabolism. In this case two mechanisms that can trigger immunogenicity can operate: somatic mutations of p53 or overexpression of the entire protein. As in the Ras model, specific T cell–mediated responses are found against both the mutated and the wild-type peptides [54,55]. These responses were obtained in healthy donors and in some patients whose tumors overexpressed p53 as a result of a somatic mutation in the gene. However, no solid evidence exists to support the recognition of human neoplastic cells by peptide-specific T cells. The failure to recognize neoplastic cells could originate from the low affinity exerted by these anti-p53 effectors. In fact Theobald et al. [56] showed that high-affinity anti-p53 effector lymphocytes can be generated only in p53-deficient HLA-A2 transgenic Kb mice, while p53 expressing mice deleted high-affinity effectors. In these animals only low-affinity p53 specific T cells occurred. Since baseline expression of p53 (in the absence of malignancy) appears to be sufficient to delete all high-affinity effector cells, the implications for immunotherapy using p53 as the target are not encouraging. Furthermore Theobald showed that increased expression of p53 did not translate into increased presentation of peptide by MHC molecules. The increased expression is, in fact, due to decreased catabolism and reduced proteasome activity, so that fewer p53 peptides reach the endoplasmic reticulum for incorporation into MHC molecules.

VI. RECOGNITION OF TRANSFORMATION-RELATED ANTIGENS IN MALIGNANT MELANOMA

Malignant melanoma represents the human solid tumor that provides the strongest evidence for involvement of the immune system in an antitumor response. Most melanoma antigens so far identified are lineage-specific proteins, or belong to the MAGE family, which have no known function. Only two studies on T-cell recognition of melanoma cells have identified antigenic molecules potentially linked to the transforming event. Woelfel et al. describe a patient in whom anti-melanoma CTLs recognized a mutated peptide from a cyclin-dependent kinase (CDK-4). This mutation abrogated the binding of the inhibitory molecule p16ink 4a to CDK4 and determined recognition by HLA-A2.1-restricted CTLs [57]. Thus, unusually, the same molecule that contributed to the malignant phenotype also rendered the malignant cell immunogenic. However, since these studies were performed on a cell line, it cannot be proved that the same mutation occurred in the original tumor. In this case the mutation could have arisen following the administration to the patient of DTIC, a known mutagenic agent.

Robbins et al. isolated lymphocytes from a patient with melanoma that recognize a peptide from a mutated form of β-catenin [58]. β-catenin is involved in cell adhesion and forms complexes with α-catenin, which, in turn, binds to intracellular actin filaments. Mutations in α- and β-catenins have been found in several cancers [58] and are associated with loss of cell adhesiveness. The mutation described changed ser37 into Phe and created a new binding site for HLA-A24. These two examples represent exceptions to the general rule that most T-cell responses to melanoma involve proteins present in both normal and malignant cells [59].

VII. RELATIONSHIP BETWEEN GRAFT-VERSUS-LEUKEMIA (GVL) EFFECT AND T-CELL RECOGNITION OF OFP

The dramatic remissions observed in patients with CML treated for relapse after marrow transplantation with donor lymphocyte infusions is strong evidence for a powerful allogenic T cell–mediated immune response against the leukemia. The possibility that the immune response is directed against the Bcr/Abl fusion protein has attracted much interest. Such a response would theoretically be separable from graft-versus- host (GVH) reactions because donor T cells would recognize only those leukemia cells bearing the Bcr/Abl tumor marker. In clinical practice, the GVH and GVL effects overlap considerably, and attempts to dissect out leukemia-specific T cells are not yet completely successful (see Chapter 14). Unfortunately there is no conclusive evidence as yet for a GVL response linked directly to Bcr/Abl (see Chapter 19). The question of whether fusion proteins make any contribution to what is undeniably a strong and effective antitumor response is clearly of great significance for designing antileukemic immunotherapy strategies in the future.

VIII. SUMMARY AND CONCLUSIONS

Table 2 summarizes current data on the development of immunotherapy strategies against OFP targets. It is now clear that oncogenic proteins are recognized by human lymphocytes, with the development of CD4, CD8, and antibody responses. The main unresolved question is whether the immunogenicity of these proteins has biological relevance and could be exploited in the development of new immunotherapy treatments. Although proteins bearing structural alterations following point mutations or translocation have the highest potential for immunogenicity, they suffer from the limitation that the number of epitopes is restricted to a small fragment of mutated or translocated protein. Molecules that become overexpressed apparently bypass these obstacles, inducing T-cell responses. In these cases, however, tolerance to the protein may occur. Finally, the cancer patient's frequent immune incompetence represents a significant obstacle to generating tumor-specific T-cell responses. Patients may be nonspecifically immunodepressed by treatment or disease progression or show specific unresponsiveness to the malignancy. This problem is particularly prevalent in leukemias. The diseases in which immunotherapeutic strategies seem most likely to succeed at present are those that express Her-2/Neu, and clinical studies in these conditions

Table 2 Cell–mediated Recognition of Human Oncogenic Proteins

Oncogenic Protein	Peptide-Specific Lymphocytes	Recognition of Malignant Cells by T-cell lines/Clones	Peptide-Specific Lymphocytes in Patients
PML/RARa	Yes	No	No
BCR/ABL	Yes	Yes	No
HER-2NEU	Yes	Yes	Yes
RAS	Yes	Unclear	Unclear
p53	Yes	No	Yes

(breast and ovarian cancer) are now warranted. To overcome the limitations of defective immunity to antigens in the autologous setting, an alternative is to develop alloimmune strategies, using healthy donors to generate T-cell responses to alloantigens (minor histocompatibility antigens) on malignant cells (see Chapter 5).

ACKNOWLEDGMENTS

Supported in part by the Italian Association for Cancer Research (AIRC, #420.198.422), the Italian Research Council (# 95.00842, 9600225.CT04), ACRO project (92.02329.PF39/94.01273.PF39), Istituto Superiore di Sanitá (#881A/10), BIOMED-2 grants #BMH4-CT96-0848 and PL96-3058, and EU-TMR grant #ERB4001GT960277. I thank Dr. Giorgio Parmiani for helpful discussions on this manuscript.

REFERENCES

1. Barbacid M. Ras genes. Annu Rev Biochem 1987; 56:779–827.
2. Berger R, Bernheim A. Cytogenetics of Burkitt's lymphoma-leukemia: a review. IARC Sci Publ 1985; 60:65–80.
3. Bakshi A, Jensen JP, Goldman P, Wright JJ, McBride OW, Epstein AL, Korsmeyer SJ. Cloning the chromosomal breakpoint of t(14;18) human lymphomas: clustering around JH on chromosome 14 and near a transcription unit on 18. Cell 1985; 41:899–906.
4. Daley GQ, Van Etten RA, Baltimore D. Induction of chronic myelogenous leukemia in mice by the P210$^{bcr/abl}$ gene of the Philadelphia chromosome. Science 1990; 247:824–830.
5. Heisterkamp N, Jenster G, ten Hoeve J, Zovich D, Pattengale PK, Groffen J. Acute leukemia in BCR/ABL transgenic mice. Nature 1990; 344:251–253.
6. Brown D, Kogan S, Lagesse E, Weissman I, Alcalay M, Pelicci PG, Atwater S, Bishop JM. A PML-RARalpha transgene initiates murine acute promyelocytic leukemia. Proc Natl Acad Sci USA 1997; 18:2551–2556.
7. Kuefer M, Look T, Pulford K, Behm F, Pattengale PK, Mason DY, Morris SW. Retrovirus-mediated gene transfer of NPM-ALK causes lymphoid malignancy in mice. Blood 1997; 90:2901–2910.
8. Gambacorti-Passerini C. Immunogenicity of fusion proteins. An example of tumor specific/transformation-related (TSTR) antigens. Int J Clin Lab Res 1993; 23:186–191.
9. Li B, Rosen JM, McMenamin-Balano J, Muller WJ, Perkins AS. Neu/ERBB2 cooperates with p53-172H during mammary tumorigenesis in transgenic mice. Mol Cell Biol 1997; 17:3155–3163.
10. Siegel PM, Dankort DL, Hardy WR, Muller J. Novel activating mutations in the

neu protooncogene involved in induction of mammary tumors. Mol Cell Biol 1994; 14:7068–7077.

11. Nowak F, Jacquemin-Sablon A, Pierre J. Expression of the activated p185erbB2 tyrosine kinase in human epithelial cells leads to MAP kinase activation but does not confer oncogenicity. Exp Cell Res 1997; 231:251–259.
12. Heim S, Mitelman F. Cancer Cytogenetics. New York: Alan R Liss, 1987.
13. Gambacorti-Passerini C, Radrizzani M, Marolda R, Belli F, Sciorelli G, Galazka AR, Schindler JD, Cascinelli N, Parmiani G. In vivo activation of lymphocytes in melanoma patients receiving escalating doses of recombinant interleukin-2. Int J Cancer 1998; 41:700–706.
14. Gambacorti-Passerini C, Sondel PM. Problems, controversies and perspectives on the clinical use of interleukin-2. Curr Opin Oncol 1990; 2:1139–1143.
15. Sibille C, Chomez P, Wildmann C, Van Pel A, De Plaen E, Maryanski JL, de Bergeyck V, Boon T. Structure of the gene of turn-transplantation antigen P198: a point mutation generates a new antigenic peptide. J Exp Med 1990; 172:35–45.
16. Traversari C, Van der Bruggen P, Luescher I, Lurquin C, Chomez P, Van Pel A, de Plaen E, Amar-Costesec A, Boon T. A nonapeptide encoded by human gene MAGE-1 is recognized on HLA-A1 by cytotoxic t lymphocytes directed against tumor antigens MZ2-E. J Exp Med 1992; 176:1453–1459.
17. Van der Bruggen P, Traversari C, Chomez P, Lurquin C, De Plaen E, Van den Eynde B, Knuth A, Boon T. A gene encoding an antigen recognized by cytolytic T lymphocytes on human melanoma. Science 1991; 254:1643.
18. Jager E, Ringhoffer M, Karbach J, Arnand M, Oesch F, Knuth A. Inverse relationship of melanocyte differentiation antigen expression in melanoma tissues and CD8+ cytotoxic T cell responses: evidence for immunoselection of antigen-loss variants in vivo. Int J Cancer 1996; 66:470–476.
19. Rabbits TH. Chromosomal translocations in human cancer. Nature 1994, 372:143–149.
20. Look AT. Oncogenic transcription factors in the human leukemias. Science 1997; 278:1059–1065.
21. Gambacorti-Passerini C, Grignani F, Arienti F, Pandolfi PP, Pelicci PG, Parmiani G. Human CD4 lymphocytes specifically recognize a peptide representing the fusion region of the hybrid protein pml/RARα present in acute promyelocytic leukemia cells. Blood, 1993; 81:1369–1375.
22. Dermime S, Bertazzoli C, Marchesi E, Ravagnani F, Blaser K, Corneo GM, Parmiani G, Gambacorti-Passerini C. Inefficient T cell mediated recognition of the fusion region of the pml/RARα hybrid protein by lymphocytes of acute promyelocytic leukemia patients. Clin Cancer Res 1996; 2:593–600.
23. Gambacorti-Passerini C, Bertazzoli C, Dermime S, Schende D, Parmiani G. Mapping HLA class I binding motifs in forty four fusion proteins involved in human cancer. Clin Cancer Res 1997; 6:675–684.
24. Hagemeijer A, Bootsma D, Spurr NK, Heisterkamp N, Groffen J, Stevenson JR. A cellular oncogene is translocated to the Philadelphia chromosome in chronic myelocytic leukemia. Nature 1982; 300:765–767.
25. Hermans A, Heisterkamp N, von Lindern M, van Baal S, Meijer D, van der Plas D, Wiedemann LM, Groffen J Bootsma D, Grosveld G. Unique fusion of bcr and

c-abl genes in Philadelphia chromosome positive acute lymphoblastic leukemia. Cell 1987; 51:33–40.

26. Bocchia, M, Wentworth PA, Southwood S, Sidney J, McGraw K, Scheinberg DA, Sette A. Specific binding of leukemia oncogene fusion protein peptides to HLA class I molecules. Blood 1995; 85:2680–2684.
27. Bocchia M, Korontsvit T, Xu Q, Mackinnon S, Yang SY, Sette A, Scheinberg DA. Specific human cellular immunity to BCR-ABL oncogene derived peptides. Blood 1996; 87:3587–3592.
28. Ten Bosch GJA, Joosten AM, Kessler, JH, Melief CJM, Leeksma OC. Recognition of BCR-ABL positive leukemic blasts by human CD4+ T cells elicited by primary in vitro immunization with a BCR-ABL breakpoint peptide. Blood 1996; 88:3522–3527.
29. Ten Bosch GJA, Kessler JH, Joosten AM, Bres-Vloemans AA, Blom J, Godthelp BC, Melief CJM, Leeksma OC. BCR-ABL oncoprotein p210^{b2a2} contains an epitope for HLA-DR restricted cytotoxic T lymphocytes (abstr 870). 39th meeting of the American Society of Hematology, San Diego, CA, Dec 5–9, 1997. Blood 1997; 90.
30. Pawelec G, Max H, Halder T, Bruserud O, Merl A, da Silva P, Kalbacher H. BCR/ABL leukemia oncogene fusion peptides selectively bind to certain HLA-DR alleles and can be recognized by T cells found at low frequency in the repertoire of normal donors. Blood 1996; 88:2118–2124.
31. Labarriere N, Diez E, Pandolfino MC, Viret C, Guillox Y, Le Guiner S, Fonteneau JF, Dreno B, Jotereau F. Optimal T cell activation by melanoma cells depends on a minimal level of antigen transcription. J Immunol 1997; 158:1238–1245.
32. Ohminami H, Yasukawa M, Kaneko S, Yakushijin Y, Fujita S. Fas-independent and non-apoptotic cytotoxicity mediated by an HLA-DRB4*0103-restricted CD4+ cytotoxic T cell clone directed against DEK-CAN fusion protein produced by translocation (6;9)(p23;q34) (abstr 601). 39th Meeting of the American Society of Hematology, San Diego, CA, Dec 5–9, 1997. Blood. 1997; 6.
33. Yotnda P, Garcia F, Even J, Kourilsky P, Lemonnier F, Langlade-Demoyen P, Vilmer F, Lehn P. Cytotoxic T cell response against the chimeric TEL-AML1 protein in childhood acute lymphoblastic leukemia (abstr 837). 38th Meeting of the American Society of Hematology, Orlando, FL, Dec 6–10, 1996. Blood 1996; 88.
34. Posthuma EFM, Falkenburg JHF, Apperley JF, Jeannet M, Schipper RF, Schreuder GMT, D'Amaro J, v Biezen JH, Hermans J, Willemze R, Niederwieser D. HLA-A3 and HLA-B8 may protect against acquiring chronic myeloid leukemia (abstr 1102). 39th Meeting of the American Society of Hematology, San Diego, CA, Dec 5–9, 1997. Blood 1997; 90.
35. Kraus MH, Popescu NC, Ambaugh SC, King CR. Overexpression of the EGF-related proto-oncogene erbB-2 in human mammary tumor cell lines by different molecular mechanisms. EMBO J 1987; 6:605–610.
36. Bouchard L, Lamarre L, Tremblay PJ, Jolicoeur P. Stochastic appearance of mammary tumors in transgenic mice carrying the MMTV/c-neu oncogene. Cell 1989; 57:931–936.
37. Li B, Rosen JM, McMenamin-Balano J, Muller WJ, Perkins AS. neu/ERB2 cooper-

ates with p53-172H during mammary tumorigenesis in transgenic mice. Mol Cell Biol 1997; 17:3155–3163.
38. Fisk B, Blevins TL, Wharton TW, Ioannides C. Identification of an immunodominant peptide of HER-2/neu proto-oncogene recognized by ovarian tumor-specific cytotoxic lymphocyte lines. J Exp Med 1995; 181:2109–2117.
39. Peoples GE, Geodegebuure PS, Smith R, Linehan DC, Yoshino I, Eberlein TJ. Breast and ovarian cancer-specific cytotoxic T lymphocytes recognize the same HER2/neu-derived peptide. Proc Natl Acad Sci USA 1995; 92:432–436.
40. Peiper M, Goedegebuure PS, Linehan DC, Ganguly E, Douville CC, Eberlein TJ. The HER2/neu-derived peptide p654–662 is a tumor-associated antigen in human pancreatic cancer recognized by cytotoxic T lymphocytes. Eur J Immunol 1997; 27: 1115–1123.
41. Kono K, Halapi E, Hising C, Petersson M, Gerdin E, Vanky F, Kiessling R. Mechanisms of escape from CD8+ T-cell clones specific for the HER-2/neu proto-oncogene expressed in ovarian carcinomas: related and unrelated to decreased MHC class 1 expression. Int J Cancer 1997; 70:112–119.
42. Disis M, Pupa S, Gralow J, Dittadi R, Menard S, Cheever MA. High-titer HER-2/neu protein-specific antibody can be detected in patients with early-stage breast cancer. J Clin Oncol 1997; 15:3363–3367.
43. Disis ML, Smith JW, Murphy AE, Chen W, Cheever MA. In vitro generation of human cytolytic T-cells specific for peptides derived from the HER-2/neu proto oncogene protein. Cancer Res 1994; 15:54:1071–1076.
44. Almoguera C, Shibata D, Forrester K, Martin J, Arnheim N, Perucho M. Most human carcinomas of the exocrine pancreas contain mutant c-k-Ras genes. Cell 1988; 53: 549–554.
45. Bos JL. Ras oncogenes in human cancer: a review. Cancer Res 1989; 49:4682–4689.
46. Scarpa A, Capelli P, Villanueva A, Zamboni G, Lluis F, Accolla R, Mariuzzi G, Capella G. Pancreatic cancer in Europe: Ki-Ras gene mutation pattern shows geographical differences. Int J Cancer 1994; 57:167–171.
47. Bertazzoli C, Marchesi E, Dermime S, Ravagnani F, Parmiani G, Gambacorti-Passerini C. HLA binding characteristics and generation of cytotoxic lymphocytes against peptides derived from oncogenic proteins. Tumori 1997; 83:847–855.
48. Fossum B, Olsen AC, Thorsby E, Gaudernack G. CD8+ T cells from a patient with colon carcinoma, specific fo a mutant p21-Ras-derived peptide (Gly 13 Asp), are cytotoxic towards a carcinoma cell line harboring the same mutation. Cancer Immunol Immunother 1995; 40:165–172.
49. Juretic A, Jürgen-Göbel J, Schaefer C, Noppen C, Willimann TE, Kocher T, Zuber M, Harder F, Heberer M, Spagnoli GC. Cytotoxic T-lymphocyte responses against mutated p21 Ras peptides: an analysis of specific T-cell-receptor gene usage. Int J Cancer 1996; 68:471–478.
50. Gjertsen MK, Bakka A, Breivik J, Aseterdal I, Solheim B, Soereide O, Thorsby E, Gaudernack G. Vaccination with mutant Ras peptides and induction of T-cell responsiveness in pancreatic carcinoma patients carrying the corresponding ras mutation. Lancet 1995; 346:1399–1400.
51. Qin H, Chen W, Takahashi M, Disis ML, Byrd DR, McCahill L, Bertram KA, Fenton

RG, Peace DJ, Cheever MA. CD4+ T-cell immunity to mutated Ras protein in pancreatic and colon cancer patients. Cancer Res 1995; 55:2984–2987.
52. Cheever MA, Disis ML, Bernhard H, Gralow JR, Hand SL, Huseby ES, Qin HL, Takahashi M, Chen W. Immunity to oncogenic proteins. Immunol Rev 1995; 145: 33–59.
53. Levine AJ, Momand J, Finlay CA. The p53 tumor suppressor antigen Nature 1991; 351:453–456.
54. Nijman HW, Van der Burg SH, Vierboom MP, Houbiers JG, Kast WM, Melief CJ. p53, a potential target for tumor-directed T cells. Immunol Lett 1994; 40:171–178.
55. Tilkin AF, Lubin R, Soussi T, Lazar V, Janin N, Mathieu MC, Lefrere I, Carlu C, Roy M, Kayibanda M, et al Primary proliferative T cell response to wild-type p53 protein in patients with breast cancer. Eur J Immunol 1995; 25:1765–1769.
56. Theobald M, Biggs J, Hernandez J, Lustgarten J, Labadie C, Sherman LA. Tolerance to p53 by A2.1-restricted cytotoxic T lymphocytes. J Exp Med 1997; 185:833–841.
57. Wolfel T, Hauer M, Schneider J, Serrano M, Wolfel C, Klehmann-Hieb E, De Plaen E, Hankeln T, Meyer zum Buschenfelde KH, Beach D. A p16INK4a-insensitive CDK4 mutant targeted by cytolytic T lymphocytes in a human melanoma. Science 1995; 269:1281–1284.
58. Robbins PF, El-Gamil M, Li YF, Kawakami Y, Loftus D, Appella E, Rosenberg SA. A mutated beta-catenin gene encodes a melanoma-specific antigen recognized by tumor infiltrating lymphocytes. J Exp Med 1996; 183:1185–1192.
59. Castelli C, Rivoltini L, Mazzocchi A, Parmiani G. T-cell recognition of melanoma antigens and its therapeutic applications. Int J Clin Lab Res 1997; 27:103–110.

8

GVL Effects in Human Marrow Stem-Cell Transplants

John Barrett
National Institutes of Health
Bethesda, Maryland

I. HISTORICAL BACKGROUND

It had long been suspected that in the process of a graft-versus-host reaction, bone marrow allografts could exert an antileukemic effect [1]. The idea was clearly in place in the 1960s, Georges Mathé was the first to describe a graft-versus-leukemia (GVL) effect in a patient undergoing bone marrow transplant (BMT) for leukemia in 1959 [2]. By the 1980s, sufficiently large numbers of BMTs had been carried out to make possible the statistical evaluation of the long suspected favorable impact of graft-versus-host disease (GVHD) on relapse of leukemia. Weiden et al. were the first to show that survivors from severe, acute GVHD had a lower relapse rate than comparable patients who did not develop severe GVHD [3]. This clinical confirmation of an equivalence between GVHD and the GVL effect was largely interpreted negatively: the therapeutic antileukemic benefit of severe GVHD went hand in hand with high mortality [4]. This view was modified following the publication of a key study by the International Bone Marrow Transplant Registry (IBMTR) [5]. Data from 2254 BMTs for leukemia were analyzed. Results showed that relapse was indeed related to clinically significant GVHD, both acute and chronic. However, when relapse rates of patients developing grade 0–I GVHD were compared in T cell–depleted transplant recipients and recipients of T cell–replete BMT, there was a statistically significant lower relapse, probability in recipients of T cell–replete transplants. This analysis also included a small group of individuals receiving transplants from identical twin donors. Surprisingly, in chronic myelogenous leukemia (CML), the relapse probability of T cell–depleted transplants exceeded that of the twin recipients who received unmanipulated (T cell–replete) marrow (Figure 1). Here, for the first time, there was strong clinical evidence for lymphocyte-mediated GVL effects independent from clinically significant GVHD. A further important observation was that the GVL effect varied according to the type of disease transplanted. Patients with CML appeared to be most susceptible to a lymphocyte/GVHD–mediated GVL effect; acute myelogenous leukemia (AML) recipients were intermediately susceptible; and acute lymphoblastic leukemia (ALL) recipients were least susceptible if at all. In the same year, the publication by Kolb et al. of three patients with CML, which had relapsed after BMT, in whom transfusions of donor lymphocytes produced durable remissions was further confirmation of the GVL potential of alloreacting lymphocytes [6].

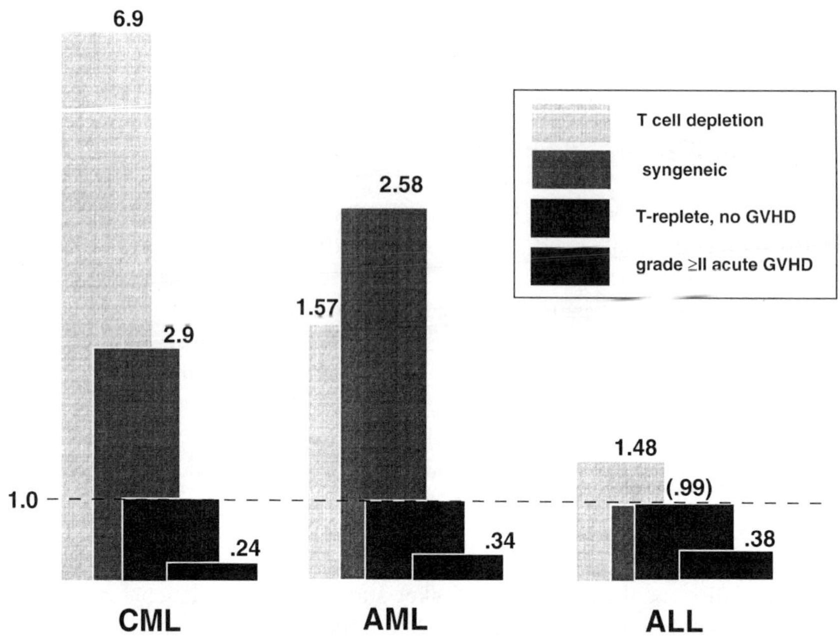

Figure 1 IBMTR study of relapse risk after bone marrow transplantation for leukemia. (From Ref. 5.) Vertical bars show relapse risk (RR) relative to a reference group of patients who had T cell–replete transplants but did not develop more than grade 0–I acute GVHD (RR = 1.0). All groups showed a beneficial effect on relapse from acute and chronic GVHD. The greatest relapse risk from T-cell depletion was observed in CML. In ALL, the difference between RR following syngeneic transplant and the reference group was not significant (figure in brackets).

In the subsequent decade, greater definition of the GVL effect in various disease categories and transplant situations has been achieved. We can now predict reasonably accurately the effect on relapse of specific degrees of donor-recipient matching, disease type, and pre- and posttransplant treatment. This chapter describes clinical features of GVL from the perspective of the leukemia as a target, the alloresponse to the leukemia, and manipulations of the transplant conditions that positively or negatively affect the GVL response.

II. GVL AND THE LEUKEMIA TARGET

The GVL immune response is determined by the nature of the effector cells and the characteristics of the target. Malignant cells vary widely in their susceptibility to immune attack, and key surface molecules on the leukemia cell determining the quality of the immune response are beginning to be better characterized (see Chapter 4). However, clinical results indicate that other features play a role in determining the overall response rate of a particular malignancy to the allograft effect. They include the proliferation rate of the malignant cells, the state of disease progression, and the site of disease. Thus GVL effects are best identified in slowly progressing diseases such as CML, chronic lymphocytic leukemia (CLL), and myeloma, while the effect in acute leukemia is less clear. In CML, GVL effects are greatest when the disease is in chronic phase. The probability of remaining in remission after BMT, and efficacy of donor lymphocyte transfusion (DLT), falls with progression to accelerated phase and again with blastic transformation. The individual biology and proliferation kinetics of leukemias translate into very wide differences in the ability of allogeneic transplants to cure the malignancy. Figure 2 displays malignant diseases where a GVL effect has been identified and ranks hematological malignancies according to their approximate susceptibility to GVL.

A. Minimal Residual Disease (MRD) Detection

The number of leukemia subtypes that can be characterized on the basis of a chromosomal translocation continues to grow (see Chapter 7). This extends the possibility of using polymerase chain reaction (PCR) techniques to quantify MRD after transplantation to more leukemias. Detailed evaluation of MRD and correlation with relapse, MRD, and cure has so far been possible only in CML. However cure (disease-free survival for more than 5 years) as a general rule equates with absence of MRD detection. The ability of the allograft to achieve a disease-free state in situations where autografts or non-myeloablative treatments (such as interferon for CML) fail to eradicate MRD is an indication of the potency of the GVL effect. It should be borne in mind, however, that failure to detect MRD,

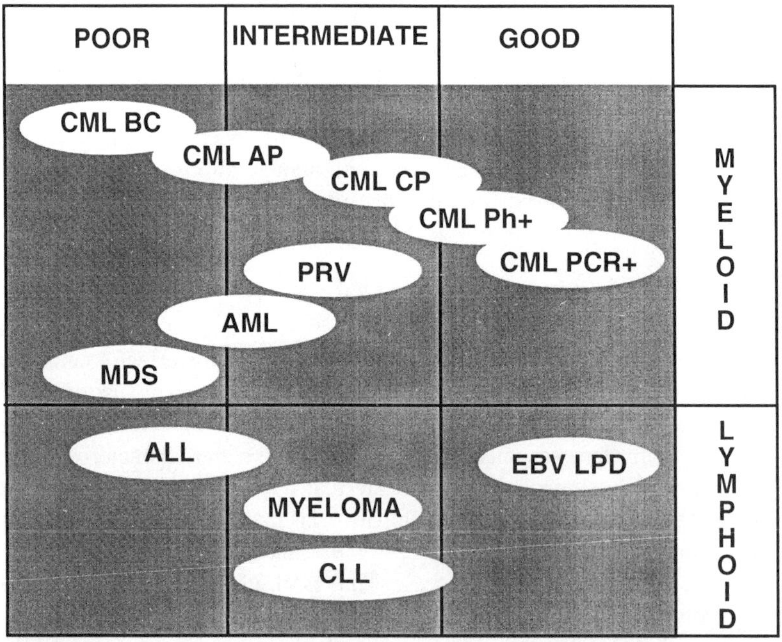

Figure 2 Schema representing the relative susceptibilities of hematological malignancies to a GVL effect from donor lymphocyte transfusions. Most susceptible diseases are CML in molecular, karyotypic, or hematological chronic-phase relapse and EBV lympho proliferative disease (EBV LPD) (usually occurring in donor cells). Least susceptible are acute leukemias and CML in blast crisis. *Key:* CML BC: Chronic myelogenous leukemia in blast crisis; AP: accelerated phase; CP: chronic phase; Ph+: karyotypic relapse; PCR+ molecular relapse; PRV: polycythemia rubra vera; AML: acute myelogenous leukemia; MDS: myelodysplastic syndrome; ALL: acute lymphoblastic leukemia; CLL: chronic lymphocytic leukemia; EBV LPD: Epstein-Barr-virus-induced lymphoproliferative disease.

even using PCR, does not imply that the last leukemic cell has been eliminated. The most sensitive competitive PCR techniques detect as few as $1/10^6$ leukemic cells. However, this level still indicates a residual leukemia burden in the body of about 10^4–10^5 cells (assuming a total marrow volume of 2 L and a cellularity of 50×10^9/L). Figure 3 illustrates the leukemic burden in overt hematological relapse, Ph+ chromosome–positive leukemia and bcr-abl PCR–positive leukemia and its relationship to curative mechanisms of GVHD and immunosuppression after allogeneic BMT. The fundamental question of whether cure equates

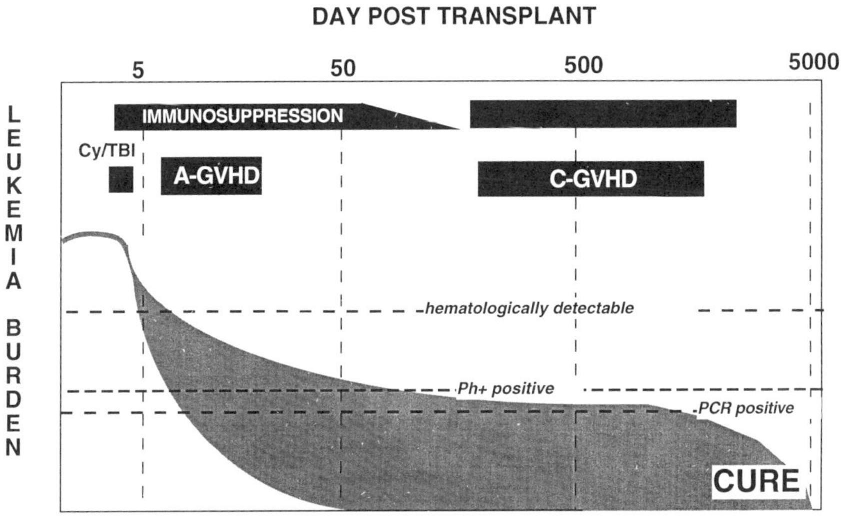

Figure 3 Relationship of leukemia burden and events following marrow transplantation for CML. Shaded area shows range of leukemia burden, which falls rapidly after the preparative regimen of Cy/TBI (cyclophosphamide and total body irradiation) but remains detectable, initially by karyotype analysis and later by PCR probes for the bcr-abl mRNA transcript. Significant events that may increase the GVL effect after transplant are the onset of acute or chronic GVHD and the termination of cyclosporine immunosuppression. Cure corresponds to a permanent PCR-negative state.

with the elimination of the last leukemic cell or is a dynamic state maintained by a continual suppression of residual disease by the GVL effect remains unresolved.

B. GVL in CML

The GVL response in transplants for CML is the best characterized because presence of the Ph+ chromosome and the detection of subclinical disease by sensitive PCR methods has facilitated the tracking of leukemia elimination and its recurrence at the level of minimal residual disease states. The characteristics of GVL in CML are therefore well known. After allogeneic BMT, PCR analysis of the bcr-abl mRNA transcript shows that leukemia can persist at the minimal disease level for up to a year posttransplant without signifying an eventual failure to cure the leukemia. In contrast, recurrence of a PCR- positive state after a period of negative measurements, PCR persisting positive beyond 1 year from transplant, or detection of increasing PCR message by quantitative PCR all signify an inevitable progression to karyotypic and subsequently hematological relapse [7–9]. These observations indicate that the curative GVL effect in CML is a slow process and that the balance between immune suppression and leukemia proliferation can change after transplant. The notion that GVL is most effective when the tumor burden is lowest is supported by the favorable results of treating MRD (PCR-positive Ph+ chromosome–negative) with donor lymphocytes [10]. Most patients treated at this stage of relapse will revert to a PCR-negative state, whereas DLT for overt hematological relapse has lower success in achieving permanent regression of CML. GVL effects in more advanced CML are much smaller; the relapse rate of transplants in accelerated-phase CML is around 40% and for blastic-phase CML 70%; compared with less than 15% for chronic phase CML [11]. These results are mirrored in the responses of CML to DLT, where only occasional and frequently temporary responses are seen in patients relapsing with accelerated- or blast-phase CML [12]. The particular susceptibility of CML to T cell–mediated effects has raised the question of whether peptides from the bcr-abl p210 protein are the targets of GVL attack. Disappointingly and despite considerable efforts, it remains unproven that GVL is mediated through this mechanism (see Chapter 19).

C. GVL In Acute Myeloid Leukemia

In AML, comparison of allo-transplants with transplants from identical twins shows that an allograft effect from donor immune function could account for about 20% of the curative effect of BMT [13]. Although the IBMTR study showed a protective effect of GVHD on relapse of AML, data are conflicting on the role of T lymphocytes in the cure of AML. Following T cell—depleted BMT for AML, Papadopoulos et al. reported extremely low relapse rates (3.2% for 31 patients in first remission and 12.5% for 8 patients in second remission) despite the fact that the grafts had been rigorously depleted by sheep red cell rosetting [14]. Recent analyses of large series of AML transplants show that different AML subtypes have differing outcomes after BMT [15]. In general, prognostic features defined in the context of response to chemotherapy also apply to the transplant situation, suggesting that non-immunological factors largely shape the responsiveness of AML to curative treatment. In general, GVL effects are greater if transplants are carried out in early rather than advanced disease [5]. There are at present no data to show whether GVL effects differ between AML subtypes. In this regard it is an open question whether GVL is mediated by chromosomal translocations causing the AML cell to present leukemia-specific fusion peptides to donor T cells. Gambacorti-Passerini failed to demonstrate t(15;17) peptide-specific T-cell cytotoxicity to promyelocytic AML cells [16]. However, an increasing number of chromosomal translocations are being identified in acute leukemias and the possibility exists that at least some specific leukemia subtypes may initiate powerful T-cell responses against fusion protein targets.

Where it is possible to use chromosome translocation fusion genes as a PCR tool to investigate residual disease, as in AML M3 t(15;17) and AML with t(8;21) translocation and inversion 16, the general rule follows the observations made in CML—namely, cure corresponds to eventual disappearance of a PCR signal for residual disease and relapse is heralded by reemergence of MRD [17–19]. The less dramatic GVL effect in AML compared with CML following the transplant is also seen following DLT to treat AML relapse. The rate of response is lower and its duration often brief [12]. AML relapse has a tendency to occur in extramedullary sites, which are less susceptible to control from DLT. This suggests that sites such as the skin and kidney could represent ''sanctuaries'' where residual leukemia can escape from contact with donor T cells [20].

D. GVL in ALL

Of all the leukemias, ALL is the most disappointing disease in terms of identifying GVL effects. The existence of a GVL effect in ALL is supported by the lower relapse rates seen in ALL recipients developing GVHD after BMT. However, although a trend was apparent, a significant GVL effect independent of GVHD was not identified in the IBMTR study (Figure 1) [5]. The GVL effect occurring without GVHD may also be weaker when compared with myeloid leukemias: a comparison of relapse rates between identical twin and allogeneic BMT did not show a significant difference [13]. However, conclusions drawn from this analysis are limited by the wide confidence limits of the very small twin transplant group (n = 40) and possible differences in the patient and disease characteristics of the twin and allograft group. It is possible that ALL subtypes differ in their susceptibility to GVL. Notably Ph+ ALL, which has a notoriously high relapse risk following autologous BMT, can be cured by allogeneic BMT, suggesting a GVL effect [21,22]. Again PCR techniques to monitor minimal residual disease of the bcr-abl fusion gene [23] or rearranged immunoglobulin genes [24] demonstrate a correlation of prolonged remission and possible cure with molecular remission.

The distinct ontogenic origins of T cells and B cells raises the question whether T-ALL and B cell–derived ALL have different susceptibilities to a GVL effect. To address this question, a recent IBMTR study compared GVL effects in B-cell (common ALL) and T-ALL [19]. These two ALL subtypes differ immunologically in important ways: T-ALL blasts lack MHC class II and fas; B-ALL express fas and MHC class II. We argued that such differences in phenotype might translate into different susceptibilities of ALL to GVL mechanisms. Interestingly, although T-ALL had a slightly lower relapse rate, the relapse in patients with and without GVHD were not significantly different in B- versus T-ALL.

Definable characteristics of ALL that determine outcome remain to be identified. In this regard, the recent description of a B cell–specific minor histocompatibility antigen by Dolstra et al. raises the exciting possibility that some ALL subtypes may be potential targets of a tissue-restricted alloresponse [26].

E. GVL in Other Hematological Malignancies

It is becoming clear that the GVL effect can make a substantial contribution to the cure of indolent lymphoid malignancies such as CLL [27–29], multiple myeloma [30–33], and low-grade lymphomas [34] (see Chapter 10). A GVL effect has also been reported in transplants for myeloproliferative disorder and probably also occurs in myelodysplastic syndrome (MDS), but no data to quantify the effect are available at present [12].

F. Graft Versus-Tumor (GVT) Effects

One of the most exciting conceptual developments in the field of allogeneic transplantation is the possibility that stem-cell allografts might be used to confer a GVT effect. There are preliminary data supporting GVT effects in breast cancer [35,36] and also renal cell carcinoma supporting this possibility. GVT effects are discussed in Chapter 11.

G. GVL and Leukemia Escape

The establishment of a potentially hostile immune system by allogeneic stem-cell transplantation may provide a powerful selective pressure on the recipient's leukemia to escape from immune control. Immune escape following allogeneic BMT was first suggested by Sondel et al. [37]. Table 1 lists some of the changes in leukemia phenotype and function that could contribute to immune escape. We recently studied five patients relapsing after allogeneic BMT; the immunogenicity of their leukemia samples obtained prior to transplant was compared with that of leukemia obtained at relapse. Relapsed leukemias were in general less capable of initiating alloimmune proliferative responses and less susceptible to destruction by alloreacting cytotoxic T lymphocytes (CTLs) or Natural Killer (NK) cells than the pretransplant leukemia [38]. These effects were accompanied by variable changes in surface expression of MHC class I and costimulatory molecules as well as other evidence of mutation in the malignant clone. The findings support the hypothesis that leukemias can escape from the GVL effect. The implications are of importance, since attempts to explain the failure of GVL have hitherto focused mainly on defects in the immune response rather than on mechanisms developed by the target to evade immune control.

Table 1 Mechanisms of Leukemia Escape from a GVL Effect

Characteristic	Effect on GVL
Down-regulation of	
MHC class I	Prevents CD8+-mediated effector function (but may enhance NK susceptibility).
MHC class II	Leukemia cell can no longer behave as an antigen-presenting cell to CD4+ T cells. Also loses susceptibility to CD4+ cell cytotoxicity.
CD80, CD86	Induction of anergy in responding T cells.
LFA-1, ICAM 1	Reduced stimulator function and effector susceptibility.
Fas	Resistant to fas ligand–mediated cytotoxicity.
Loss of susceptibility to cytokines (e.g., TNF, IFN)	Resistant to antiproliferative effects of cytokines produced by T cells, NK cells, and macrophages.
Proliferation rate	Increase in proliferation rate may outstrip pace of responding T-cell clonal expansion

III. THE ALLORESPONSE TO LEUKEMIA

Many factors interact positively and negatively to influence the GVL effect, and many of the interactions are linked. Figure 4 illustrates treatment and donor-recipient factors that influence GVHD, which are discussed in detail below.

A. GVHD

The IBMTR study of 1990 showed a close relationship between relapse and the incidence and severity of acute GVHD. Furthermore, it showed that chronic GVHD also added a GVL effect [5]. However, several issues remain unclear: How long does the GVHD need to be active in order to exert a GVL effect? What is the impact on the GVL response of the immunosuppressive agents used to treat GVHD? Do acute and chronic forms of GVHD differ in their mechanisms and effect on residual leukemia? The IBMTR study showed that acute and chronic GVHD had an additive effect on the probability of staying in remission. These findings, supported by other observations [3,4], emphasize that GVL reactivity is exerted over a prolonged period and coexists with both acute and chronic GVHD. Studies with Tk gene–transfected lymphocytes may soon provide the answer to the first question: lymphocytes tagged with a suicide gene can be destroyed at a chosen threshold of acute GVHD, abrogating the progression of the reaction [39]. If the GVL effect is prompt, it may be possible to achieve the long sought after goal of causing GVL without GVHD. The most recent clinical trials show that

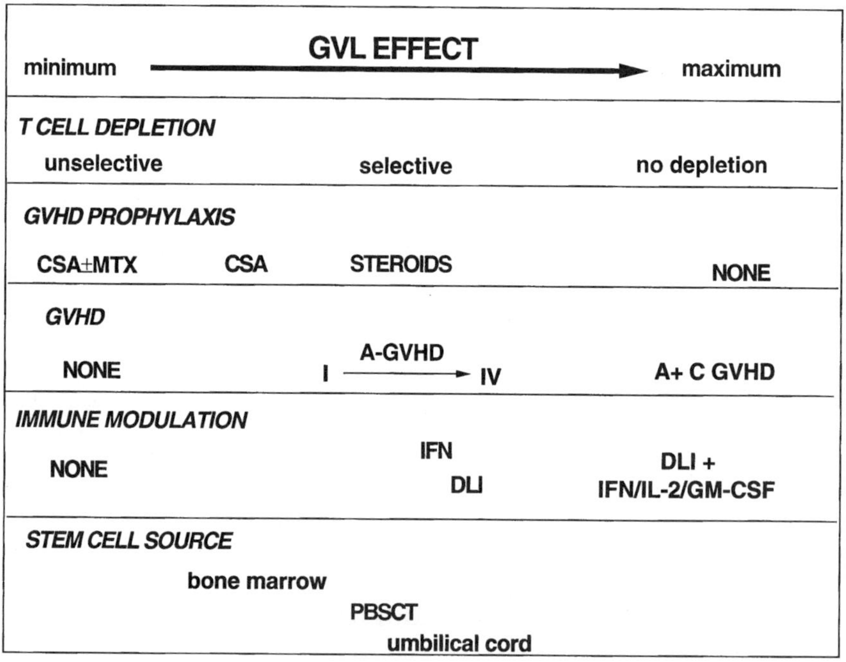

Figure 4 Schema showing the impact of treatment-related factors on the GVL effect.

the strategy of abrogating GVHD from Tk-marked T cells is feasible [39,40]. However, we do not yet know whether the GVL effect is conserved. The established fact that survivors from the most severe forms of acute GVHD have low relapse rates presents, on closer scrutiny, an intriguing paradox: Patients developing severe GVHD receive large amounts of steroids, and their survival of GVHD suggests that the immunosuppression achieved was sufficient to abort the GVHD reaction. What the effect of steroids is on the GVL reaction is therefore unclear. Does the alloreaction cause more rapid and complete damage to the leukemia than to other tissues, or do steroids have only a modest anti-GVL action? What is the role of cyclosporine in modifying GVL in this context? Currently there are no clear answers.

B. Histocompatibility Differences

Numerous animal experiments have confirmed the assumption that, in general, the more disparate the tissue match between recipient and donor, the more it is likely that a GVL effect will be observed. In clinical transplantation, significantly higher relapse rates in syngeneic and autologous transplants can be attributed largely to a lack of an allogeneic GVL effect, although it must be remembered that persistence of residual disease in the graft can contribute to the relapse after autologous BMT [5,13,41].

C. Minor Histocompatibility Antigen (mHA) Differences

The importance of mHA differences in exerting GVL effects can be studied by comparing the outcome of HLA-identical sibling BMT in genetically homogeneous and genetically diverse populations. In this situation, patient and donor are genotypically matched at the MHC loci but the genetically homogeneous group should have a lower diversity in the mHA gene repertoire. The question of mHA disparity effects on GVL were studied by comparing comparable CML patients transplanted with HLA-identical siblings in Japan (genetically homogeneous) and the United Kingdom (genetically diverse). In the United Kingdom, BMT recipients had twice as much acute GVHD (50 versus 25%) and became PCR-negative more rapidly than comparable Japanese patients. However, the overall relapse rate in both groups was low (10 versus 12%) and comparable in the two groups [42].

D. Major Histocompatibility Antigen Differences

Comparison of relapse rates between HLA-identical siblings and haploidentical family transplants should identify contribution of differences in major histocompatibility antigen to the GVL effect. At present there are no good data comparing GVL between matched and mismatched transplants to make reliable comparisons. Furthermore, any comparisons are complicated by inevitable differences in GVHD prevention approaches, most mismatched BMT being T cell–depleted. However, two studies are of interest. A report from Polchi et al. comparing HLA-identical sibling BMT with parental BMT in children with high-risk ALL showed a lower relapse rate in the parental transplant recipients [43]. This apparent GVL effect was sufficiently strong to outweigh a higher transplant-related mortality and confer a disease-free survival comparable to that of HLA-identical sibling recipients. Studies from the Perugia group have shown extremely low or zero relapse rates in AML (but not ALL) recipients of rigorously T cell–depleted haploidentical transplants for high-risk disease [44]. Nevertheless, relapse is still a major complication of mismatched transplants, and a beneficial GVL effect is probably often outweighed by the need to aggressively deplete such transplants of T cells to prevent lethal GVHD [45]. That haploidentical alloimmune effects against leukemia can be very powerful is borne out by anecdotal reports of complete remission accompanied by lethal GVHD in the treatment of relapse with haploidentical DLT [46].

E. HLA-Identical Unrelated Transplants

The GVL potential of HLA-identical unrelated donor transplants should be greater than that of HLA-identical sibling transplants because of a greater likelihood of minor histocompatibility antigen (mHA) disparity in the unrelated transplants as well as differences in nonclassic MHC antigens and cryptic variations in DNA sequences of HLA molecules, apparently identical by serotyping. The assumption that relapse rates following unrelated donor BMT are lower than comparable transplants from HLA-identical sibling donors, however, remains unconfirmed. Comparisons are complicated by the greater degree of immunosuppression given to unrelated transplant recipients. Nevertheless, one report of T cell–depleted unrelated BMT for leukemia suggests that the effect on GVL of histocompatibility differences outweighs the deleterious effect of T-cell depletion on relapse [47]. A comparison of unrelated versus related donor DLT to treat relapse of CML showed a more rapid disappearance of residual disease but an overall response rate similar to that of the unrelated donor transplants, indicating that the GVL effect in unrelated donor BMT may be more rapid but has strength comparable to that of identical sibling BMT [48].

F. Source of Transplant Cells

The 1990s have seen the growing use of granulocyte colony-stimulating factor (G-CSF), mobilized peripheral blood stem-cell transplants (PBSCT), and cord blood transplants (CBT) as the means of reconstituting hematopoiesis and immune function. The lymphocyte component of these transplant tissues is distinctly different from that of bone marrow. G-CSF–mobilized PBSCT contain some tenfold more T cells. Furthermore, they contain more helper cells of the Th2 phenotype, which direct immune responses away from cytotoxic functions associated with GVHD [49]. It is not obvious whether the combined effect of these features of PBSCT could affect the GVHD and the GVL response positively or negatively. Good comparative clinical data on PBSCT versus BMT are still scanty. Several comparisons between unmanipulated BMT and PBSCT indicate that the incidence of acute GVHD is comparable, but chronic GVHD is more frequent after PBSCT. There are intriguing data from the Calgary BMT group suggesting that relapse rates following PBSCT are lower for both high- and standard-risk leukemia transplants [50]. In a comparison of relapse rates in 30 cases of PBSCT for high-risk leukemia with 31 cases of BMT as historical controls, there was a 25% relapse risk versus 50% for the historical BMT group. Confirmation that PBSCT exerts a greater GVL effect than PBSCT awaits the outcome of several large randomized comparisons of blood versus marrow allografts.

Because very few CBTs have so far been carried out, to what degree such stem cell sources differ in their GVL potential from BMT and PBSCT is even less clear. Results of CBT in high-risk leukemias do, however, suggest the presence of a strong GVL effect [51].

G. Donor-Recipient Chimerism

The use of sensitive PCR techniques to identify donor- and recipient-specific DNA minisatellite sequences has shed new light on the complex balance between donor and recipient hematopoiesis and immune function after BMT [52]. In particular it has become clear that mixed donor-recipient chimerism is a frequent finding after T cell–depleted transplants [53–58]. and after nonmyeloablative preparative regimens [59]. The state of mixed chimerism is associated with a lower risk of GVHD and a higher risk of leukemia relapse. However, the interpretation of chimerism is not straightforward: the occurrence of mixed chimerism could signify either residual recipient leukaemia cells, immune cells, hematopoietic cells, or combinations of these. Only by characterizing chimerism in myeloid and lymphoid compartments separately can the exact donor-recipient conditions be defined. When individual populations have been studied after BMT, there is evidence that the presence of residual host lymphocytes favors relapse and also predicts a lower response of relapsed leukemia to DLT. The coexistence of donor and host T cells suggests that a state of tolerance exists that may, in turn, be unfavorable for a GVL effect. However, it may be that the significance of chimerism per se has been overstated: low-intensity preparative regimens can predispose to persistence of both residual leukemia cells and nonmalignant lymphohematopoietic cells. Similarly, T-cell depletion of the donor marrow could diminish the immune elimination of both recipient leukemia and normal lymphohematopoietic tissues. Thus identification of chimerism is best considered as a marker of other mechanisms that directly lead to incomplete eradication of normal and leukemic host tissues.

IV. AUTOLOGOUS GVL

The possibility of a GVL effect occurring after autologous stem-cell transplants has been investigated by several groups. Such an effect presupposes the existence of autologous effector cells, either NK cells or T cells, with antileukemia effects. There is some evidence for autologous NK cell–mediated effects, and several investigators have succeeded in generating strong LAK cell–type reactivity against leukemia targets (reviewed in Ref. 60). However, evidence for MHC-restricted T cell-mediated effects against autologous leukemia is more tenuous: in CML, Pawelec et al. succeed in generating eight CD4+ T-cell clones that showed restricted recognition of an autologous CML target [61]. Coleman et al. recently described T cells with specific cytotoxicity against autologous CML

[62], and Choudhury et al. were able to generate leukemia-specific CTLs using autologous dendritic cells from CML patients [63]. In contrast, Lewalle et al. studied 15 patients with CML for evidence of a precursor frequency of patients' lymphocytes to autologous marrow cells. While a low autologous Helper T lymphocyte precursor (HTLP) frequency was identified (<1/500,000), identical low frequencies were found in normal individuals [64]. These results do not support the existence of a functional T-cell response to leukemia in CML. In AML, Lowdell et al. have identified CD8+ T cells cytotoxic to autologous leukemia in several patients following autologous BMT [65].

A skin rash identical to acute GVHD both clinically and on biopsy is seen occasionally following both autologous and syngeneic BMT [66]. The basis for this autoimmune response is a CD4+ T cell–mediated response to an undefined autoantigen presented by MHC class II–bearing cells [67]. Using cyclosporine with or without IL-2, it is possible to reproducibly generate autologous GVHD following autologous bone marrow or stem-cell transplantation [68]. This has stimulated clinical trials to evaluate a possible antitumor effect in lymphoma [69], breast cancer [70], and myeloma [71]. Only in myeloma has a possible antitumor response so far been identified.

A. Syngeneic GVL

There is a small amount of evidence supporting a syngeneic GVL effect in identical twin transplants in humans. First, syngeneic GVHD is a frequently described occurrence [66,72]. Second, comparisons in CML of relapse after T-cell depletion and identical twin BMT show a lower risk of relapse in the (T-replete) twin BMT, suggesting that there is a lymphocyte-mediated effect from syngeneic BMT [5]. A similar finding was made in a recent analysis of BMT in multiple myeloma by the European Group for Blood and Marrow transplantation (EBMT): relapse rates were lower in recipients of an identical twin BMT than in those who received an allogeneic BMT and did not develop GVHD. Unlike the syngeneic recipients, the allograft recipients would have received immunosuppressive therapy to prevent GVHD (G. Gahrton, personal communication).

V. IMMUNE MODULATION AND GVL

As cell separation techniques become more sophisticated and more agents that either suppress or stimulate immune responses become available, possibilities increase for favoring GVL by altering the transplant and posttransplant conditions. T-cell depletion and add-back of lymphocytes either prophylactically or to treat relapse is currently an active area of clinical investigation. More attention to the effect of GVHD prophylaxis on relapse may improve posttransplant immunosuppressive regimens, and the successful use of agents such as IL-2, IFN-α, and GM-CSF may open up new ways of stimulating the GVL response. Figure 4 summarizes the positive and negative impacts of immune manipulations on GVL and relapse.

A. Lymphocyte Depletion

Early experience with T cell–depleted BMT to prevent GVHD made it rapidly clear that the beneficial effect of GVHD reduction was offset by an increased relapse rate [73]. The effect is most marked in CML; in acute leukemia, the role of T-cell depletion is less clear (see above). In CML, the effect of T-cell depletion on relapse has been confirmed in a detailed analysis of different T cell–depletion approaches [74]. The reduction of a GVL effect from T-cell depletion extends to unrelated transplants but is less marked when techniques with narrow-spectrum antibodies and techniques are used. Significantly some T cell–depletion techniques—such as the use of Campath monoclonal antibody—result in depletion of both T cells and NK cells, whereas other approaches and especially the rosetting technique deplete mainly T cells [75]. The lower relapse rates reported following narrow-spectrum T-cell depletion could therefore result from the conservation of an NK cell–mediated GVL effect. In support of a role for NK cells in GVL is the finding that NK-cell recovery but not T-cell recovery predicts relapse in CML transplants [76]. However, a role for NK cells in GVL for other leukemias has not been shown.

B. Donor Lymphocyte Transfusion (DLT)

The powerful antileukemic effect of DLT in the treatment of relapsed leukemia is fully covered in Chapter 9. Possible outcomes of relapsed leukemia following DLT are illustrated in Figure 5. The time course to a response following DLT varies but typically requires several months, during which time donor lymphocyte clones with GVL reactivity are expanding. Acute leukemias tend to escape from immune control during this period by virtue of a more rapid proliferation rate. More slowly proliferating diseases tend to be more susceptible to DLT. The outcome depends upon the susceptibility of the disease to the alloimmune effect. Diseases treated at the stage of MRD still require a similar time period to response but are more likely to be controlled by the GVL effect of DLT. That donor lymphocytes given after the graft can have a stronger antileukemic effect than the original T cell–replete transplant is surprising. There are several possible explanations: first, DLT may break a state of tolerance. In favor of this possibility is the observation that mixed chimerism can be abolished by DLT [77]. Alternatively, it has been argued that the ability of DLT to exert a GVL effect where the transplant has failed relates to the low precursor frequency of leukemia-reactive T cells,

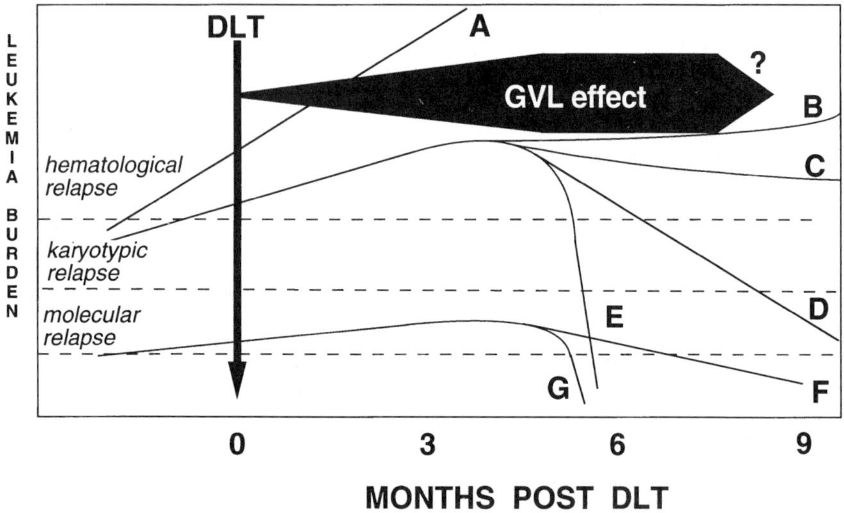

Figure 5 Changes in leukemia burden following donor lymphocyte transfusion (DLT) for leukemia. The maximum GVL effect is not achieved until about 3–6 months after DLT. A. escape of rapidly proliferating acute leukemia from GVL. B–C. Failure to control leukemia (e.g., chronic-phase CML) with eventual progression (B). D–E. Slow and rapid elimination of detectable disease following treatment of hematological relapse. E–F. slow and rapid loss of PCR message following treatment of PCR+ state. Note that the time to molecular remission is still almost as prolonged as for hematological relapse.

necessitating large numbers of T cells in the DLT to ensure the establishment of growing clones of leukemia-reactive donor cells. In this regard there is good evidence supporting a dose response of DLT in CML [78]. As confidence in the antileukemic potential and relative safety of carefully dosed lymphocyte transfusions has grown, several investigators have used DLT successfully to treat CML in a minimal residual disease state before overt hematological relapse [10]. A further extension to this strategy is to give donor lymphocytes as prophylaxis against relapse in high-risk leukemias [79]. Johnson and Truitt showed that, in mice, T cell–depleted stem-cell transplants could be reconstituted with spleen cells 21 days after transplantation without causing GVHD but with a conserved GVL ability [80]. In a similar transplant design in humans, we evaluated T-cell depletion followed by delayed lymphocyte add-back to achieve the two goals of GVHD prevention and prophylaxis of leukemic relapse. In 45 patients receiving a BMT depleted of T cells by elutriation, acute grade >II GVHD occurred in 20% of recipients between days 0–30 posttransplant. After add-back of up to 5×10^7CD3 + cells per kilogram, there was a further 20% risk of developing grade II acute GVHD. However, in 12 evaluable patients with CML, the relapse rate was 15%, comparable with that of T cell–replete rather than T cell–depleted transplants. Further studies of planned T-cell add-back are warranted [81].

C. Role of GVHD Prophylaxis and Immune Suppression

The need to prevent GVHD after unmanipulated BMT must inevitably compromise the allograft response to residual leukemia. However in the absence of any studies where no GVHD prophylaxis is used, the contribution of immunosuppressive prophylaxis to leukemic relapse can only be inferred indirectly. The standard approach of combining methotrexate with cyclosporine has been widely accepted as representing an optimum control of GVHD without a high relapse rate [82]. However, reports where leukemic relapse has been reversed by withdrawal of

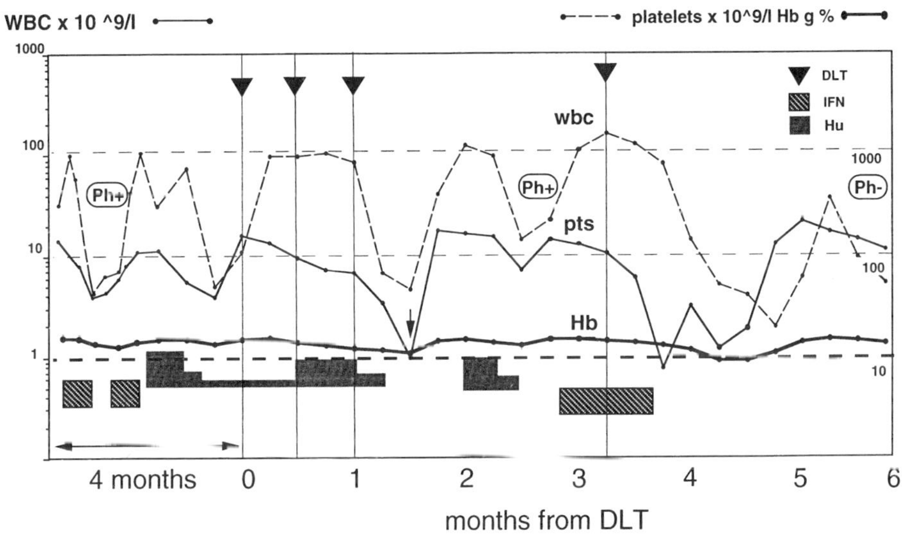

Figure 6 Treatment of a patient (male, age 51) relapsing 3 years after HLA-identical sibling transplant for CML in chronic phase. Initial treatment with interferon-α(IFN) cause temporary pancytopenia but no induction of remission. Subsequently three donor lymphocyte transfusions (DLT) of 1–5 × 107 CD3+ cells per kilogram produced transient cytopenia requiring platelet transfusion (arrow). However a Ph+ chromosome recovery occurred, requiring hydroxyurea (Hu) to control blood counts. Two months after these treatments, IFN and 5 × 10^7/kg DLT were given simultaneously, with a prompt fall in blood counts and recovery to a normal count with 100% Ph+ chromosomes in the marrow. Subsequent testing of PCR for bcr-abl was negative. The patient has remained in sustained molecular remission for over 18 months.

cyclosporine suggest that cyclosporine does exert a negative effect on GVL reactivity [83,84]. The role of FK506 in this regard is not known. In contrast, steroids, even in high doses, to treat GVHD do not block the GVL effect from clinically significant GVHD, since no study has shown an increased relapse rate with acute and chronic GVHD. Nevertheless, immunosuppression posttransplant should be minimized to reduce the risk of leukemic relapse.

D. Immune Modulators

Several agents have been evaluated for an antileukemic effect with or without donor lymphocyte transfusions. Interferon-alpha (IFN-α) has an antiproliferative antileukemic effect in its own right and can achieve remissions in CML relapsing after BMT [85]. We recently observed a possible synergistic effect of IFN-α with DLT in a patient relapsing with chronic-phase CML after BMT who failed to respond to IFN-α or donor lymphocytes alone but achieved a durable remission with the combination (Figure 6). IFN has also been used following DLT for acute leukemias, with some possible efficacy [86–88]. IL-2 has been less widely used, probably because of its reputation for inducing GVHD [88]. Slavin's group used IL-2 or in vitro IL-2–activated lymphocytes with some success in the prophylaxis and treatment of relapse of malignant disease (see Chapter 12). Finally, some data support a role for GM-CSF in the treatment of relapsed leukemia after BMT. Again, there appears to be a benefit from combining DLT with the cytokine. Kolb has recently reported durable remission in 9/12 AML recipients relapsing after BMT following DLT and GM-CSF (H.J. Kolb, personal communication). The mechanisms involved in these interactions of donor lymphocytes with cytokines are not known. The action of IFN-α and GM-CSF may be mediated as much by rendering the target more susceptible to immune destruction as by a direct effect on the donor lymphocytes.

VI. CONCLUSIONS

Clinical observations over the last decade have greatly extended our understanding of the factors that determine GVL reactivity. Specific clinical situations provide insight into mechanisms of GVL that can, in turn, lead to new approaches to enhance GVL reactivity. In the ensuing chapters, these effects and ways to isolate and control the GVL component of allograft immunity are examined in detail.

REFERENCES

1. Barnes DWH, Loutit JF. Treatment of murine leukemia with x-rays and homologous bone marrow. Br Med J 1956; 2:626–627.

2. Mathé G. L'immunotherapie des cancers humains. Nouv Presse Med 1975; 4:1333–1336.
3. Weiden PL, Fluornoy N, Thomas ED, Prentice R, Fefer A, Buckner CD, Storb R. Antileukemic effects of graft versus host disease in human recipients of allogeneic marrow grafts. N Engl J Med 1969; 300:1068–1072.
4. Sullivan K, Storb R, Buckner C, Fefer A, Fisher L, Weiden PL, Witherspoon RP, Appelbaum FR, Banaji M, Hansen J, Clift RA, Thomas ED. Graft versus host disease as adoptive immunotherapy in patients with advanced hematologic malignancics. N Eng J Med 1989; 320:828–834.
5. Horowitz MM, Gale RP, Sondel PM, Goldman JM, Kersey J, Kolb H-J, Rimm AA, Ringden O, Rozman C, Speck B, Truitt RL, Zwaan FE, Bortin MM. Graft-versus-leukemia reactions after bone marrow transplantation. Blood 1990; 75:555–562.
6. Kolb H-J, Mitmuller J, Clemm Ch, Holler H, Ledderose G, Brehm G, Heim M, Wilmanns W. Donor leukocyte transfusions for treatment of recurrent chronic myelogenous leukemia in marrow transplant patients. Blood 1990; 76:2462–2465.
7. Lin F, van Rhee F, Goldman JM. Kinetics of increasing BCR-ABL transcript numbers in chronic myeloid leukemia patients who relapse after bone marrow transplantation. Blood 1996; 87:4473–4478.
8. Frassoni F, Martinelli G, Saglio G, Sessarego M, Podesta M, Piaggio G, Farabegoli P, Zaccaria A, TestoniN, Remiddi C, Zaccaria A, Testoni N, Remiddi C, Marmont AM. bcr/abl chimeric transcript in patients in remission after marrow transplantation for chronic myeloid leukemia: higher frequency of detection and slower clearance in patients grafted in advanced disease as compared to patients grafted in chronic phase. Bone Marrow Transplant 1995; 16:595–601.
9. Radich JP, Gehly G, Gooley T, Bryant E, Clift RA, Collins S, Edmands S, Kirk J, Lee A, Kessler P, Schoch S, Buckner CD, Sullivan KM, Appelbaum FR, Thomas ED. Polymerase chain reaction detection of the BCR-ABL fusion transcript after allogeneic marrow transplantation for chronic myeloid leukemia: results and implications in 346 paticnts. Blood 1995; 85:2632–2638.
10. Van Rhee F, Feng L, Cullis JO, Spencer A, Cross NPC, Chase A, Garicochea B, Bungay J, Barrett AJ, Goldman JM. Relapse of chronic myeloid leukemia after allogeneic bone marrow transplantation: the case for giving donor leucocyte transfusions before the onset of hematological relapse. Blood, 1994; 83:3377–3383.
11. Clift RA, Buckner CD, Thomas ED, Bryant TE, Anasetti C, Bensinger WI, Bowden R, Deeg HJ, Doney KC, Fisher LD, Hansen JA, Martin P, Mcdonald GB, Saunders JE, Singer J, Storb R, Sullivan KM, Witherspoon RP, Appelbaum FR. Marrow transplantation for patients in accelerated phase of chronic myeloid leukaemia. Blood 1994; 84:4368–4373.
12. Kolb HJ, Schattenberg A, Goldman JM. Hertenstein B, Jacobsen N, Arcese W, Ljungman P, Ferrant A, Versdonk L, Niederwieser D, van Rhee F, Mittmuller J, de Witte T, Holler E, Ansari H. Graft-versus-leukemia effect of donor lymphocyte transfusions in marrow grafted patients. Blood 1995; 86:2041–2050.
13. Gale RP, Horowitz MM, Ash RC, Champlin RE, Goldman JM, Rimm AA, Ringden O, Veum Sone J, Bortin MM. Identical twin bone marrow transplants for leukemia. Ann Intern Med 1994; 120:646–652.
14. Papadopoulos EB, Carabasi MH, Castro-Malaspina H, Childs BH, Mackinnon S,

Boulad F, Gillio AP, Kernan NA, Small TN, Szabolcs P, Taylor J, Yahalom J, Collins NH, Bleau SA, Black PM, Heller G, O'Reilly RJ, Young JW. T cell–depleted allogeneic bone marrow transplantation as postremission therapy for acute myelogenous leukemia: freedom from relapse in the absence of graft-versus-host disease. Blood 1998; 91:1083–1090.

15. Gale RP, Horowitz MM, Weiner RS, Ash RC, Atkinson R, Babu R, Dicke KA, Klein JP, Lowenberg B, Reiffers J. Impact of cytogenetic abnormalities on outcome of bone marrow transplants in acute myelogenous leukemia in first remission, Bone Marrow Transplant 1995; 16:203–208.
16. Gambacorti-Passerini C, Grignani F, Arienti F, Pandolfi PP, Pelicci P, Parmiani G. Human CD4+ lymphocytes specifically recognize a peptide representing the fusion region of the hybrid protein PML/RARa present in acute promyelocytic cells. Blood 1993; 81:1369–1375.
17. Román J, Martín C, Torrés A, Jiminéz MA, Andrés P, Florés R, de la Torre MJ, Sanchéz J, Serrano J, Falcón M. Absence of detectable PML-RARa fusion transcript in long term remission patients after bone marrow transplant for acute promyelocytic leukemia. Bone Marrow Transplant 1997; 19:679–685.
18. Kusec R, Laczika K, Knobl P, Friedl J, Greinix H, Kahls P, Linkesch W, Schwarzinger I, Mitterbauer G, Purtscher B, et al AML1/ETO fusion mRNA can be detected in remission blood samples of all patients with t(8;21) acute myeloid leukemia after chemotherapy or autologous bone marrow transplantation. Br J Haematol 1993; 84: 67–74.
19. Elmaagacli AH, Beelen DW, Kroll M, Trzensky S, Stein C, Schaefer UW. Detection of CBFbeta/MYH11 fusion transcripts in patients with inv(16) acute myeloid leukemia after allogeneic bone marrow or peripheral blood progenitor cell transplantation. Bone Marrow Transplant 1998; 21:159–166.
20. Singhal S, Powles R, Kulkarni S, Treleaven J, Mehta J. Immunotherapy of acute leukemia relapsing after allogeneic transplantation: the inseparability of GVHD and graft-vs-leukemia, and the problem of extramedullary relapse. Blood 1997; 90 (suppl 1):547.
21. Barrett AJ, Horowitz MM, Ash RC, Atkinson K, Ehninger G, Gajewski J, Gale RP, Henslee-Downey PJ, Herzig RH, Kolb HJ, Masaoka T, O'Reilly RJ, Speck B, Zwaan FE and Bortin MM. Bone marrow transplantation for Philadelphia chromosome positive acute lymphoblastic leukaemia. Blood 1992; 11:3067–3070.
22. Stockschläder M, Hegewisch-Becker S, Krüger W, tom Dieck A, Mross K, Hoffknecht M, Berger, C, Kohlschütter B, Martin H, Peters S, Kabisch H, Kuse R, Weh H, Zandler A. Bone marrow transplantation for Philadelphia-chromosome-positive acute lymphoblastic leukemia. Bone Marrow Transplant 1995; 16:663–667.
23. Radich J, Gehly G, Lee A, Avery R, Bryant E, Edmands S, Gooley T, Kessler P, Kirk J, Ladne P, Thomas ED, Appelbaum FR. Detection of bcr-abl transcripts in Philadelphia chromosome–positive acute lymphoblastic leukemia after marrow transplantation. Blood 1996; 88:2228–2235.
24. Radich J, Ladne P, Gooley T. Polymerase chain reaction–based detection of minimal residual disease in acute lymphoblastic leukemia predicts relapse after allogeneic BMT. Bone Marrow Transplant 1995; 16:663–667.
25. Passweg J, Tiberghien P, Cahn JY, Vowles MR, Camitta BM, Gale RP, Herzig RH,

Hoelzer D, Horowitz MM, Ifrah N, Klein JP, Marks DI, Ramsay NKC, Rowlings PA, Weisdorf DJ, Zhang M-J, Barrett AJ. Graft-versus-leukemia effects in T-lineage and B-lineage acute lymphoblastic leukaemia. Bone Marrow Transplant 1998; 21: 153–158.

26. Dolstra H, Fredrix H, Preijers F, Goulmy E, Figdor CG, de Witte TM, van de Wiel-van Kemenade E. Recognition of a B cell leukemia-associated minor histocompatibility antigen by CTL. J Immunol 1997; 158:560–565.
27. Provan D, Bartlett-Pandite L, Zwicky C, Neuberg D, Maddocks A, Corradini P, Soiffer R, Ritz J, Nadler LM, Gribben JG. Eradication of polymerase chain reaction-detectable chronic lymphocytic leukemia cells is associated with improved outcome after bone marrow transplantation. Bone Marrow Transplant 1996; 17:643–647.
28. Jarque I, Palau J, Sanz GF, Guinot M, Gomis F, Martin G, Martinez J, Sanz MA. Delayed complete response after allogeneic bone marrow transplantation in chronic lymphocytic leukemia. Blood 1993; 82:1036–1038.
29. Mehta J, Powles R, Singhal S, Iveson T, Treleaven J, Catovsky D. Clinical and hematologic response of chronic lymphocytic and prolymphocytic leukemia persisting after allogeneic bone marrow transplantation with the onset of acute graft-versus-host disease: possible role of graft-versus-leukemia. Bone Marrow Transplant 1996; 17:371–375.
30. Tricot G, Vesole D, Jagannath S, Hilton J, Munshi N, Barlogie B. Graft-versus-myeloma effect: proof of principle. Blood 1996; 87:1196–1198.
31. Verdonck LF, Lokhorst HM, Dekker AW, Nieuwenhuis HK, Petersen EJ. Graft-versus-myeloma effect in two cases. Lancet 1996; 347:800–801.
32. Bertz H, Burger JA, Kunzmann R, Mertelsmann R, Finke J. Adoptive immunotherapy for relapsed multiple myeloma after allogeneic bone marrow transplantation (BMT): evidence for a graft-versus-myeloma effect. Leukemia 1997; 11:281–283.
33. Lokhorst HM, Schattenberg A, Cornelissen JJ, Thomas LLM, Verdonck LF. Donor leukocyte infusions are effective in relapsed multiple myeloma after allogeneic bone marrow transplantation. Blood 1997; 90:4206–4211.
34. Jones RJ, Ambinder RF, Piantadosi S, Santos GW. Evidence of a graft-versus-lymphoma effect associated with allogeneic bone marrow transplantation. Blood 1991; 77:649–653.
35. Eibl B, Schwaighofer H, Nachbaur D, Marth C, Gachter A, Knapp R, Bock G, Gassner C, Schiller L, Petersen F, Niederwieser D. Evidence for a graft-versus-tumor effect in a patient treated with marrow ablative chemotherapy and allogeneic bone marrow transplantation for breast cancer. Blood 1996; 88:1501–1508.
36. Ueno NT, Rondon G, Mirza NQ, Geisler DK, Anderlini P, Giralt SA, Andersson BS, Claxton DF, Gajewski JL, Khouri IF, Korbling M, Mehra RC, Przepiorka D, Rahman Z, Samuels BI, van Besien K, Hortobagyi GN, Champlin RE. Allogeneic peripheral-blood progenitor-cell transplantation for poor-risk patients with metastatic breast cancer. J Clin Oncol 1998; 16:986–993.
37. Sondel PM, Hank JA, Molanda J, Blank, J, Borcherding W, Longo W, Trigg ME, Hong R, Bozdech MJ. Relapse of host leukaemic lymphoblasts following engraftment by an HLA-mismatched marrow transplant: mechanisms of escape from the "graft versus leukaemia" effect. Exp Hematol 1985; 13:782–790.

38. Dermime S, Hensel N, Jiang YZ, Mavroudis D, Molldrem, Barrett AJ. Does immune escape from a graft-versus-leukemia effect play a role in the relapse of myelogenous leukemias following allogeneic bone marrow transplantation? Bone Marrow Transplant 1997; 19:989–999.
39. Bonini C, Verzeletti S, Servida P, Zappone F, Ruggieri L, Ponzoni M, Rossini S, Mavilio F, Traversari C, Bordignon C. HSV-TK gene transfer into donor lymphocytes for control of allogeneic graft-versus-leukemia. Science 1997; 276: 1719–1723.
40. Thiberghien P, Reynolds CW, Keller J, Spence S, Deschaseaux M, Certoux J-M, Contassot E, Murphy WJ, Lyons R, Chiang Y, Herve P, Longo D, Ruscetti FW. Ganciclovir treatment of herpes simplex thymidine kinase-transduced primary T lymphocytes: an approach for specific in vivo donor T-cell depletion after bone marrow transplantation? Blood 1994; 84:1333–1334.
41. Brenner MK. The contribution of marker gene studies to hemopoietic stem cell therapies. Stem Cells 1995; 13:453–461.
42. Miyamura K, Barrett AJ. Kodera Y, Saito H. Minimal residual disease after bone marrow transplantation for chronic myelogenous leukemia and implications for graft-versus-leukemia effect: a review of recent results. Bone Marrow Transplant 1994; 14:201–210.
43. Polchi P, Lucarelli G, Galimberti M, Giardini C, Baronciani D, Angelucci E, Sparaventi G, Capponi D, Talevi N, Debiagi M, Manna M, Nesci S, Andreani MD. Haploidentical bone marrow transplantation from mother to child with advanced leukemia. Bone Marrow Transplant 1995; 16:529–535.
44. Aversa F, Tabilio A, Terenzi A, Velardi A, Falzetti F, Giannoni C, Iacucci R, Zei T, Martelli MP, Gambelunghe C. Successful engraftment of T-cell depleted haploidentical "three-loci" incompatible transplants in leukemia patients by addition of recombinant human granulocyte colony-stimulating factor–mobilized peripheral blood progenitor cells to bone marrow inoculum. Blood 1994; 84:3948–3955.
45. Henslee-Downey PJ, Abhyankar SH, Parrish PRS, Pati AR, Godder KT, Neglie WJ, Goon-Johnson KS, Geier SS, Lee CG, Gee AP. Use of partially mismatched related donors extends access to allogeneic marrow transplant. Blood 1997; 89:384–387.
46. Pati AR, Godder K, Parrish R, Lamb L, Gee A, Henslee-Downey PJ. Pre-emptive therapy with donor leukocyte infusions to prevent relapse following partially mismatched related donor bone marrow transplantation. Blood 1996; 88(suppl 1):259.
47. Hessner M, Endean D, Casper J, Horowitz MM, Keever-Taylor CA, Roth M, Flomenberg N, Drobyski WR. Use of unrelated marrow grafts compensates for reduced graft-versus-leukemia reactivity after T-cell-depleted allogeneic marrow transplantation for chronic myelogenous leukemia. Blood 1995; 86:3987–3996.
48. van Rhee F, Savage D, Blackwell J, Orchard K, Dazzi F, Lin F, Chase A, Bungey J, Cross NC, Apperley J, Szydlo R, Goldman JM. Adoptive immunotherapy for relapse of chronic myeloid leukemia after allogeneic bone marrow transplant: equal efficacy of lymphocytes from sibling and matched unrelated donors. Bone Marrow Transplant 1998; 21:1055–1061.
49. Bensinger W, Clift R, Martin P, et al. Allogeneic peripheral blood stem cell transplantation in patients with advanced hematologic malignancies: a retrospective comparison with marrow transplantation. Blood 1996; 88:2794–2800.

50. Russell JA. Allogeneic blood stem cell transplantation for hematological malignancies: Preliminary comparison of outcome with bone marrow transplantation. Bone Marrow Transplant, 1996, 17:703–709.
51. Kurtzberg J, Laughlin M, Graham ML, Smith C, Olson JF, Halpertin BC, Cioeci G, Carrier C, Stevens CS, Rubinstein P. Placental blood as a source of hematopoietic stem cells for transplantation into unrelated recipients. N Engl J Med 1996; 335: 157–161.
52. Mackinnon S, Barnett L, Bourhis JH, Black P, Heller G, O'Reilly RJ. Myeloid and lymphoid chimerism after T-cell depleted bone marrow transplantation: evaluation of conditioning regimens using the polymerase chain reaction to amplify human minisatellite regions of genomic DNA. Blood 1992; 80:3235–3242.
53. Costello RT, Kirk J, Gabert J. Value of PCR analysis for long term survivors after allogeneic bone marrow transplant for chronic myelogenous leukemia: a comparative study. Biol Blood Marrow Transplant 1995; 1:24–31.
54. McKinnon S, Barnett L, Heller G, O'Reilly RJ. Minimal residual disease is more common in patients who have mixed T-cell chimerism after bone marrow transplantation for chronic myelogenous leukemia. Blood 1994; 83:3409–3416.
55. Kogler G, Hernandez A, Heyll A, Wolf HH, Wernet P. Qualitative assessment of mixed chimerism after allogeneic bone marrow transplantation with regard to leukemic relapse. Cancer Detect Prev 1996; 20:601–609.
56. Roux E, Helg C, Dumont-Girard F, Chapuis B, Jeannet M, Roosnek E. Analysis of T-cell repopulation after allogeneic bone marrow transplantation: significant differences between recipients of T-cell depleted and unmanipulated grafts. Blood 1996; 87:3984–3992.
57. Gardiner N, Lawler M, O'Riordan J, DeArce M, Humphries P, McCann SR. Persistent donor chimaerism is consistent with disease-free survival following BMT for chronic myeloid leukaemia. Blood 1997; 90:1321–1325.
58. Mackinnon S, Barnett L, Heller G. Polymerase chain reaction is highly predictive of relapse in patients following T cell–depleted allogeneic bone marrow transplantation for chronic myeloid leukemia. Leuk Lymph 1996; 20:239–243.
59. Giralt S, Estey E, Albitar M, van Biesen K, Rondori G, Anderlini P, O'Brien S, Khouri I, Gajewski J, Mehra R, Claxton D, Andersson B, Beran M, Przepiorka D, Koller C, Kornblau S, Korbling M, Keating M, Kantarjian H, Champlin R. Engraftment of allogeneic hematopoietic progenitor cells with purine analog containing chemotherapy: harnessing graft-versus-leukemia without myeloablative therapy. Blood 1997; 89:12–20.
60. Ashman KL, O'Keefe ED, Michaels SR. Autologous responses to human leukemia cells. Immunol Immunother 1986; 22:95–99.
61. Pawelec G, Kalbacher H, Bruserud O. Tumor-specific antigens revisited: presentation to the immune system of fusion peptides resulting solely from tumor-specific chromosomal translocations. Oncol Res 1992; 4:315–320.
62. Coleman S, Fisher J, Hoy T, Burnett AK, Lim SH. Autologous MHC-dependent leukaemia-reactive T lymphocytes in a patient with chronic myeloid leukaemia. Leukemia 1996; 10:483–487.
63. Choudhury A, Gajewski JL, Liang JL, Popat U, Claxton DF, Kliche K-O, Andreef M, Champlin RE. Use of leukemic dendritic cells for the generation of antileukemic

cellular cytotoxicity against Philadelphia-chromosome positive chronic myelogenous leukemia. Blood 1997; 89:1133–1142.
64. Lewalle P, Hensel N, Guimarães A, Couriel D, Jiang YZ, Mavroudis D, Barrett AJ. Helper and cytotoxic T lymphocyte responses to chronic myeloid leukemia: implications for adoptive immunotherapy with T cells. Br J Haemat 1996; 92:587–594.
65. Lowdell MW, Deane M, Ray N, Craston R, Prentice HG. In vitro antileukemia activity after autologous bone marrow transplantation for acute leukemia correlates with clinical remission. Bone Marrow Transplant 1997; 19:891–897.
66. Hess AD, Thoburn CJ. Immunobiology and immunotherapeutic implications of syngeneic/autologous graft-versus-host disease. Immunol Rev 1997; 157:111–123.
67. Hess AD, Bright EC, Thoburn C, Vogelsang GB, Jones RJ, Kennedy MJ. Specificity of effector T lymphocytes in autologous graft-versus-host disease: role of the major histocompatibility complex class II invariant chain peptide. Blood 1997; 89:2203–2209.
68. Yeager AM, Vogelsang GB, Jones RJ, Farmer ER, Hess AD, Santos GW. Cyclosporine-induced graft-versus-host disease after autologous bone marrow transplantation for acute myeloid leukemia. Leuk Lymph 1993; 11:215–220.
69. Gryn J, Johnson E, Goldman N, Devereux L, Grana G, Hageboutros A, Fernandez E, Constantinou C, Harrer W, Viner E, Goldberg J. The treatment of relapsed or refractory intermediate grade non-Hodgkin's lymphoma with autologous bone marrow transplantation followed by cyclosporine and interferon. Bone Marrow Transplant 1997; 19:221–226.
70. Kennedy MJ, Vogelsang GB, Jones RJ, Farmer ER, Hess AD, Altomonte V, Huelskamp AM, Davidson NE. Phase I trial of interferon gamma to potentiate cyclosporine-induced graft-versus-host disease in women undergoing autologous bone marrow transplantation for breast cancer. J Clin Oncol 1994; 12:249–257.
71. Byrne JL, Carter GI, Ellis I, Haynes AP, Russell NH. Autologous GVHD following PBSCT, with evidence for a graft-versus-myeloma effect. Bone Marrow Transplant 1997; 20:517–520.
72. Wolin MJ, Rigor RL. Acute graft-versus-host disease in a recipient of a twin blood cell transplant. Bone Marrow Transplant 1996; 17:125–126.
73. Apperley JF, Jones L, Hale G, Goldman JM. Bone marrow transplantation for chronic myeloid leukaemia: T cell depletion with Campath-1 reduces the incidence of acute graft-versus-host disease but may increase the risk of leukaemic relapse. Bone Marrow Transplant 1986; 1:53–66.
74. Marmont AM, Horowitz MM, Gale RP, Sobocinski K, Ash RC, Van Bekkum DW, Champlin RE, Dicke KA, Goldman JM, Good RA, Horowitz MM, Rimm AA, Bortin NM. T-cell depletion of HLA-identical transplants in leukaemia. Blood 1991; 78: 2120–2130.
75. Champlin RE, Passweg JR, Zhang M-J, Rowlings PA, Pelz CJ, Atkinson KA, Barrett AJ, Cahn J-Y, Drobyski WR, Gale RP, Goldman JM, Gratwohl A, Gordon-Smith EC, Henslee-Downey J, Herzig RH, Klein JP, Marmont AM, O'Reilly RJ, Ringden O, Slavin S, Sobocinski KA, Speck B, Weiner RS, Horowitz MM. T-cell depletion of bone marrow transplants for leukemia from donors other than HLA-identical sib-

lings: advantages of T-cell antibodies with narrow specificities. Blood 1998. *In press*.

76. Jiang YZ, Barrett AJ, Goldman JM, Mavroudis DA. Evidence for natural killer cell modulation of a graft-versus-leukaemia effect without graft-versus-host disease following allogeneic bone marrow transplantation. Ann Hematol 1997; 74:1–6.
77. Bader P, Beck J, Schlegel PG, Handgretinger R, Niethammer D, Klingebiel T. Additional immunotherapy on the basis of increasing mixed hematopoietic chimerism after allogeneic BMT in children with acute leukemia: is there an option to prevent relapse? Bone Marrow Transplant 1997; 20:79–81.
78. Mackinnon S, Papadopoulos EB, Carabasi MH, Reich L, Collins NH, O'Reilly RJ. Adoptive immunotherapy using donor leukocytes following bone marrow transplantation for chronic myeloid leukemia: is T cell dose important in determining biological response? Bone Marrow Transplant 1995; 15:591–594.
79. Naparstek E, Or R, Nagler A, et al. T-cell depleted allogeneic bone marrow transplantation for acute leukaemia using Campath-1 antibodies and posttransplant administration of donor's peripheral blood lymphocytes for prevention of relapse. Br J Haematol 1995; 89:506–515.
80. Johnson BD, Truitt R. Delayed infusion of immunocompetent donor cells after bone marrow transplantation breaks graft-host tolerance and allows for persistent antileukemic reactivity without severe graft-versus-host disease. Blood 1995; 85:3302–3306.
81. Barrett J, Mavroudis D, Tisdale J, Molldrem J, Dunbar C, Cottler-Fox M, Phang S, Carter C, Okunnieff P, Young NS, Read EJ. T-cell depleted bone marrow transplantation followed by delayed T-cell add-back to prevent severe acute GVHD. Bone Marrow Transplantation 1998; 21:543–521.
82. Ringden O, Labopin M, Gluckman E, Reiffers J, Vernant JP, Jouet JP, Harrousseau JL, Fiere D, Bacigalupo A, Frassoni F, Gorin NC. Graft-versus-leukemia effect in allogeneic marrow transplant recipients with acute leukemia is maintained using cyclosporin A combined with methotrexate as prophylaxis. Acute Leukemia Working Party of the European Group for Blood and Marrow Transplantation. Bone Marrow Transplant, 1996; 18:921–929.
83. Higano CS, Brixey M, Bryant EM, et al. Durable complete remission of acute nonlymphoblastic leukaemia associated with discontinuation of immunosuppression following relapse after allogeneic bone marrow transplantation: a case report of a probable graft-versus-leukaemia effect. Transplantation 1990; 50:175–177.
84. Collins RH Jr, Rogers ZR, Bennett M, Kumar V, Niekein A, Fay JW. Hematologic relapse of chronic myelogenous leukemia following allogeneic bone marrow transplantation: apparent graft-versus-leukemia effect following abrupt discontinuation of immunosuppression. Bone Marrow Transplant 1992; 10:391–395.
85. Higano CS, Chielens D, Raskind W, Bryant E, Flowers MD, Radich J, Clift R, Appelbaum F. Use of α-2a-interferon to treat cytogenetic relapse of chronic myeloid leukemia after marrow transplantation. Blood 1997; 90:2549–3554.
86. Mehta J, Powles RL, Singhal S, Tait D, Sawnsbury J, Treleaven J. Cytokine-mediated immunotherapy with or without donor leukocytes for poor-risk acute myeloid leukemia relapsing after allogeneic bone marrow transplantation. Bone Marrow Transplant 1995; 16:133–138.

87. Singhal S, Powles R, Treleaven J, Mehta J. Sensitivity of secondary acute myeloid leukemia relapsing after allogeneic bone marrow transplantation to immunotherapy with interferon-2b. Bone Marrow Transplant 1997; 19:1151–1153.
88. Giralt S, O' Brien S, Talpaz M, et al. Alpha interferon and interleukin-2 as treatment for leukemia relapse after allogeneic bone marrow transplantation. Cytokines Mol Ther 1995; 1:115–122.

9

The GVL Effect in Donor Lymphocyte Transfusion

Frits van Rhee
University of South Carolina
Columbia, South Carolina

Hans-Jochem Kolb
Ludwig Maximilian's University
Munich, Germany

I. INTRODUCTION

The existence of an immunologic antileukemia effect mediated by donor cells after bone marrow transplantation (BMT) was first found more than four decades ago in murine transplant models [1]. However, it was only in the 1980s that the presence of an antitumor effect, also referred to as the graft-versus-leukemia effect (GVL), in human bone marrow grafting was first shown from the statistical analyses of large cohorts of patients transplanted at single institutions or reported to the International Bone Marrow Transplant Registry (IBMTR) [2–4]. These studies found that absence of graft-versus-host disease (GVHD) after BMT or removal of immunocompetent lymphoid cells from the marrow inoculum increased leukemia relapse rates. The first attempts to induce immunological effects in bone marrow graft recipients by transfusing lymphocytes from the donor were carried out in the early 1980s. The purpose of these studies was to prevent graft rejection in aplastic anemia and to reduce the relapse rate in advanced hematological malignancies [5–7]. These studies were abandoned due to an increased incidence of GVHD attributed to the fact that donor lymphocyte transfusions (DLTs) were given at or shortly after BMT. Animal studies demonstrated that delayed transfusion of donor cells resulted in considerably less GVHD [8]. Several investigators provided the first clear evidence that transfused donor lymphoid cells exert a direct antileukemic effect in patients with relapse of leukemia after BMT with acceptable toxicity. Komori et al. [9] described a patient with frank relapse of acute lymphoblastic leukemia (ALL) 18 months after an HLA-identical transplant who responded to transfusions of donor lymphocytes activated with IL-2. However, the response proved transient, and this patient eventually succumbed to leukemia. Kolb et al. [10] first induced lasting, complete remissions in three patients with clinical relapse of CML after allografting by transfusing donor lymphocytes and administering interferon-alpha (IFN-α). Slavin et al. [11] reported a patient with persistent ALL, treated in the 1980s, who obtained a remission with DLT given between 1 and 3 months post-DLT. Several other investigators have since reported similar results with lymphocyte therapy for relapse after transplant [12–17]. This chapter describes the clinical results and complications of DLT therapy for relapse of hematological malignancies after allografting. It seeks to determine the overall place of DLT in the management of relapse and addresses the role of adjuvant therapies such as chemotherapy, IL-2, and IFN-α. DLT is not only a important new addition to our therapeutic arsenal but also serves as an in vivo model of adoptive immunotherapy that can be used to test new strategies for inducing leukemia-specific T-cell responses. The final section of the chapter discusses some of the current clinical and preclinical efforts to develop specific anti-leukemic T-cell immunotherapy.

II. RESULTS OF IMMUNOTHERAPY WITH DLT

A. Chronic Myeloid Leukemia (CML)

Two large series representing the collective European [18] and North American [19] experiences with DLT have now been reported. The principal findings of these studies, including response rates and incidence of GVHD, were very similar. Both series reported that patients with CML in cytogenetic relapse or CML relapsing into chronic phase had the best response to DLT, with complete cytogenetic remission rates of 84 and 76% for the European and American cohorts respectively. These responses were complete not only at the cytogenetic level but also by molecular criteria, since nearly all patients studied were negative for BCR-ABL mRNA by sensitive two-step polymerase chain reaction (PCR) techniques. The majority of remissions were stable, with second relapse rates of only 6–12%. However, the results for transformed-phase CML were considerably worse, both in the European and American series, with complete response rates of only 13 and 28% respectively. The time to cytogenetic remission after DLT is on average between 3–4 months, but delayed cytogenetic responses after several months have been described [19,20]. The long interval from infusion of donor lymphocytes to response presumably reflects the period required for the activation and expansion of the GVL effector cells. The time interval to molecular remission is even longer, on average 10 months, which indicates that even a successful response to DLT can be slow [20]. More rapid responses have been observed when the transfusate contains a high frequency of alloreactive or Epstein-Barr virus (EBV)–specific T cells (e.g., with DLT from haploidentical donors or DLT for EBV lymphoproliferative disorders [21–23].

In multivariate analysis, transformation of CML was the most significant predictor of a poor response to DLT in both patient series (Table 1). Absence of acute or chronic GVHD after the primary transplant procedure was associated with response in the European Group for Blood and Marrow Transplantation (EBMT) cohort. One explanation for this observation may be that in some patients, both GVHD and GVL were abrogated after transplant by suppression or removal of alloreactive T cells and that GVL could be reestablished in these patients by DLT. In contrast, patients who had already experienced GVHD after BMT, and by inference GVL, were less likely to benefit from further transfusion of donor lymphocytes. In contrast, Collins et al. [19] found that chronic GVHD post-BMT was associated with an increased response. The reason for this disparity is not clear, but it can probably be attributed to different characteristics of the study cohorts. The North American patients were more likely to have received a T cell–depleted allograft and few CML patients developed chronic GVHD,

Table 1 Pre-DLT Factors Found to Influence Response in Multivariate Analysis in the EBMT Study (Kolb et al 1995) and North-American Study (Collins et al 1997); percent of patients responding indicated.

	% of patients responding	
Pre-DLT factor	EBMT study	North-American study
Type of relapse		
cytogenetic	82	100
chronic phase	78	74
transformed phase	12 (0.0001*)	28 (0.02*)
GVHD post BMT (yes vs no)		
acute or chronic	64 vs 84 (0.03)	NT
acute	NT	NS
chronic	NT	87 vs 65 (0.03)
Recipient sex (male vs female)	NS	64 vs 85 (0.02)

p Value in Multivariate Analysis in Parentheses. NT = not tested, NS = not significant, *transformed versus cytogenetic/hematologic which may have biased the statistical analysis. Both multicenter studies also shed some light on the role of adjuvant therapy with IFN-α. The first studies of DLT combined transfusions of donor cells with IFN-α, although several investigators have since reported complete remissions with use of lymphocyte transfusions alone [13,17]. Both the European and American studies failed to demonstrate an improved response rate with use of IFN-α, suggesting that DLT alone is adequate first-line therapy [18,19]. However, a definitive answer regarding the role of IFN-α still awaits a prospective randomized trial. A further issue that remains unresolved is the cell dose for immunotherapy. In neither series was a correlation between cell dose transfused and response rate found. However, the mean number of mononuclear cells transfused was high (3 to 4 $\times$ 10^8/kg), and it may be that a cell dose–response relationship is seen only when substantially lower cell doses are transfused.

B. Acute Leukemias and Myelodysplastic Syndrome

The AMLs and myelodysplastic syndromes are less responsive to immunotherapy with DLT. The contribution of DLT to the induction of remission is not always clear in the relapsed acute leukemias, since many patients receive DLT after or in conjunction with intensive chemotherapy [24,25]. The studies of Kolb et al. [18] and Collins et al. [19] reported responses in 15 and 29% of patients who either received DLT as sole therapy or received DLT after failing to achieve remission with chemotherapy. However, the remissions appear to be less stable and the rate of second relapse is increased. No pre-DLT parameters have been recognized that predict response in the acute leukemias. Reports in the literature of DLT for myelodysplastic syndrome are few, but the limited data available suggest that responses are observed in approximately 20% of patients.

In general, the results of DLT in relapsed ALL have been disappointing, with response rates of 3–18% [18,19]. However, there are a number of reports of successful therapy with DLT in ALL [11,19,26]. This supports the existence of a GVL effect in ALL at least in some patients. These observations are also consistent with IBMTR data showing an increased risk of relapse in ALL patients transplanted with T cell–depleted marrow [4]. Interestingly, several recent case reports suggest that ALL positive for the Philadelphia chromosome (Ph) in relapse after BMT may respond to DLT [27–30]. This is perhaps surprising, since Ph-positive ALL is an aggressive leukemia that might be expected to respond poorly to immune manipulation. It is at present not clear if Ph-positive ALL responds better to DLT than other types of ALL or whether these reports merely reflect a bias toward reporting successful cases. Some of these Ph-positive cases responded to DLT only after the infusion of large numbers of cells and have been complicated by severe GVHD.

C. Other Hematological Malignancies

There is some evidence to suggest that donor lymphocytes also mediate an antitumor effect in chronic lymphoid malignancies. Hematological responses coinciding with the onset of de novo GVHD post-BMT or GVHD induced by DLT have been observed in patients with persistent chronic lymphoid leukemia or prolymphocytic leukemia [31,32]. A graft-versus-myeloma effect has been demonstrated in three patients with progressive myeloma treated with lymphocyte transfusions after T cell–depleted transplants [33,34]. All three patients had progressive myeloma prior to transplant and achieved a durable complete remission coincided with the development of GVHD. In contrast, the collective North American data suggest that DLT has little efficacy in non-Hodgkin's lymphoma and Hodgkin's disease [19]. There have been incidental cases of other malignant disorders, including Fanconi's anemia and Polycythemia Rubra Vera (PRV), which have been successfully treated with DLT [18,19].

1. Adjuvant Therapies

The possible benefits of combining chemotherapy with DLT in patients with relapsing acute leukemia are presently not clear. Many patients have rapidly proliferating disease and require some form of cytoreductive treatment prior to immunotherapy in order to control the disease and allow time for response to DLT to occur. Combined analysis of the European and North American data suggest that patients who receive both chemotherapy and DLT do somewhat better than patients who receive only DLT (Table 2). However, the follow-up is still short in some cases and the higher response rates may be due to disease that is still chemotherapy-sensitive but cannot be cured. It remains to be seen whether any true synergism between DLT and chemotherapy exists. Recently, intensive chemotherapy has been combined with transfusions of granulocyte-macrophage colony-stimulating factor (GM-CSF)–mobilized peripheral blood stem cells. The rationale of this approach is to control the tumor burden by intensive chemotherapy, followed by transfusions of a combination of stem cells and lymphocytes in order to reinforce donor hematopoiesis and induce a GVL effect [35]. Cytokine enhancement of immunotherapy of DLT by administering IFN-α or interleukin-

Table 2 Benefits of Combining DLT with Chemotherapy

Disease	DLT alone	DLT & chemotherapy
AML	11/56(20%)	4/13(30%)
ALL	2/23(9%)	6/16(38%)

2 (IL-2) has also been used in order to increase response rates in acute leukemias and resistant CML [11,36]. IFN-α can potentially increase the immunogenicity of leukemia cells by up-regulating HLA and accessory molecule expression, while IL-2 enhances leukemia cell killing by activating T cells and natural killer (NK) cells [37]. Post-DLT administration of IFN-α did not increase the response rate in the two large multicenter studies [18,19]. However, the actual number of patients treated was relatively small and case reports suggest some efficacy [36]. IL-2 has been used both in vivo and in vitro to increase the GVL effect after DLT [9,11,36]. One study reported responses in five of six patients with hematologic relapse of ALL or CML resistant to prior therapy with DLT alone [11]. The exact role of IFN-α and IL-2 therapy in the management of patients with acute leukemia or CML resistant to DLT alone requires further exploration.

III. COMPLICATIONS OF IMMUNOTHERAPY WITH DONOR LYMPHOCYTES

A. Graft-Versus-Host Disease

Acute and chronic GVHD is the most important complication of DLT, occurring in approximately 60% of patients [18,19]. Immunosuppressive therapy for acute GVHD of grade II–IV severity is required in 41% of patients, and severe GVHD (III–IV) is observed in 22% [19]. The overall mortality associated with DLT approaches 20% and can be attributed to GVHD or infectious complications during marrow aplasia. The risk factors predisposing to GVHD after DLT have not been clearly delineated and conflicting observations have been made. Non-Caucasians appear to have a greater risk of GVHD after DLT [19]. Treatment with DLT for relapse after T cell–depleted BMT was a significant risk factor for the development of GVHD in multivariate analysis only in the European BMT study [18]. One explanation might be that T-cell depletion permitted patients to survive who would have succumbed to severe GVHD after T-replete BMT. Chronic GVHD after BMT was predicted for GVHD after DLT in the North American cohort, but this association was not detected in the European data [18,19]. IFN-α given in conjunction with DLT significantly increased the risk of GVHD in the European BMT cohort, but, surprisingly, the opposite was found in the North American patients.

B. Marrow Aplasia

Marrow aplasia develops in 19–33% of patients treated in hematologic relapse with DLT [18,19]. Aplasia is a potentially fatal complication and mortality was usually due to infection and/or bleeding. The marrow aplasia post-DLT is reminiscent of pancytopenias described in transfusion-associated GVHD. However, aplasia in transfusion-associated GVHD occurs much more rapidly, with pancytopenia developing within a month of blood transfusion. It is likely that transfusion-associated GVHD is caused by the transfusion of high-frequency alloreactive lymphocytes that recognize antigenic disparities at major HLA loci, while aplasia post-DLT is probably due to low precursor frequencies of donor lymphocytes reacting against minor histocompatibility antigens presented by leukemic cells. A further difference is that, in contrast to transfusion-associated GVHD, aplasia post-DLT may be followed by spontaneous recovery, which is virtually always of donor origin. It is thought that hematopoietic reconstitution is derived from donor stem cells in the marrow that persist despite the recurrence of leukemia.

Marrow aplasia usually indicates response to therapy with concurrent suppression or eradication of the leukemia clone. In the EBMT study reported by Kolb et al. [18], 45 of 135 patients treated for a variety of leukemias developed marrow aplasia. Aplasia resolved spontaneously in 30 patients while 5 required a second marrow infusion; 10 patients were not evaluable for recovery because of early death due to infections or hemorrhage. In the North American data set, 13 of 26 patients with marrow aplasia had spontaneous recovery. A further 10 patients recovered either after treatment with G-CSF (n = 8) or a marrow boost from the donor [19]; while 3 patients did not recover and 4 deaths were attributed to pancytopenia. These data would suggest that the initial management of aplasia can be supportive, with the administration of blood products and growth factors. However, a second stem-cell infusion should not be unduly delayed in order to reduce the period of pancytopenia and prevent serious complications.

C. Strategies for Preventing Marrow Aplasia

Several studies suggest that aplasia is rare in patients treated for cytogenetic relapse of CML [14,17–19]. This implies that the presence of a sizable stem-cell pool of donor origin at the time of DLT can prevent any fall in blood cell counts during full reconstitution of the marrow by donor hematopoiesis. It is important to identify which patients with hematological relapse will develop aplasia after DLT and which patients will repopulate their marrow with donor cells without a period of pancytopenia. Patients with hematologic relapse at risk of developing persistent aplasia could be either treated with G-CSF–mobilized stem cells in conjunction with lymphocytes or, alternatively, receive a second stem-cell infusion as soon as aplasia occurs. The ability to predict aplasia is particularly relevant to unrelated donors, who will require counseling regarding a possible request for a second stem-cell donation. The detection of residual donor hematopoiesis by molecular methods in the marrow does not reliably predict recovery from aplasia [13,15,38]. It has recently been reported that assessment of chimerism of the CD34+ cell population may be of help for the prediction of marrow aplasia.

Four of six patients in whom donor-derived CD34-positive cells could be detected did not develop aplasia, while 2 patients with no residual donor CD34+ cells became aplastic and required stem-cell support [39].

IV. IMMUNOTHERAPY FOR LEUKEMIA RELAPSE AFTER TRANSPLANTATION FROM UNRELATED AND MISMATCHED FAMILY DONORS

The initial experience with adoptive immunotherapy with donor lymphocytes was mainly confined to patients who relapsed after allogeneic transplantation from an HLA-matched sibling donor. There is reason to expect a more powerful GVL effect using allogeneic lymphocytes from matched unrelated donors. First, allogeneic transplantation with T cell–depleted marrow cells from unrelated donors for CML is associated with a low risk of relapse. This is in clear contrast to the high relapse rates observed after T-depleted sibling BMT [44,41]. Second, a recent study suggests that use of a matched unrelated donor also reduces the relapse risk of CML when the transplant is carried out with marrow cells that are not T cell–depleted [42]. The enhanced GVL effect exerted by lymphocytes from matched unrelated donors might be explained by differences in fine specificities at HLA loci and increased mismatching for minor histocompatibility antigens. It seems reasonable to assume, therefore, that this increase in alloreactivity between unrelated donors and recipients would also lead to a higher response rate to lymphocyte transfusions administered for relapse after transplant. However, two recent studies suggest that immunotherapy for leukemia relapse with allogenic lymphocytes collected from unrelated marrow donors does not result in higher response rates. One single-center study compared the outcome of patients treated with lymphocyte transfusions for relapse of CML after unrelated (n = 12) and sibling donor (n = 18) transplantation [20]. In all cases the lymphocytes had been collected from the original marrow donor by leukapheresis. Both groups were well matched for a number of parameters including disease stage, patient/donor age and patient sex, incidence of acute and chronic GVHD post-BMT, interval from first detection of relapse to DLT, and cell dose transfused, although the unrelated donor group was more likely to have received ex vivo or in vivo T-cell depletion at the time of the original transplant procedure. The probability of attaining a complete remission in the sibling and unrelated donor group was not significantly different (73 versus 64% respectively) (Figure 1). This unexpected result might be explained by the fact that all volunteer donor-recipient pairs were closely matched at HLA loci not only by serological typing but also by isoelectric focusing and by DRβ1 analysis. This premise is further supported by the observation that there were no significant differences in either acute or

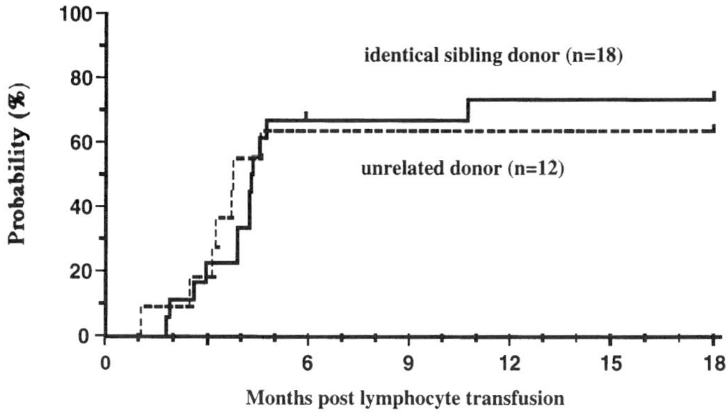

Figure 1 Probability of complete remission according to donor type.

chronic GVHD between volunteer and sibling donor groups. The second study, which involved the analysis of 71 patients treated for relapse of leukemia or EBV-lymphoproliferative proliferative disease with lymphocytes collected from donors provided by the National Marrow Donor Program, recorded similar results with response rates, incidence of GVHD and marrow aplasia comparable with that described for DLT from sibling donors [43]. These results indicate that patients who relapse after unrelated donor BMT should be considered for lymphocyte transfusion, especially when donor and recipient are phenotypically matched. There have been a few reports of DLT for relapse of leukemia after BMT from partially matched family donors [19,21,23]. The limited experience available suggests that remissions can be induced but that there is an increase risk of severe GVHD, particularly when using lymphocytes from two or three antigen-mismatched family donors.

V. MANAGING RELAPSED CML:DLT OR IFN-α?

A. Natural History of Relapsed CML Postallogeneic BMT

There is little doubt that the ability to treat relapsed leukemia with DLT has had a major impact on the overall effectiveness of allogeneic BMT for CML. A recent study of 188 patients transplanted for CML at a single institution showed that DLT administered to 57 patients with relapsing leukemia increased the long-term leukemia-free survival of the whole cohort by approximately 10% (C. Craddock, personal communication). However, it is also important to remember that DLT has considerable toxicity and that the immediate prognosis of relapsed CML is not necessarily poor. This point is highlighted by a study of the European Group for Blood and Marrow Transplantation (EBMT), which reported overall 6-year survivals of 53 and 39% for patients with CML in cytogenetic relapse and hematological relapse respectively [44]. Furthermore, a recent study compared the outcome of 89 CML patients relapsing after allogeneic BMT and reported to the IBMTR with a cohort of 344 CML patients treated conservatively with chemotherapy according to trials of the Italian Co-operative Study Group [45]. The transplant group had a median survival advantage of 21 months, which suggests that allogeneic BMT alters the natural course of CML even when it fails to cure. Alternative strategies—such as simple chemotherapy, IFN-α for CML, or a second marrow transplant procedure—therefore also deserve consideration for relapsed leukemia after allogeneic BMT.

B. Efficacy of IFN-α for Hematological Relapse of CML

IFN-α has an established track record in the pretransplant management of CML and the results of recent large multicenter studies indicate that treatment with IFN-α improves survival [46,47]. IFN-α can even restore normal marrow function in a minority of patients by suppressing leukemic hematopoiesis completely. The encouraging results obtained with IFN-α therapy in chronic-phase CML has prompted several centers to explore its efficacy in controlling CML in relapse post-BMT. Two studies have reported complete cytogenetic remission in approximately 33% of patients [48,49]. One study reported durable complete cytogenetic remissions in 10 patients with a median follow-up of 5 years [49]. Five of these patients tested negative for the BCR-ABL gene rearrangement by RT/PCR. However, a EBMT study of 130 patients with relapsed CML found that IFN-α only improved short-term survival and that the response to treatment was eventually lost [44]. The survival advantage at 2 years was approximately 20% for patients who were treated with IFN-α for cytogenetic relapse compared with patients who were managed with oral chemotherapy, but this advantage was lost over time and there was no difference in the 6-year probability of survival. Similar observations were made for patients with hematologic relapse.

C. Should IFN-α Be Given Instead of DLT for Molecular and Cytogenetic Relapse of CML?

The question whether IFN-α should be preferred to DLT for the management of early recurrence of CML (i.e., relapse at the molecular or cytogenetic stage) is difficult and remains unresolved. Several factors require careful consideration when weighing the advantages and disadvantages of DLT and IFN-α therapy, including the efficacy and toxicity of both treatment options, durability of response, the accuracy with which relapse can be predicted at the molecular or chromosomal level in individual patients, and the incidence of transient relapse. It has been suggested that IFN-α therapy is more efficacious when administered for cytogenetic rather than frank relapse. However, several studies have found similar complete cytogenetic response rates for patients treated in hematological and cytogenetic relapse [44,48,49]. A recent study from a single institution contradicts these findings: complete cytogenetic remissions were observed in 12 of 14 patients with cytogenetic relapse of CML managed with IFN-α, although durable remissions were recorded in only 8 individuals [50]. Although randomized comparative studies of DLT versus IFN-α have not been performed, it appears that DLT is more efficacious in inducing remissions. In addition, most remissions induced by DLT are stable and second relapses are relatively rare [51,52]. However, a strong argument in favor of initial therapy with IFN-α for early relapse is its relative safety and lack of life-threatening toxicity. Severe exacerbations of GVHD have been reported on only few occasions [17,48].

1. Transient Relapse

A further consideration is that Ph-positive cells identified in the marrow post-transplant may disappear spontaneously, a phenomenon referred to as *transient relapse* [53,54]. A significant incidence of transient relapse would suggest IFN-α as the preferred treatment, since early DLT would expose these patients to the possibility of severe morbidity and even death. A recent study of 26 patients with cytogenetic recurrence of CML reported four (15%) transient relapses [55]. However, during further follow-up, 2 of the 4 patients with transient relapse eventually progressed to frank relapse, while the other 2 remained in cytogenetic remission but are still strongly positive for BCR-ABL transcripts and are presumably still at risk for relapse. These data suggest that true transient cytogenetic relapses are comparatively rare and that early DLT for cytogenetic relapse will not result in the treatment of a significant number of patients who were never destined to relapse.

2. Prediction of Relapse by Molecular Methods

There has been much interest in the PCR detection of small numbers of CML cells after allografting, and many investigators have sought to establish whether RT/PCR for BCR-ABL mRNA can predict relapse in patients who are in remission by conventional criteria. Several studies suggest that the PCR detection of residual disease more than 6 to 12 months post-BMT defines a group of patients with an increased risk of relapse, but the predictive value of PCR positivity for individual patients is limited and would argue against the use of DLT on the basis of molecular data [56–59]. Radich et al. [60] studied a large cohort of 346 patients after BMT with unmanipulated marrow cells and found that PCR positivity was a strong predictor of relapse independent of donor type, disease stage, and acute or chronic GVHD. However, the probability of relapse for patients with a positive PCR test at 6 months, although increased, was only 42%. Furthermore, the ability to predict relapse progressively decreased with time posttransplant and late PCR positivity is associated with a low risk of relapse [60–62]. These data suggest that qualitative PCR is insufficient to predict relapse accurately, at least after non-T cell–depleted transplant. This may not necessarily apply to PCR studies after T cell–depleted transplant, where qualitative PCR studies appear to have greater prognostic value [63,64]. Sequential PCR analyses or the introduction of an element of semiquantitation by noting whether amplified BCR-ABL product is present after the first step of a nested PCR may be strategies to improve the predictive power of qualitative PCR. Several investigators have sought to facilitate the monitoring of the leukemia clone by enumerating the number of BCR-ABL transcripts in RNA derived from blood or bone marrow cells. Quantitation of the BCR-ABL transcripts levels by competitive PCR in series of 28 patients, all PCR-positive post-BMT, showed that a progressive increase of BCR-ABL mRNA in serial samples accurately identified those individuals with incipient relapse. In contrast, patients who remained in remission had persistently low or falling levels of BCR-ABL mRNA [65]. The criteria for ''PCR or molecular relapse'' post-BMT have not been well defined but might include serial positivity after T cell–depleted BMT or persistent positivity on a one-step PCR after T-replete allografting. It seems likely the introduction of real-time PCR techniques will make quantitative PCR more widely available in the future [66]. A suggested quantitative PCR criterion for molecular relapse could be an increase of more than 1 log in the number of BCR-ABL transcripts by at least three consecutive assays or the detection of more than 100 BCR-ABL transcripts per microgram of RNA by competitive PCR.

3. Algorithm

Taken together, these considerations suggest that a conservative approach is to treat molecular relapses first with IFN-α reserving DLT for those patients who clearly have progressive disease recurrence. This would also be an ideal setting to explore investigational approaches to prevent or reduce GVHD (e.g., gradual escalation of the lymphocyte dose). The efficacy of IFN-α for the treatment of CML in molecular relapse post-BMT is not known and this issue is the subject of a prospective trial organized by EBMT. The argument for treating cytogenetic relapse of CML with DLT rather than IFN-α is substantially stronger, since most patients progress to frank relapse and DLT is more effective at inducing a remission that is both complete and stable. Furthermore, early treatment of cytogenetic relapse will prevent marrow aplasia.

VI. ROLE OF SECOND ALLOGRAFTS

A second transplant can induce lasting remissions in a minority of patients with relapsed leukemia. A number of favorable prognostic factors have been identified, including a remission of more than 6 months after the first transplantation, a transplant for chronic-phase CML or acute leukemia in first remission, good performance status, and a prolonged interval between first and second BMT [67–69]. However, second transplants are associated with increased transplant-related mortality, and the reported leukemia-free survival after second BMT for CML in these series was 19–49%. It is of interest to note that the best results of second transplants in CML were observed when the intensity of the conditioning was reduced by using busulphan as the sole preparative agent [69]. This suggests that the benefit of a second transplant at least in the case of CML, depends more on the potency of immunologically mediated antileukemia effects than the efficacy of the conditioning regimen.

The results of DLT in relapsed acute leukemias are disappointing, with the majority of patients failing to respond. At first sight, it would seem that DLT and second transplant procedures have similar efficacy in treating relapsed acute leukemia, salvaging 20 to 30% of patients [67,68]. However, only a small and highly selected proportion of patients with relapsed leukemia actually receive a second allograft, while immunotherapy may be more readily available [70]. Second allografts are poorly tolerated, particularly by patients who were not in first complete remission at the time of transplant or who relapse less than 6 months post-BMT [68,70]. Relapse of leukemia after BMT indicates that resistant leukemia stem cells survived the intensive chemoradiotherapy regimen. Second transplant procedures are more likely to succeed by establishing a GVL effect, which failed during the primary transplant, rather than by eradication of leukemia cells by yet more drug therapy. It would therefore be reasonable to first try lymphocyte therapy before subjecting the patient to the increased toxicity of a second transplant procedure. Second relapse rates are high both after second allografts and DLT [70,71].

VII. LEUKEMIA-SPECIFIC IMMUNOTHERAPY

The aim of future immunotherapy studies should be to limit the toxicity of DLT for cytogenetic and chronic-phase relapse of CML and to augment the GVL activity of donor lymphocytes transfused for relapse of advanced phase CML and the acute leukemias. This calls for immunotherapeutic strategies that either harness GVHD after DLT or induce leukemia-specific T-cell activity. There are clinical data to support the notion that it is possible to develop such approaches and separate GVHD from GVL. First, a comparison of the relapse rates after undepleted allogeneic and syngeneic marrow transplant has provided evidence for an antileukemic effect mediated by allogeneic donor cells that is independent of GVHD [4]. Second, some patients treated with DLT attain complete remission without developing any GVHD [18]. Current clinical studies center around the infusion of incremental doses of lymphocytes, lymphocyte subset depletion strategies, and control of GVHD by inserting suicide genes into donor cells prior to DLT. The aim of most preclinical studies is to raise leukemia-specific CLTs in vitro by stimulation with leukemia cells that have been modified to enhance immunogenicity. Efforts are also in progress to identify the peptides and proteins that are the targets for the GVL response. For further details, the reader is referred to Chapters 6 to 8.

A. Dose Escalation

A clear relationship between lymphocyte dose, response, and GVHD has not been established. Most investigators have transfused large numbers of donor lymphocytes ($>1 \times 10^8$/kg) for adoptive immunotherapy. However, there has been considerable variation in the cell dose, and some patients have responded to smaller doses. It is likely that a threshold exists for the induction of GVL and GVHD after DLT. It is well established that there is a critical cell dose ($>1 \times 10^5$ clonable T cells) for the induction of GVHD after BMT [72]. This threshold for GVHD may not necessarily apply to therapy with DLT, since studies in murine MHC-matched and haploidentical models show that the timing of lymphocyte transfusion after BMT is an important determinant of the risk of GVHD [73]. Clinical studies suggest that the timing of lymphocyte transfusion also plays an important role in humans. A recent trial found that the delayed add-back of 10^7 T cells per kilogram 30 days after T-depleted BMT under CyA cover is associated with a high risk of acute GVHD, while the transfusion of five times as many cells only 15 days later is relatively safe and largely prevents acute GVHD while retaining GVL [74]. Stepwise escalation of the number of lymphocytes transfused has been employed in order to find a cell dose that is both effective and minimizes GVHD. This is based on the premise that the frequency of leukemia reactive T cells in collections of donor lymphocytes is greater than the frequency of cells causing GVHD. The aim of dose-escalation studies is to find the therapeutic window in a particular recipient/donor pair where remission can be restored without GVHD. Two dose-finding studies point to a threshold of 1 to 5×10^7 T cells per kilogram for the induction of GVHD using DLT from matched sibling donors. Mackinnon et al. [75] reported remissions in eight patients receiving 1.0×10^7 T cells per kilogram, with GVHD developing in only a single patient. However, 11 patients required higher T-cell doses, ranging from 5×10^7 to 5×10^8 T cells per kilogram, and 8 of these developed GVHD. In a series of 10 patients, Bagicalupo et al. [76] observed GVHD in one patient at dose level of 2×10^6 T cells per kilogram and in 6 patients at dose level of 2×10^7 T cells per kilogram. Retrospective comparison with a comparable group treated with unquantitated larger amounts of DLT at the same institution showed that dose escalation reduced the incidence of severe GVHD and improved outcome. These preliminary data suggests that gradual dose escalation can induce remissions in some patients without causing GVHD, while in other patients the incidence of severe GVHD was reduced. However, disadvantages are that some patients may still require large doses or develop severe acute or chronic GVHD at lower dose levels. In addition, the number of dose levels that can be attempted is limited and is dictated by the tempo of leukemic relapse. It is also likely that the optimum dose of lymphocytes is influenced by other factors in given donor/recipient pairs (e.g., leukemia burden at relapse, proliferative potential of the leukemia cells, degree of matching for major and minor histocompatibility antigens, and abrogation of GVL by immunosuppressive drugs).

B. CD8 Depletion

Selective depletion of the cytotoxic/suppressor CD8-positive subset of lymphocytes from bone marrow grafts reduces the incidence of severe GVHD, but does not increase relapse rates in patients transplanted for acute leukemias and CML [77,78]. This approach has been extended to immunotherapy with DLT for relapse. Transfusions of CD8-depleted donor lymphocytes appear to retain GVL activity, since 6 of 7 patients treated for cytogenetic or hematological relapse responded [79]. However, these data should be interpreted with some caution, since 3 responders developed acute or chronic GVHD. Furthermore, it cannot be ruled out that residual CD8-positive cells in the marrow grafts or lymphocyte transfusions expand rapidly in vivo and mediate both GVHD and GVL. Additional studies are required to determine if CD8 depletion of donor lymphocyte transfusion improves overall outcome (see Chapter 15).

C. Generation of CTLs by Stimulating with Leukemia Cells

1. CML-Specific T-Cell Lines

It is at present not clear if the GVL effect is initiated directly by host leukemia cells or by persisting host- or donor-derived professional antigen presenting cells (APCs), which process and present antigens from normal host tissues and leukemia cells. The observation that all the target organs of GVHD harbor professional APCs suggests that the alloresponses against the host tissues and perhaps also the host leukemia cells are initiated by professional APCs. CML differs from the acute leukemias in that the malignant clone differentiates and generates mature monocyte-macrophages that can function as APCs. The ability of CML cells to elicit normal alloresponses in mixed lymphocyte cultures can be explained by the expression of HLA-DR and costimulatory molecules such as B7.1 and ICAM-1 on CD33+ cells [80,81]. The CD33+ population also contains cells that capture, process, and present soluble antigen to antigen-specific T-cell clones [82]. It has been shown that dendritic cells, which are the most potent inducers of alloresponses, can be readily isolated from the peripheral blood of CML patients or alternatively cultured in vitro from CD34+ progenitor cells. These dendritic cells are Ph-positive and appear to have normal function [83,84]. A recent report suggests that it may be possible to generate autologous antileukemic cytotoxic T cells using Ph-positive dendritic cells [83], but this has not found clinical application as yet.

The currently available techniques for the induction T-cell lines or clones to CML cells with lymphocytes collected from HLA-identical sibling donors are imperfect, and it has proved difficult to obtain sufficient cells for clinical application. It has recently been shown that it is possible to generate leukemia-reactive T-cell lines in a modified limiting dilution assay by screening individual wells for antileukemic activity. This technique has been used to generate CTLs that induced remission in a patient with accelerated-phase CML who was resistant to standard DLT (Ref. 85; also see Chapter 18). The raising of T-cell lines and clones is less problematic in HLA mismatched donor-recipient pairs and could potentially be used to identify alloreactive donor cells. Screening of clones against recipient leukemia cells and Phytohaemagglutinin (PHA) lymphoblasts allows for the identification of leukemia-reactive clones that could be studied for Vβ T-cell receptor expression by RT/PCR. Using immunomagnetic beads coated with antibodies to specific Vβ families, it may prove possible in future to select from donor lymphocyte collections only the T cells with antileukemic activity [86].

2. T-Cell Lines Specific to Acute Leukemias

The immunological mechanisms responsible for the relative resistance of the acute leukemias to immunotherapy require further elucidation. One explanation may be that the proliferative rate of acute leukemia cells simply outstrips the capacity for T-cell expansion and that the leukemia ''overgrows'' any antileukemic T cells. Alternatively, it is possible that acute leukemia cells are either inept at stimulating antileukemia responses or, alternatively, are resistant to T or NK cell–mediated cytotoxicity. T cells require two signals for activation: the first is antigen-specific and results from the interaction of the peptide-MHC complex with the T-cell receptor, while the second or costimulatory signal depends on the interaction of members of the B7 family on the antigen presenting cell with the CD28 receptor on the T cell. Presentation of antigen to T cells in the absence of costimulation via the B7 pathway usually results in anergy. Lack of HLA-

DR expression has been correlated with poor allostimulatory capacity of acute leukemia cells [87]. A study of 54 patients with acute myeloid leukemia showed expression of B7.1 on the leukemia cells of only 1 individual, while B7.2 was present in 15 cases [88]. A recent paper demonstrates that pre-B acute lymphoblastic leukemia cells lack B7 and cannot induce proliferation of allogeneic mismatched lymphocytes but instead induce alloantigen-specific unresponsiveness [89].

Strategies to enhance the immunogenicity of acute leukemia cells include coinfusion of APCs with donor lymphocytes, transfection of leukemia cells with costimulatory molecules, and the induction of costimulatory molecules on leukemia cells by CD40 ligation or recombinant cytokines. Transfusion of marrow or GM-CSF-mobilized stem cells followed by treatment of the patient with GM-CSF to enhance presentation of leukemia antigens has already found clinical application. A preliminary report described responses in 6 of 9 patients treated for recurrent AML post-BMT [51]. Treatment of normal donors with Flt3 ligand increases the percentage of dendritic cells in the blood, and these could potentially be infused in conjunction with donor lymphocytes collected by leukapheresis [90]. Transfection of costimulatory or other immunomodulatory molecules enhances the ability of leukemia cells to stimulate responses from donor cells. Gene-modified cells could be used ex vivo to generate CTLs or injected into the patient in a vaccine approach. The importance of B7.1-mediated costimulation of myeloid leukemia cells has been demonstrated in a syngeneic murine model using a BCR-ABL–transformed cell line. Protective immunity to the transformed cell line was conferred only if the line had been co-transfected with B7.1, while mice challenged with unmodified leukemia cells rapidly died of leukemia [91]. Several studies suggest that CD40 ligation can upregulate B7 expression and repair APC function of B-lymphoid malignancies [89,92,93]. CD40 ligation restores the ability of pre-B ALL cells to stimulate allogeneic T-cell proliferation [92]. Furthermore, CD40-ligated ALL cells have been used to generate leukemia-specific T-cell lines using autologous lymphocytes collected from the bone marrow [92] Preliminary studies suggest that it may also be possible to improve the APC function of acute myeloid leukemia cells by incubation with recombinant cytokines. Incubation with GM-CSF and IL-4 can differentiate the AML cells of some patients toward dendritic cells with upregulation of HLA-class II, B7.1, and B7.2 [94,95]. These differentiated AML cells could also stimulate autologous cytotoxic T-cell responses.

VIII. FUTURE PERSPECTIVES

It is clear that the next decade will be an exciting time for BMT physicians and hematoimmunologists. New advances in graft engineering and stem-cell mobilization have already made it possible to increase the stem-cell dose for allogeneic transplantation. Studies are currently in progress to determine whether an increased stem-cell dose permits a reduction in the intensity of the conditioning regimen and limit regimen-related toxicity. A better understanding of the interactions between leukemia cells and T cells offers the prospect of developing specific immunotherapy and selectively reconstituting the immune systems of allograft recipients. The basic techniques for the identification of leukemia antigens—such as T-cell cloning, peptide elution, and mass tandem spectrometer, expression of leukemic cDNA in libraries, and knowledge of peptide binding motifs of individual HLA molecules—are now well established, and it is likely that in the ensuing years many more leukemia and minor histocompatibility antigens will be identified. Techniques have also been developed to obtain professional antigen-presenting cells (APCs), such as dendritic cells or activated B cells. The availability of well-defined leukemia antigens and professional APCs for the presenting of these antigens will facilitate the expansion of leukemia-specific T cells for therapeutic purposes.

REFERENCES

1. Barnes D, Loutit J. Treatment of murine leukemia with x-rays and homologous bone marrow. Br J Dermatol 1957; 3:241–252.
2. Weiden PL, Flournoy N, Thomas ED, et al. Antileukemic effects of graft-versus-host disease in human recipients of allogeneic marrow grafts. N Engl J Med 1979; 300:1068–1073.
3. Weiden P, Sullivan K, Flournoy N, et al. Antileukemic effect of chronic graft-versus-host disease: contribution to improved survival after allogeneic marrow transplantation. N Engl J Med 1981; 304:1529–1531.
4. Horowitz MM, Gale RP, Sondel PM, et al. Graft-versus-leukemia reactions after bone marrow transplantation. Blood 1990; 75:555–562.
5. Storb R, Doney KC, Thomas ED, et al. Marrow transplantation with or without buffy coat cells for 65 patients with aplastic anemia. Blood 1982; 59:236–246.
6. Niederwieser D, Pepe M, Storb R, et al. Factors predicting chronic graft-versus-host disease and survival after marrow transplantation for aplastic anemia. Bone Marrow Transplant 1989; 4:151–156.
7. Sullivan KM, Weiden PL, Storb R, et al. Influence of acute and chronic graft-versus-host disease after relapse and survival after bone marrow transplantation from HLA identical siblings as treatment of acute and chronic leukemia. Blood 1989; 73:1720–1728.
8. Kolb H-J, Beisser K, Holler E, et al. Donor buffy coat transfusions for adoptive immunotherapy in human canine chimeras. Period Biol 1991; 93:81–85.
9. Komori T, Sugiyama H, Ogawa H, et al. Treatment of a patient in relapse after bone marrow transplantation for acute lymphoblastic leukemia with the systemic

administration of allogeneic lymphokine activated killer cells and recombinant interleukin 2. Eur J Hematol 1989; 43:184–185.
10. Kolb H-J, Mittermüller J, Clemm Ch, et al. Donor leukocyte transfusions for treatment of recurrent chronic myelogenous leukemia in marrow transplant patients. Blood 1990; 76:2462–2465.
11. Slavin S, Naparstek E, Nagler A, et al. Allogeneic cell therapy with donor peripheral blood cells and recombinant interleukin 2 to treat leukemia relapse after allogeneic bone marrow transplantation. Blood 1996; 87:2195–2204.
12. Cullis JO, Jiang YZ, Schwarer AP, et al. Donor leukocyte infusions for chronic myeloid leukemia in relapse after allogeneic bone marrow transplantation. Blood 1992; 79:1379–1381.
13. Drobyski W, Keever C, Roth M, et al. Salvage immunotherapy using donor leukocyte infusions as treatment for relapsed chronic myelogenous leukemia after allogeneic bone marrow transplantation: efficacy and toxicity of a defined T-cell dose. Blood 1993; 82:2310–2318.
14. Bär BMAM, Schattenberg A, Mensink EJBM, et al. Donor leukocyte infusions for chronic myeloid leukemia after allogeneic bone marrow transplantation. J Clin Oncol 1993; 11:513–519.
15. Hertenstein B, Wiesneth M, Novotny J, et al. Interferon-α and donor buffy coat transfusions for treatment of relapsed chronic myeloid leukemia after allogeneic bone marrow transplantation. Transplantation 1993; 56:1114–1118.
16. Porter DL, Roth MS, McGarigle C, et al. Induction of graft-versus-host disease as immunotherapy for relapsed chronic myeloid leukemia. N Engl J Med 1994; 330: 100–106.
17. van Rhee F, Feng L, Cullis JO, et al. Relapse of chronic myeloid leukemia after allogeneic bone marrow transplantation: the case for giving donor leukocyte transfusions before the onset of hematologic relapse. Blood 1994; 83:3377–3383.
18. Kolb H-J, Schattenberg A, Goldman JM et al. Graft-versus-leukemia effect of donor lymphocyte transfusions in marrow grafted patients. Blood 1995; 86:2041–2050.
19. Collins RH Jr, Shpilberg O, Drobyski WR, et al. Donor leukocyte transfusions in 140 patients with relapsed malignancy after allogeneic bone marrow transplantation. J Clin Oncol 1997; 15:433–444.
20. van Rhee F, Savage D, Blackwell J, Orchard K, Dazzi F, Lin F, Chase A, Bungey J, Cross NCP, Apperley J, Szydlo R, Goldman JM. Adoptive immunotherapy for relapse of chronic myeloid leukemia after allogeneic bone marrow transplant: equal efficacy of lymphocytes from sibling and matched unrelated donors. Bone Marrow Transplant. In press.
21. Ferster A, Bujan W, Mouraux T, et al. Complete remission following donor leukocyte transfusion after haplo-identical bone marrow transplantation. Bone Marrow Transplant 1994; 14:331–332.
22. Papadopoulos EB, Lananyi M, Emmanuel D, et al. Infusions of donor leukocytes to treat Epstein-Barr virus-associated lymphoproliferative disorders after allogeneic bone marrow transplantation. N Engl J Med 1994; 330:1185–1191.
23. Pati AR, Godder K, Lamb L, Gee A, Henslee-Downey P. Immunotherapy with donor leukocyte transfusions for patients with relapsed acute myeloid leukemia following

partially mismatched related donor bone marrow transplantation. Bone Marrow Transplant 1995; 15:979–981.

24. Szer J, Grigg AP, Phillips GL, Sheridan WP. Donor leukocyte transfusions after chemotherapy for patients relapsing with acute leukemia following allogeneic BMT. Bone Marrow Transplant 1993; 11:109–111.
25. Porter D, Roth MS, Lee SJ, et al. Adoptive immunotherapy with donor mononuclear cell infusions to treat relapse of acute leukemia or myelodysplasia after allogeneic bone marrow transplantation. Bone Marrow Transplant 1996; 18:975–980.
26. Dunlop L, Powles R, Singhal S, et al. Bone marrow transplantation for Philadelphia chromosome–positive acute lymphoblastic leukemia. Bone Marrow Transplant 1996; 17:365–369.
27. Azuno Y, Kaneko T, Nishimura M, et al. Donor leukocyte transfusions and discontinuation of immunosuppressants to achieve an initial remission after allogeneic bone marrow transplantation in a patient with primary refractory acute leukemia. Bone Marrow Transplant 1996; 18:257–259.
28. Atra A, Millar B, Sheperd V, et al. Donor lymphocyte infusion for childhood acute lymphoblastic leukemia relapsing after bone marrow transplantation. Br J Hematol 1997; 97:165–168.
29. Keil F, Kalhs P, Haas OA, et al. Relapse of Philadelphia chromosome positive acute lymphoblastic leukemia after marrow transplantation: sustained molecular remission after early and dose-escalating infusion of donor leukocytes. Br J Hematol 1997; 97:161–164.
30. Saw HM, Teh A, Wong HC, et al. Haematological remission induced by donor leukocytes infusion in a case of Philadelphia positive acute lymphoblastic leukemia relapsing after allogeneic bone marrow transplantation. Int J Hematol 1997; 65:173–178.
31. Mehta J, Powles R, Singhal S, et al. Clinical and hematologic response of chronic lymphocytic and prolymphocytic leukemia persisting after allogeneic bone marrow transplantation with the onset of acute graft-versus-host disease: possible role of graft-versus-leukemia. Bone Marrow Transplant 1996; 17:371–375.
32. Róndon G, Giralt S, Huh Y, et al. Graft-versus-leukemia effect after allogeneic bone marrow transplantation for chronic lymphocytic leukemia. Bone Marrow Transplant 1996; 18:669–672.
33. Tricot G, Vesole D, Jagannath S, et al. Graft-versus-myeloma effect: proof of principle. Blood 1996, 87:1196–1198.
34. Verdonck LF, Lokhorst HM, Dekker AW, Nieuwenhuis HK, Petersen EJ. Graft-versus-myeloma effect in two cases. Lancet 1996; 347:800–801.
35. Bernasconi P, Alessandrino ES, Caldera D, et al. Intensive chemotherapy followed by donor PBSC in ANLL relapsed after allogeneic BMT. Bone Marrow Transplant 1995; 15:643–645.
36. Mehta J, Powles RL, Singhal S, Tait D, et al. Cytokine-mediated immunotherapy with or without donor leukocytes for poor-risk acute myeloid leukemia relapsing after allogeneic bone marrow transplantation. Bone Marrow Transplant 1995; 16: 133–138.
37. Balkwill FR. Interferons. Lancet 1989; 1:1060–1063.
38. Garicochea B, van Rhee F, Spencer A, et al. Aplasia after donor lymphocyte transfu-

sion (DLI) in relapse after sex-mismatched BMT: recovery of donor-type haematopoiesis predicted for by non-isotopic in situ hybridisation. Br J Hematol 1994; 88: 400–402.
39. Keil F, Haas OA, Fritsch G, et al. Donor leukocyte infusion for leukemic relapse after allogeneic marrow transplantation: lack of residual donor hematopoiesis predicts aplasia. Blood 1997; 89:3113–3331.
40. McGlave P, Bartsch G, Anasetti C, et al. Unrelated donor marrow transplantation for chronic myelogenous leukemia: initial experience of the National Marrow Donor program. Blood 1993; 81:543–550.
41. Drobyski WR, Ash RC, Casper JT, et al. Effect of T-cell depletion as graft-versus-host disease prophylaxis on engraftment, relapse, and disease-free survival in unrelated marrow transplantation for chronic myelogenous leukemia. Blood 1994; 83: 1980–1987.
42. Enright H, Davies S, DeFor T, et al. Relapse after non-T-cell-depleted allogeneic bone marrow transplantation for chronic myelogenous leukemia: early transplantation, use of an unrelated donor and chronic graft-versus-host disease are protective. Blood 1996; 88:714–720.
43. Porter D, Collins R, Mick R, et al. Unrelated donor leukocyte infusions (U-DLI) to treat relapse or EBV-lymphoproliferative disease (EBV-LPD) after unrelated donor bone marrow transplantation (abstr 2622). Blood 1997; 90(suppl 1):590a.
44. Arcese W, Goldman JM, D'Arcangelo E, et al. Outcome for patients who relapse after allogeneic bone marrow transplantation for chronic myeloid leukemia. Blood 1993; 82:3211–3219.
45. Zhang M-J, Baccarani M, Gale RP, et al. Survival of patients with chronic myelogenous leukemia relapsing after bone marrow transplantation: comparison with patients receiving conventional chemotherapy. Br J Hematol 1997; 99:23–29.
46. Allan NC, Richards SM, Shepherd PCA, et al. UK Medical Research Council randomised, multicentre trial of interferon-an1 for chronic myeloid leukemia: improved survival irrespective of cytogenetic response. Lancet 1995; 345:1392–1397.
47. Hehlmann R, Heimpel H, Hossfeld DK, et al. Randomized study of the combination of hydroxyurea and interferon alpha versus hydroxyurea monotherapy during the chronic phase of chronic myelogenous leukemia (CML Study II). Bone Marrow Transplant 1996; 17:(suppl 3):S21–S24.
48. Higano CS, Raskind WH and Singer JW. Use of α-interferon for the treatment of relapse of chronic myelogenous leukemia in chronic phase after allogeneic bone marrow transplantation. Blood 1992; 80:1437–1442.
49. Pigneux A, Devergie A, Potchitaloff M, Rio B, et al. Recombinant alpha-interferon as treatment for chronic myelogenous leukemia in relapse after allogeneic bone marrow transplantation: a report of the French Sociétié Française De Greffe de Moelle. Bone Marrow Transplant 1995; 15:819–824.
50. Higano CS, Chielens D, Rashkind W, et al. Use of interferon-α to treat cytogenetic relapse of chronic myeloid leukemia after marrow transplantation. Blood 1997; 90: 2549–2554.
51. Kolb H-J, Menzel H, Holler E, et al. Donor cell transfusion for the treatment of recurrent leukemia after allogeneic bone marrow transplantation (abstr 2434). Blood 1997; 90(suppl 1):546a.

53. Zaccaria A, Rosti G, Sessarego M, et al. Relapse after allogeneic bone marrow transplantation for Philadelphia chromosome positive chronic myeloid leukemia: cytogenetic analysis of 24 patients. Bone Marrow Transplant 1988; 3:413–423.
54. Arthur CK, Apperley JF, Guo AP, et al. Cytogenetic events after bone marrow transplantation for chronic myeloid leukemia in chronic phase. Blood 1988; 71:1179–1186.
55. Lin F, Kirkland MA, van Rhee F, et al. Molecular analysis of transient cytogenetic relapse after allogeneic bone marrow transplantation for chronic myeloid leukemia. Bone Marrow Transplant 1996; 18:1147–1152.
56. Delage R, Soiffer RJ, Dear K, Ritz J. Clinical significance of BCR-ABL gene rearrangement detected by polymerase chain reaction after allogeneic bone marrow transplantation in chronic myelogenous leukemia. Blood 1991; 78:2759–2767.
57. Roth MS, Antin JH, Ash R, et al. Prognostic significance of Philadelphia chromosome–positive cells detected by the polymerase chain reaction after allogeneic bone marrow transplant for chronic myelogenous leukemia. Blood 1992; 79:276–282.
58. Arnold R, Janssen JWG, Heinze B, et al. Influence of graft-versus-host disease on the eradication of minimal residual disease detected by polymerase chain reaction in chronic myeloid leukemia patients after bone marrow transplantation. Leukemia 1993; 7:747–751.
59. Cross NCP, Hughes TP, Lin F, et al. Minimal residual disease after allogeneic bone marrow transplantation for chronic myeloid leukemia in first chronic phase: correlations with acute graft-versus-host disease and relapse. Br J Hematol 1993; 84:67–74.
60. Radich JP, Gehly G, Gooley T, et al. Polymerase chain-reaction detection of the bcr-abl fusion transcript after allogeneic marrow transplantation for chronic myeloid leukemia—results and implications in 346 patients. Blood 1995; 85:2632–2638.
61. Guerrasio A, Martinelli G, Saglio G, et al. Minimal residual disease status in transplanted chronic myelogenous leukemia patients: low incidence of polymerase chain reaction positive cases among 48 long disease free subjects who received unmanipulated allogeneic bone marrow transplantation. Leukemia 1992; 6:507–512.
62. Miyamura K, Tahara T, Tanimoto M, et al. Long persistent bcr-abl positive transcript detected by polymerase chain reaction after marrow transplant for chronic myelogenous leukemia without clinical relapse: a study of 64 patients. Blood 1993; 81:1089–1093.
63. MacKinnon S, Barnett L, Heller G, et al. Polymerase chain reaction is highly predictive of relapse in patients following T cell-depleted allogeneic bone marrow transplantation for chronic myeloid leukemia. Bone Marrow Transplant 1996; 17:643–647.
64. Drobyski WR, Endean DJ, Klein JP, et al. Detection of BCR/ABL RNA transcripts using the polymerase chain reaction is highly predictive for relapse in patients transplanted with unrelated marrow grafts for chronic myelogenous leukemia. Br J Hematol 1997; 98:458–466.
65. Cross NCP, Lin F, Chase A, et al. Competitive polymerase chain reaction to estimate the number of BCR-ABL transcripts in chronic myeloid leukemia after bone marrow transplantation. Blood 1993; 82:1929–1936.
66. Mandigers CMPW, Meijerink JPP, Schattenberg AVMB, et al. Quantitative analysis

of t(14;18) carrying lymphoma cells correlates with relapse after BMT and graft-versus-lymphoma effect of donor leukocyte infusions (abstr 2433). Blood 1997; 90(suppl 1):546a.

67. Barrett AJ, Locatelli F, Treleaven JG, et al. Second transplants for leukaemic relapse after bone marrow transplantation: high early mortality but favourable effect of chronic GVHD on continued remission. Br J Hematol 1991; 79:567–574.
68. Mrsic M, Horowitz MM, Atkinson K, et al. Second HLA-identical sibling transplants for leukemia recurrence. Bone Marrow Transplant 1992; 9:269–275.
69. Cullis JO, Schwarer AP, Hughes TP, et al. Second transplants for patients with chronic myeloid leukemia in relapse after original transplant with T-depleted marrow: feasibility of using busulphan alone for re-conditioning. Br J Hematol 1992b; 80:33–39.
70. Mehta J, Powles R, Treleaven J, et al. Outcome of acute leukemia relapsing after bone marrow transplantation: utility of second transplants and adoptive immunotherapy. Bone Marrow Transplant 1997; 19:709–719.
71. Porter DL, Collins R, Drobyski W, et al. Long term follow-up of 55 patients who achieved complete remission (CR) after donor leukocyte infusions (DLI) for relapse after allogeneic bone marrow transplantation (BMT) (abstr 2444). Blood 1997; 90(suppl 1):549a.
72. Kernan NA, Collins NH, Juliano L, et al. Clonable T-lymphocytes in T-cell depleted bone marrow transplants correlate with development of graft-versus-host disease. Blood 1986; 68:770–773.
73. Johnson BD and Truitt RL. Delayed infusion of immunocompetent donor cells after bone marrow transplantation breaks graft-host tolerance and allows for persistent antileukemic reactivity without severe graft-versus-host disease. Blood 1995; 85: 3302–3312.
74. Barrett AJ, Mavroudis D, Tidsdale J, et al. T-cell depleted bone marrow transplantation followed by delayed T-cell add-back to prevent severe acute GVHD Bone Marrow Transplant 1998, 21:543–551.
75. Mackinnon S, Papadopoulos E, Carabasi M, et al. Adoptive immunotherapy evaluating escalating doses of donor leukocytes for relapse of chronic myeloid leukemia after bone marrow transplantation: separation of graft-versus-leukemia responses from graft-versus-host disease. Blood 1995; 86:1261–1268.
76. Bagicalupo A, Soracco M, Vassallo F, et al. Donor lymphocyte infusions (DLI) in patients with chronic myeloid leukemia following bone marrow transplantation. Bone Marrow Transplant 1997; 19:927–932.
77. Nimer SD, Giorgi J, Gajewski JL, et al. Selective depletion of CD8+ cells for prevention of graft-versus-host disease after bone marrow transplantationn. Blood 1994; 57:82–87.
78. Champlin R, Ho W, Gajewski J, et al. Selective depletion of CD8+ T lymphocytes for prevention of graft-versus-host disease after allogeneic bone marrow transplantation. Blood 1990; 76:418–423.
79. Giralt S, Hester J, Huh Y, et al. CD8-depleted donor lymphocyte infusion as treatment for relapsed chronic myelogenous leukemia after allogeneic bone marrow transplantation. Blood 1995; 86:4337–4343.
80. Lewalle P, Hensel N, Guimarães A, et al. Helper and cytotoxic T lymphocyte re-

sponses to chronic myeloid leukemia: implications for adoptive immunotherapy with T cells. Br J Hematol 1996; 92:587–594.

81. Dermime S, Mavroudis D, Jiang Y-Z, et al. Does immune escape from a graft-versus-leukemia effect play a role in the relapse of chronic myelogenous leukemia following allogeneic bone marrow transplantation? Bone Marrow Transplant 1997; 10:989–989.
82. Jiang YZ, Mavroudis D, Dermime S, et al. Alloreactive CD4+ T lymphocytes can exert cytotoxicity to chronic myeloid leukemia cells processing and presenting exogenous antigen. Br J Hematol 1996; 93:606–612.
83. Choudhury A, Gajewski JL, Liang JL, et al. Use of leukemic dendritic cells for the generation of antileukemic cellular cytotoxicity against Philadelphia-chromosome positive chronic myelogenous leukemia. Blood 1997; 89:1133–1142.
84. Smit WM, Rijnbeek M, van Bergen CAM, et al. Generation of dendritic cells expressing bcr-abl from CD34-positive chronic myeloid leukemia cells. Hum Immunol 1997; 53:216–223.
85. Falkenburg JHF, Wafelman AR, van Bergen CAM, et al. Leukemia-reactive cytotoxic T-cells (CTL) induce complete remission in a patient with refractory accelerated phase chronic myeloid leukemia. Blood 1997; 90(suppl 1):589a.
86. Jiang YZ, Mavroudis D, Dermime S, Hensel N, Barrett AJ. Preferential usage of T cell receptor (TCR) Vβ by allogeneic T cells recognising myeloid leukemia cells: implications for separating GVL from GVHD. Bone Marrow Transplant 1997; 19: 899–903.
87. Delain M, Tiberghien P, Racadot E, et al. Variability of the alloreactive T-cell response to human leukemic blasts. Leukemia 1994; 8:642–647.
88. Hirano N, Takahashi T, Takahashi T, et al. Expression of costimulatory molecules in human leukemias. Leukemia 1996; 10:1168–1176.
89. Cardoso AA, Schultze JL, Boussiotis VA, et al. Pre-B acute lymphoblastic leukemia cells may induce T-cell anergy to alloantigen. Blood 1996; 88:41–48.
90. Maraskovsky E, Roux E, Teepe M, et al. Flt3 ligand increases peripheral blood lymphocytes in healthy volunteers (abstr. 2585), Blood 1997; 90(suppl 1):581a.
91. Matulonis UA, Dosiou CD, Lamont C, et al. Role of B7.1 in mediating an immune response to myeloid leukemia cells. Blood 1995; 85:2507–2515.
92. Cardoso AA, Seamon MJ, Afonso HM, et al. Ex-vivo generation of human anti-pre B leukemia-specific cytolytic T cells. Blood 1997; 2:549–561.
93. Shultze JL, Seamon MJ, Michalak S, et al. Autologous tumor infiltrating T-cells cytotoxic for follicular lymphoma cells can be expanded in vitro. Blood 1997; 89: 3806–3816.
94. Choudhury A, Agusala K, Sutaria S, et al. Leukemic dendritic cells derived in vitro from AML patients can stimulate anti-leukemic activity in autologous T-cell populations (abstr 2263). Blood 1997; 90(suppl 1):508a.
95. Strunk D, Linkesh W. Acute myelogenous leukemia cells can differentiate into dendritic cells in vitro (abstr 829). Blood 1997; 90(suppl 1): 188a.

10
The Graft-Versus-Myeloma Effect

Jayesh Mehta
Richland Memorial Hospital and South Carolina Cancer Center
Columbia, South Carolina

I. INTRODUCTION

Although high-dose therapy and autologous transplantation confer a survival benefit in multiple myeloma [1,2], eventual disease progression is almost universal and few patients are cured [1–3]. Disease recurrence rates after purged autografts do not appear to be different from those seen with unpurged grafts [4], and relapse rates after syngeneic transplantation are also high [5,6]. This situation is unlike that in hematological malignancies such as the acute leukemias and the lymphomas, where a number of patients are cured with autologous or syngeneic transplantation [7], suggesting that currently available conditioning regimens alone are incapable of eradicating myeloma. Although relapse rates are high after allogeneic bone marrow transplantation (BMT) in myeloma [8–10], some patients do attain sustained molecular remissions [11] and become long-term disease-free survivors [8–10,12,13]. This suggests that an immunological graft-versus-tumor effect similar to the well-characterized graft-versus-leukemia [GVL] reactions [14] operates in the setting of allogeneic transplantation for myeloma.

II. CLINICAL EVIDENCE

A number of reports have described the exploitation of a graft-versus-myeloma (GVM) reactions in clinical practice [15–22]. The first attempt at harnessing GVM was reported by Or et al. [15] in a patient with recurrent multiple extramedullary plasmacytomas and IgA paraproteinemia. The patient received a T cell–

depleted allograft from her sibling, followed by graded increments of donor T cells at weekly intervals, to achieve a graft-versus-tumor effect. The treatment resulted in complete eradication of all tumor masses and normalization of serum immunoglobulin levels. The patient was in complete remission (CR) 4 years after transplantation [15] and remains in continuous CR at 10 years (Reuven Or, personal communication).

Pavord et al. [16] administered interferon-α2b to a patient with IgA myeloma relapsing three months after T-cell nondepleted allogeneic BMT from an HLA-identical sibling. The patient developed cutaneous GVHD after 2 weeks of interferon (IFN). The paraprotein level remained stable, and GVHD resolved after IFN was discontinued. Collins et al. [17] described a patient with primary refractory myeloma who did not respond to a T-cell nondepleted allograft from an HLA-identical sibling. Four months after transplant, 1.63×10^8 mononuclear cells per kilogram were infused, followed 4 weeks later by IFN-α. CR was attained 4 months after the cell infusion. Although the patient relapsed 2 months later, the disease burden remained low, and the patient was reportedly alive with disease 2 years after immunotherapy [17].

Verdonck et al. [18] reported two patients who experienced recurrent myeloma after T cell–depleted BMT. Both had received 10^5 T cells per kilogram at the time of the original graft. CR was attained in both patients in conjunction with GVHD after administration of $>10^8$ T cells per kilogram. Both the patients were reportedly alive in CR at 2 years and 8 months [18].

Tricot et al. [19] reported a patient who experienced recurrent disease after a T cell–depleted transplant from an HLA-identical unrelated donor. An initial infusion of a small amount of cryopreserved peripheral blood containing 10^6 total nucleated cells per kilogram resulted in no apparent antitumor effect. Subsequently, an infusion of 1.2×10^6 T cells per kilogram in 100 mL of donor blood resulted in acute GVHD and CR. The patient eventually developed chronic GVHD and died of a fungal infection while on immunosuppressive therapy. She had recurrent disease at the time of death. Figure 1 shows the complete clinical course of this patient. A subsequent report described three more patients allografted with T cell–depleted marrow from unrelated donors at the University of Arkansas in whom responses were seen after donor leukocyte infusions (DLI), but GVHD and death due to infectious complications or toxicity was the eventual outcome in all [20].

Aschan et al. [21] described two patients who were treated with a combination of DLI and interleukin-2 (IL-2) for relapse after T-cell nondeleted BMT from HLA-identical siblings. The first had responded partially to a previous DLI without cytokines but did not respond to combined cell-cytokine therapy. No GVHD was seen in this patient. The second patient attained CR after combination immunotherapy, which resulted in GVHD.

In a multicenter study of 140 patients with malignant diseases relapsing

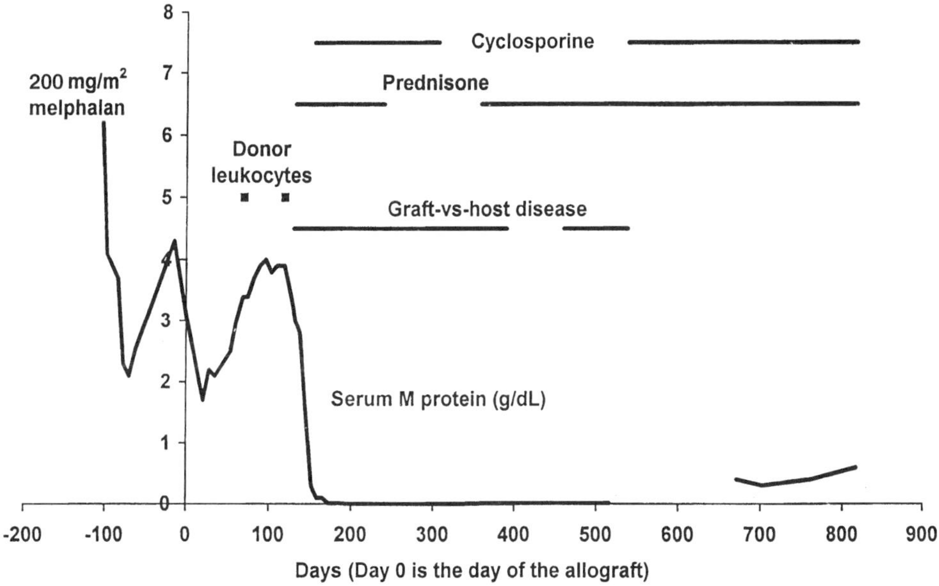

Figure 1 Correlation between graft-versus-host disease and graft-versus-myeloma [19]. The first DLI contained 10^6 nucleated cells per kilogram and the second contained 1.2×10^6 CD3+ cells per kilogram.

after allogeneic transplantation, Collins et al. [22] reported CR in two of four evaluable meyeloma patients receiving DLI from family donors.

Unlike Pavord et al. [16], Verdonck et al. [18] and Tricot et al. [19], whose patients had systemic disease recurrence with marrow plasmacytosis, Bertz et al. [23] treated a patient whose marrow was in remission but who developed multiple cutaneous plasmacytomas after T-cell nondepleted allogeneic BMT. The patient developed acute and chronic GVHD after combined intervention with cessation of immunosuppression, infusion of 6.2×10^7 T cells per kilogram, and administration of IFN-α. All the plasmacytomas disappeared with the immunotherapy, and the patient was reportedly in CR with extensive chronic GVHD [23].

In a cooperative study from the Netherlands, Lokhorst et al. [24] updated their initial report [18] of 2 patients and provided data on 11 more patients treated with DLI. All 13 had originally received T cell–depleted grafts from HLA-identical siblings. These 13 patients were treated with 29 courses of DLI containing 1×10^6 to 3.3×10^8 T cells per kilogram. CR was observed in 4 patients and partial remission (PR) in 4. A of total of 10 patients were alive at the time of the report; 2 in CR.

The infusion of CD8-depleted donor leukocytes (CD4+ cells) was reported to cause regression of relapsed disease in three of four patients who had been allografted from HLA-identical siblings using CD6-depleted marrow [25]. Response was associated with GVHD in all three patients.

Of 97 patients allografted at the University of Arkansas, 30 relapsed following transplantation [26]. While 24 died of recurrent disease or complications of further therapy (including attempts to elicit GVM) [20], 6 survive in CR or PR after various approaches to elicit GVM [24]. These approaches included, in varying combinations, withdrawal of immunosuppression, DLI, and administration of IFN-α or IL-2.

The available data suggest that it is possible to elicit GVM in patients relapsing after T cell–depleted as well as nondepleted grafts.

III. ARE GVHD AND GVM SEPARABLE?

Graft-versus-leukemia (GVL) reactions after allogeneic BMT (''primary GVL'') do operate in the absence of clinically detectable GVHD [14]. However, the relationship between GVHD and GVL is very strong in the setting of adoptive immunotherapy of relapsed disease (''salvage GVL''), especially in patients with acute leukemia [22,27,28]. Although the data are limited, a small number of allografted myeloma patients do appear to survive in CR long term without having developed GVHD [12,13]. Therefore, GVHD may not be essential for ''primary GVM'' after allografting.

However, whether this holds true for patients who undergo immunotherapy for disease recurring after allogeneic transplantation (''salvage GVM'') is not known. Table 1 outlines the correlation between GVHD and GVM in the pub-

Table 1 Relationship Between Graft-Versus-Myeloma and Graft-Versus-Host Disease (GVHD)

Author [Reference]	Number of Patients	GVHD	Response
Aschan [21]	2	No	1 (partial)
Bertz [23]	1	Yes	Yes
Collins [17]	1	Yes	Yes
Lokhorst [24]	13	9 (acute) 7 (chronic)	7 (1 without acute GVHD) 6 (all with chronic GVHD)
Orsini [25]	4	3	3 (all with GVHD)
Pavord [16]	1	Yes	No
Tricot [20]	4	4	4

lished reports of immunotherapy of relapsed myeloma. Clearly, the relationship between GVHD and response is very strong in the setting of salvage therapy.

Figure 1 shows the complete clinical course of the patient originally reported by Tricot et al. [19,20]. As the figure shows, GVHD continued to remain a problem, but the myeloma stayed in remission while there was active GVHD. As GVHD improved on combined immunosuppression with cyclosporine and prednisone, the disease recurred. The patient eventually died of an opportunistic infection secondary to the immunosuppressive therapy, with detectable paraprotein in the serum. The clinical course of this patient is strikingly similar to that of another patient we have treated with secondary acute myeloid leukemia whose disease recurred coincidentally with improvement in GVHD [29] and who died of relapse when GVHD resolved on intermittent methotrexate (unpublished data).

In an elegant experiment, the Dana-Farber group studied the T cell–receptor repertoire in four patients with relapsed myeloma who received CD4+ lymphocytes from HLA-identical siblings [25]. Clonal T-cell populations emerged after DLI in each of the three responding patients. Some clones appeared within 3 months after DLI, and coincident with disease response, whereas other clones appeared later, coincident with the development of GVHD. Sensitive polymerase chain reaction (PCR) studies of CDR III region sequences and a semi-quantitative hybridization assay for the junctional region of each clone showed that the early clones (temporally associated with GVM) were detectable by PCR in patient blood samples before DLI and expanded at least 10-fold in the first 3 months after DLI. In contrast, the late clones (temporally associated with GVHD) were not detectable either prior to DLI or in the first 3 months after DLI. These findings suggest that DLI may mediate antitumor activity through an indirect effect on preexisting T-cell populations, whereas the induction of GVHD may be mediated through new T-cell populations developing after DLI [25]. These data suggest that GVHD and GVM may potentially be separable.

The University of Arkansas approach to separate GVM and GVHD consists of the administration of donor cells transduced with the herpes simplex virus thymidine kinase (TK) gene after T cell–depleted BMT [30,31]. Transduction of the viral TK suicide gene permits specific cell kill on administration of ganciclovir. Laboratory data show that adequate numbers of TK-transduced lymphocytes can be selected efficiently with >90% purity and the selected cells remain functional; 24 h of exposure to ganciclovir at clinically achievable concentration kills >90% of the selected cells, and ganciclovir can kill TK-transduced cells in vivo [30]. Patients with persistent or recurrent disease after T cell–depleted allogenic BMT receive TK-marked cells followed electively by ganciclovir 3 weeks later [31]. In the absence of response or GVHD, a second DLI is administered 6 weeks after the first. Ganciclovir is then administered only if there is GVHD. Dose escalation of TK-marked cells has been planned from 1×10^6 T cells per kilogram to 5, 10, 20, and 50×10^6 T cells per kilogram in cohorts of three patients each. None of the three patients receiving both infusions at the first dose level developed GVHD, and one patient experienced a reduction of monoclonal protein and marrow plasmacytosis. The TK-marked cells were detectable 6 weeks after the second infusion in the absence of ganciclovir therapy in all patients.

The 3-week interval to ganciclovir administration was based on the phenomenon seen in one patient (Figure 1), where it was felt that the entire antitumor effect was completed in the first 2 weeks prior to the onset of GVHD [19]. However, in light of the Dana-Farber data, this assumption is not necessarily true. Also, as most other reports show, the time taken to respond is generally several weeks. A better way may be to monitor T-cell clones after DLI and withhold ganciclovir as long as no new clones appear to emerge. Ganciclovir could be administered when there is clinical evidence of GVHD or appearance of new T-cell clones.

We are currently trying to induce GVM in a patient who has relapsed after T cell–depleted BMT from an unrelated donor. Despite three infusions of TK-marked cells, one infusion of CD8-depleted cells, one infusion of a small quantity of frozen peripheral donor blood after chemotherapy, and one infusion of fresh donor buffy coat, neither GVHD nor response has been seen (unpublished data). This suggests indirectly that some amount of GVHD may be necessary for GVM.

The right balance between ongoing GVHD, with its morbidity but action against myeloma on the one hand, and treatment of GVHD with its own infectious complications, as well as compromised GVM, is difficult to achieve. One potential way of doing this is to treat only patients whose GVHD is progressive and to avoid immunosuppressive therapy when GVHD is limited. When GVHD is treated, the use of single agents other than corticosteroids may be considered to avoid severe immunosuppression. In patients with GVHD, especially those requiring intensive immunosuppression including corticosteroids, attention to broad-spectrum antimicrobial prophylaxis is critical [32] to avoid deaths [20] due to opportunistic infections.

IV. TIME TO RESPONSE

Low-grade lymphoid malignancies take time to respond after high-dose therapy and autologous or allogeneic transplantation [33,34]. Similarly, time to response after induction of GVL for relapsed disease may also be prolonged, especially with diseases such as chronic myeloid [22] or lymphocytic [35] leukemia.

Table 2 shows the time to response in relapsed myeloma from the published reports where these data are available. It appears that it could take some weeks for a response to be seen and months to attain CR. The apparently short time to response after the second DLI in the patient described by Tricot et al. [19] may have been due to the HLA disparity (unrelated donor) or due to a rapid expansion

Table 2 Time to Disease Response After Immunotherapy for Myeloma Relapsing After Allogeneic Transplantation[a]

Author [Reference]	Time to Initial Response	Time To Complete Remission
Collins [17]	Not specified	4 months
Tricot [20][b]	2 weeks	7 weeks
Lokhorst [24]	Median 6 weeks (range, 4–10 weeks)	Not specified
Bertz [23][c]	5 weeks	10 weeks

[a] All donors except the one reported by Tricot et al. are HLA-identical siblings.

[b] Unrelated donor.

[c] This patient had, sequentially, withdrawal of immunosuppression, donor-cell infusion, and IFN-α. The time shown represents time from withdrawal of immunosuppression. Donor cells were administered 3 weeks after stopping immunosuppression and IFN was started 10 days after donor cells.

of preexisting clones triggered by the first of the two infusions of donor cells [25].

V. THE EFFECT OF THE CELL DOSE ON RESPONSE

Variable cell doses have been used to elicit GVM. Although the Dutch group tried escalating cell doses, they found that the infusion of $>1 \times 10^8$ T cells per kilogram was associated with the best response rates (4 of 6 compared with 4 of 21 infusions containing $<1 \times 10^8$ T cells per kilogram). The two patients who did not respond despite getting high T-cell doses were those who did not develop GVHD. Since GVHD appears to be at least a surrogate marker for subsequent GVM (if not the actual phenomenon responsible for GVM), the correct dose of T cells would appear to be the one that causes some GVHD. Therefore, it is probably reasonable to escalate T-cell dose with each infusion until some GVHD is seen.

The four unrelated donor transplant recipients treated at the University of Arkansas received relatively modest cell doses per kilogram body weight: 1.2×10^6 T cells, 1.2×10^6 T cells, 1.1×10^6 T cells, and 6×10^6 nucleated cells. However, GVHD (and response) was seen in all, indicating that a much smaller number of T cells may be required in the unrelated donor transplant setting to cause GVHD and GVM.

Higher cell doses may be required if the histocompatibility between unrelated donors and recipients is particularly good: an unrelated donor transplant recipient we are treating currently has not developed GVHD despite having received 1×10^6 TK-marked T cells per kilogram twice, 10×10^6 CD4+ cells once, 0.8×10^6 T cells per kilogram during myelosuppression after chemotherapy, and 23×10^6 T cells per kilogram in the steady state. The donor and the recipients share two ancestral haplotypes resulting in very close HLA identity [36].

As a starting point, 0.5 to 1×10^8 T cells per kilogram may be appropriate for HLA-identical sibling transplants and 0.5 to 1×10^6 T cells per kilogram for HLA-mismatched grafts or unrelated donor transplants. Whether T cell doses required to elicit GVHD and GVM would be higher in patients relapsing after T-cell nondepleted grafts is not known.

VI. THE PROBLEM OF EXTRAMEDULLARY RECURRENCE

Isolated extramedullary relapse after allogeneic transplantation is not common in leukemia [37], although this unusual phenomenon appears to be a noticeable problem in patients with acute leukemia treated with immunotherapy for relapse after allograft [28].

The patient described by Bertz et al. [23] had isolated recurrence of extramedullary disease after BMT, which responded to immunotherapy. However, a commoner scenario is extramedullary recurrence following successful immunotherapy of relapsed myeloma, where the marrow often tends to be in CR (unpublished data) [38]. The management of this problem is unsatisfactory. Isolated lesions may be amenable to radiation or intraarterial chemotherapy. However, control of systemic disease probably needs to be maintained through ongoing GVM (GVHD) [29].

We are currently investigating the relationship between CD13 expression and the propensity to develop extramedullary deposits in patients with malignant hematological diseases—leukemia [28] and myeloma—who have been treated with immunotherapy for disease recurrence posttransplant.

VII. PROPHYLACTIC IMMUNOTHERAPY

The ideal way to exploit GVM would be to identify patients at high risk of disease progression on the basis of disease biology or other factors, such as poor immunological reconstitution [39] or lack of GVHD, and augment immune responses in them. With T cell–depleted grafts, this could be accomplished using one or more of graded T-lymphocyte repletion [40] or the administration of IFN-α [41], IFN-γ, or IL-2 [42]. With T-cell nondepleted grafts, this could be accomplished by abbreviating the duration of immunosuppression or administering cytokines. The risk of getting severe GVHD due to immune manipulations in the relatively early stages after transplantation [35] must be carefully weighed against potential benefits.

The idiotype of the myeloma monoclonal protein can be used as a unique tumor-specific antigen. Immunization of the donor with the recipient's myeloma idiotype prior to the harvest can augment T cell–mediated specific immunity against the idiotype protein [43]. There is evidence in a murine B-cell lymphoma model characterized by expression and secretion of clonal immunoglobulin that reconstitution with marrow from idiotype-immune donors can confer protection against subsequent lethal tumor challenge [44]. If the anti-idiotype response is protective in myeloma, this would be a way to selectively boost GVM. Graded infusion of lymphocytes from donors vaccinated with idiotype protein is therefore another avenue to be explored.

Infusion of dendritic cells loaded with the myeloma protein after BMT could also be used to enhance GVM effects of allogeneic transplantation by stimulating T cell–mediated specific immunity.

VIII. GRAFT-VERSUS-MYELOMA INDEPENDENT OF CONVENTIONAL ALLOGENIC TRANSPLANTATION

The high transplant-related mortality seen with allogeneic transplantation significantly decreases long-term disease-free survival [10,26]. Attempts have therefore been made to exploit allogenic GVM effects outside the setting of conventional allogeneic BMT so as to avoid morbidity and mortality [45–48].

These approaches have included conditioning with nonmyeloablative but adequately immunosuppressive regimens to achieve secure alloengraftment, albeit with mixed chimerism because of persistent host hematopoiesis (as well as, probably, persistent disease). This is followed by DLI in gradual increments to convert the mixed chimerism to full donor-type chimerism and eliminate the disease through graft-versus-tumor reactions in the process. Early results are encouraging [45,46].

Another approach has been to exploit ''hit-and-run'' [49,50] graft-versus-tumor effects by infusing haploidentical donor cells in conjunction with a conventional autograft [47]. This has been tried in a small number of patients who were being transplanted for the second or third [47] time. Fatal toxicity, including GVHD, was a serious problem in patients receiving this therapy with their third autografts. Although survival of donor cells for several weeks was seen in the few patients receiving this therapy with their second autografts, all patients eventually relapsed and sufficient data were not available to judge the efficacy of this approach.

Infusion of mononuclear cells from HLA-identical sibling donors has been tried without any preceding conditioning therapy [48]. While almost all patients had donor cells detectable immediately after infusion, a quarter had donor cells detectable more than 4 weeks after infusion and all of these developed GVHD. There appeared to be transient antitumor response in two patients (including one with myeloma) during GVHD. Again, these data are too limited to permit any conclusions about the feasibility or efficacy of this approach.

IX. AUTOLOGOUS GRAFT-VERSUS-MYELOMA

Apart from problems with toxicity, the limited availability of suitably matched donors for allogeneic transplantation makes it accessible only to a minority of patients who are relatively young and fit. Because of their safety, exploitation of graft-versus-tumor reactions in the autologous setting is potentially very attractive [51]. Although a number of studies have shown that a short course of cyclosporine given after autografting can cause a clinical and histological syndrome resembling GVHD in animal models and human beings, antitumor activity has been seen only in a rat model against a plasmacytoma cell line [52]. No antitumor activity was seen against Ia-bearing murine myeloid and lymphoid leukemias [51].

Giralt et al. [53] administered cyclosporine for 28 days after autografting to 14 myeloma patients conditioned with thiotepa, busulfan, and cyclophosphamide. One patient developed skin GVHD which responded to corticosteroids. Six patients developed histological evidence of GVHD without clinical signs. Of 11 patients with evaluable disease, 3 attained remission. One died of treatment-related toxicity, 3 experienced disease progression, and 10 patients are alive without progression at 2–14 months. This suggests that induction of autologous GVHD is feasible and reasonably well tolerated in myeloma patients. There are limited data on its efficacy [54].

Vaccination with the myeloma idiotype protein [55] and infusion of idiotype-pulsed dendritic cells once a minimal residual disease state has been attained after autotransplantation are other potential ways of exploiting immune reactions against myeloma. These responses may require enhancement with cytokines such as the interferons or IL-2.

X. UNANSWERED QUESTIONS

The fact that data are limited means that most questions about GVM, apart from the fact that it does exist, remain unanswered. Table 3 lists important issues that need to be addressed and have been discussed at various places in the text.

Table 3 Unanswered Questions

1.	Can GVHD and GVM be separated?
2.	Which myeloma patients are at high risk of relapse after allografting?
3.	What is the optimum starting cell dose for donor leukocytes for prophylaxis?
4.	What is the optimum starting cell dose for donor leukocytes for treatment of relapse?
5.	How long an interval should be left between two cell infusions?
6.	Should chemotherapy be administered prior to donor leukocytes?
7.	When should cytokines such as IFN-α or IL-2 be used?
8.	Which patients are at a high risk of isolated extramedullary relapse?
9.	How should extramedullary relapse be dealt with when systemic disease is controlled with GVM?
10.	Can GVM be exploited independent of conventional allogeneic transplantation?
11.	Does autologous GVM exist?
12.	Can GVM be exploited without a graft?

XI. APPROACH TO A PATIENT WITH RELAPSED MYELOMA AFTER AN ALLOGRAFT

The best way to treat a relapsed patient would be in the context of much-needed well-designed clinical trials evaluating one or more of the questions outlined in Table 3. In the absence of a study, a reasonable approach depends upon the patient's general condition, the nature of the graft, current immunosuppression, time from transplant, and tumor burden. Figure 2 shows a suggested approach based upon our treatment of leukemia relapsing after allogeneic transplantation [27].

The clinical condition of patients with relapsed disease who are undergoing attempts to induce graft-versus-tumor reactions is often unstable. In addition to intensive supportive therapy including broad-spectrum antimicrobial prophylaxis, the actual treatment plan may need to be changed.

In patients failing to respond to ''standard'' approaches, infusion of donor cells collected after donor vaccination with the myeloma idiotype could be tried. Dendritic cells loaded with the idiotype protein could be administered to the patient after DLI, or donor cells could be collected after stimulation of the donor with dendritic cell infusions.

XII. CONCLUSIONS

GVM effects operate in the setting of donor-cell chimerism after allogeneic BMT and are probably responsible for curing a small number of patients after alloge-

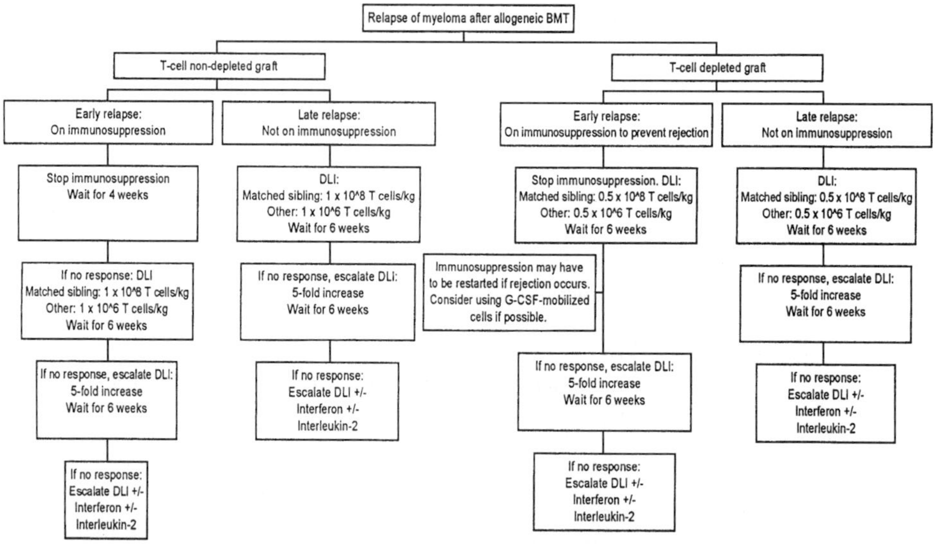

Figure 2 Suggested approach for patients with myeloma relapsing after allogeneic transplantation.

neic BMT. It is not known whether GVM is separable from GVHD in practice. The best way to exploit GVM reactions is unclear, and morbidity of GVHD remains a major problem. There is usually a time lag of a few weeks between immune intervention and disease response. There is a propensity for extramedullary disease recurrence in patients whose marrow disease is controlled with immunological manipulations. Exploration of GVM outside conventional allogeneic transplantation or after autologous transplantation is necessary to increase the number of patients likely to benefit from this phenomenon and to make it safer.

REFERENCES

1. Attal M, Harousseau JL, Stoppa AM, Sotto JJ, Fuzibet JG, Rossi JF, Casassus P, Maisonneuve H, Facon T, Ifrah N; Payen C, Bataille R. A prospective, randomized trial of autologous bone marrow transplantation and chemotherapy in multiple myeloma: Intergroupe Francais du Myeloma. N Engl J Med 1996; 335:91–97.
2. Barlogie B, Jagannath S, Vesole DH, Naucke S, Cheson B, Mattox S, Bracy D, Salmon S, Jacobson J, Crowley J, Tricot G. Superiority of tandem autologous transplantation over standard therapy for previously untreated multiple myeloma. Blood 1997; 89:789–793.

3. Singhal S, Mehta J, Barlogie B. Advances in the treatment of multiple myeloma. Curr Opin Hematol 1997; 4:291–297.
4. Singhal S, Mehta J, Jagannath S, Barlogie B. Hematopoietic stem cell transplantation for myeloma. In: Foley JF, Vose JM, Armitage JO, eds. Current Therapy in Cancer, 2d ed. Philadelphia: Saunders. In preparation.
5. Bensinger WI, Demirer T, Buckner CD, Appelbaum FR, Storb R, Lilleby K, Weiden P, Bluming AZ, Fefer A. Syngeneic marrow transplantation in patients with multiple myeloma. Bone Marrow Transplant 1996; 18:527–531.
6. Gahrton G, Svensson H, Bj''rkstrand B, Apperley J, Carlson K, Cavo M, Ferrant A, Fouillard L, Gratecos N, Gratwohl A, Guilhot F, Lambertenghi G, Milligan DW, Powles RL, Reiffers J, Samson D, Vernant JP. Syngeneic bone marrow transplantation in multiple myeloma. Bone Marrow Transplant 1997; 19(suppl 1):S88.
7. Mehta J, Powles R. Peripheral blood stem cell transplants and autotransplants. In: Whittaker JA, Holmes JA, eds. Leukaemia and Associated Diseases. Oxford: Blackwell, 1998.
8. Bensinger WI, Buckner CD, Anasetti C, Clift R, Storb R, Barnett T, Chauncey T, Shulman H, Appelbaum FR. Allogeneic marrow transplantation for multiple myeloma: an analysis of risk factors on outcome. Blood 1996; 88:2787–2793.
9. Bjorkstrand B, Ljungman P, Svensson H, Hermans J, Alegre A, Apperley J, Blad, J, Carlson K, Cavo M, Ferrant A, Goldstone AH, de Laurenzi A, Majolino I, Marcus R, Prentice HG, Remes K, Samson D, Sureda A, Verdonck LF, Volin L, Gahrton G. Allogeneic bone marrow transplantation versus autologous stem cell transplantation in multiple myeloma: a retrospective case-matched study from the European Group for Blood and Marrow Transplantation. Blood 1996, 88:4711–4718.
10. Mehta J, Tricot G, Jagannath S, Ayers D, Singhal S, Siegel D, Desikan K, Munshi N, Fassas A, Mattox S, Bracy D, Vesole D, Crowley J, Barlogie B. Salvage autologous or allogeneic transplantation for multiple myeloma refractory to or relapsing after a first line autograft? Bone Marrow Transplant 1998; 21:887–892.
11. Bird JM, Russell NH, Samson D. Minimal residual disease after bone marrow transplantation for multiple myeloma: evidence for cure in long-term survivors. Bone Marrow Transplant 1993; 12:651–654.
12. Russell NH, Miflin G, Stainer C, McQuaker JG, Bienz N, Haynes AP, Bessell EM. Allogeneic bone marrow transplant for multiple myeloma. Blood 1997; 89:2610–2611.
13. Kulkarni S, Powles R, Treleaven J, Singhal S, Sastry P, Raje N, Tait D, Mehta J. Allogeneic bone marrow transplantation for multiple myeloma. Blood 1997; 90(suppl 1):389b.
14. Mehta J. Graft-versus-leukemia reactions in clinical bone marrow transplantation. Leuk Lymph 1993; 10:427–432.
15. Or R, Mehta J, Naparstek E, Okon E, Cividalli G, Slavin S. Successful T cell-depleted allogeneic bone marrow transplantation in a child with recurrent multiple extramedullary plasmacytomas. Bone Marrow Transplant 1992; 10:381–382.
16. Pavord S, Sivakumaran M, Durrant S, Chapman C. The role of alpha interferon in the pathogenesis of GVHD. Bone Marrow Transplant 1992; 10:477.
17. Collins RH Jr, Pineiro LA, Nemunaitis JJ, Jain VK, Waxman D, Miller WV, Fay JW. Transfusion of donor buffy coat cells in the treatment of persistent or recurrent

malignancy after allogeneic bone marrow transplantation. Transfusion 1995; 35: 891–898.

18. Verdonck LF, Lokhorst HM, Dekker AW, Nieuwenhuis HK, Petersen EJ. Graft-versus-myeloma effect in two cases. Lancet 1996; 347:800–801.
19. Tricot G, Vesole DH, Jagannath S, Hilton J, Munshi N, Barlogie B. Graft-versus-myeloma effect: proof of principle. Blood 1996; 87:1196–1198.
20. Tricot G, Munshi N, Vesole D, Jagannath S, Desikan KR, Siegel D, Barlogie B. Graft versus myeloma effect: risks and benefits. In: Dicke KA, Keating A, eds. Autologous Marrow and Blood Transplantation: Proceedings of the Eighth International Symposium, Arlington, Texas. Charlottesville, TX: Carden Jennings, 1997: 225–232.
21. Aschan J, Lönnqvist B, Ringdén O, Kumlien G, Gahrton G. Graft-versus-myeloma effect. Lancet 1996; 348:346.
22. Collins RH Jr., Shpilberg O, Drobyski WR, Porter DL, Giralt S, Champlin R, Goodman SA, Wolff SN, Hu W, Verfaillie C, List A, Dalton W, Ognoskie N, Chetrit A, Antin JH, Nemunaitis J. Donor leukocyte infusions in 140 patients with relapsed malignancy after allogeneic bone marrow transplantation. J Clin Oncol 1997; 15: 433–444.
23. Bertz H, Burger JA, Kunzmann R, Mertelsmann R, Finke J. Adoptive immunotherapy for relapsed multiple myeloma after allogeneic bone marrow transplantation (BMT): evidence for a graft-versus-myeloma effect. Leukemia 1997; 11:281–283.
24. Lokhorst HM, Schattenberg A, Cornelissen JJ, Thomas LLM, Verdonck LF. Donor leukocyte infusions are effective in relapsed multiple myeloma after allogeneic bone marrow transplantation. Blood 1997; 90:4206–4211.
25. Orsini E, Alyea EP, Schlossman R, Soiffer RJ, Anderson KC, Ritz J. Expansion of pre-existing clonal populations following donor lymphocyte infusion for relapsed multiple myeloma after allogeneic bone marrow transplantation. Blood 1997; 90(suppl 1):549a.
26. Mehta J, Ayers D, Mattox S, Singhal S, Siegel D, Fassas A, Hilton J, Anaissie E, Desikan K, Munshi N, Jagannath S, Tricot G, Barlogie B. Allogeneic bone marrow transplantation in multiple myeloma: single-center experience of 97 patients. Blood 1997; 90(suppl 1):225a.
27. Mehta J, Powles R, Treleaven J, Kulkarni S, Singhal S. Induction of graft-versus-host disease as immunotherapy of leukemia relapsing after allogeneic transplantation: single center experience of 32 adult patients. Bone Marrow Transplant 1997; 20:129–135.
28. Singhal S, Powles R, Kulkarni S, Treleaven J, Mehta J. Immunotherapy of acute leukemia relapsing after allogeneic transplantation: the inseparability of GVHD and graft-vs-leukemia, and the problem of extramedullary relapse. Blood 1997; 90(suppl 1):547a.
29. Singhal S, Powles R, Treleaven J, Mehta J. Sensitivity of secondary acute myeloid leukemia relapsing after allogeneic bone marrow transplantation to immunotherapy with interferon-α2b. Bone Marrow Transplant 1997; 19:1151–1153.
30. Munshi NC, Govindarajan R, Drake R, Ding LM, Iyer R, Saylors R, Kornbluth J, Marcus S, Chiang Y, Ennist D, Kwak L, Reynolds C, Tricot G, Barlogie B. Thymidine kinase (TK) gene-transduced human lymphocytes can be highly purified, remain fully functional, and are killed efficiently with ganciclovir. Blood 1997; 89: 1334–1340.

31. Munshi NC, Tricot G, Jagannath S, Mehta J, Desikan K, Siegle S, Singhal S, Fassas A, Fink L, Schichman S, Chiang Y, Reynolds C, Barlogie B. Clinical results of thymidine kinase (TK) gene transduced donor lymphocyte infusion following allogeneic transplantation in myeloma. Blood 1997; 90(suppl 1):111a.
32. Mehta J, Powles R, Singhal S, Riley U, Treleaven J, Catovsky D. Antimicrobial prophylaxis to prevent opportunistic infections in patients with chronic lymphocytic leukemia after allogeneic blood or marrow transplantation. Leuk Lymph 1997; 26: 83–88.
33. Jarque I, Palau J, Sanz GF, Guinot M, Gomis F, Martin G, Martinez J; Sanz MA. Delayed complete response after allogeneic bone marrow transplantation in chronic lymphocytic leukemia. Blood 1993; 82:1036–1038.
34. Singhal S, Powles R, Milan S, Raje N, Viner C, Treleaven J, Cunningham D, Mehta J. Clearance of paraprotein after autografting for multiple myeloma. Bone Marrow Transplant 1995; 16:537–540.
35. Mehta J, Powles R, Singhal S, Iveson T, Treleaven J, Catovsky D. Clinical and hematologic response of chronic lymphocytic and prolymphocytic leukemia persisting after allogeneic bone marrow transplantation with the onset of acute graft-versus-host disease: possible role of graft-versus-leukemia. Bone Marrow Transplant 1996; 17:371–375.
36. Christiansen FT, Witt CS, Dawkins RL. Questions in marrow matching: the implications of ancestral haplotypes for routine practice. Bone Marrow Transplant 1991; 8:83–86.
37. Bekassy AN, Hermans J, Gorin NC, Gratwohl A. Granulocytic sarcoma after allogeneic bone marrow transplantation: a retrospective European multicenter survey. Acute and Chronic Leukemia Working Parties of the European Group for Blood and Marrow Transplantation. Bone Marrow Transplant 1996; 17:801–808.
38. Zomas A, Stefanoudaki K, Fisfis M, Papadaki T, Mehta J. Graft-versus-myeloma after donor leukocyte infusion: maintenance of marrow remission but extramedullary relapse with plasmacytomas. Bone Marrow Transplant. 1998; 21:1163–1165.
39. Powles R, Singhal S, Treleaven J, Kulkarni S, Horton C, Mehta J. Identification of patients who may benefit from prophylactic immunotherapy after bone marrow transplantation for acute myeloid leukemia on the basis of lymphocyte recovery after transplantation. Blood 1998; 91:3481–3486.
40. Naparstek E, Or R, Nagler A, Cividalli G, Engelhard D, Aker M, Gimon Z, Manny N, Sacks T, Tochner Z, Weiss L, Samuel S, Brautbar C, Hale G, Waldmann H, Steinberg SM, Slavin S. T-cell-depleted allogeneic bone marrow transplantation for acute leukaemia using Campath-1 antibodies and post-transplant administration of donor's peripheral blood lymphocytes for prevention of relapse. Br J Haematol 1995; 89: 506–515.
41. Samson D, Volin L, Schanz U, Bosi A, Gahrtron G. Feasibility and toxicity of interferon maintenance therapy after allogeneic BMT for multiple myeloma: a pilot study of the EBMT. Bone Marrow Transplant 1996; 17:759–762.
42. Soiffer RJ, Murray C, Gonin R, Ritz J. Effect of low-dose interleukin-2 on disease relapse after T-cell-depleted allogeneic bone marrow transplantation. Blood 1994; 84:964–971.
43. Kwak LW, Taub DD, Duffey PL, Bensinger WI, Bryant EM, Reynolds CW, Longo

DL. Transfer of myeloma idiotype-specific immunity from an actively immunised marrow donor. Lancet 1995; 345:1016–1020.

44. Kwak LW, Pennington R, Longo DL. Active immunization of murine allogeneic bone marrow transplant donors with B-cell tumor-derived idiotype: a strategy for enhancing the specific antitumor effect of marrow grafts. Blood 1996; 87:3053–3060.
45. Giralt S, Cohen A, Mehra R, Gajewski J, Andersson B, Przepiorka D, Khouri I, Korbling M, Davis M, van Besien K, Ippoliti C, Bruton J, Anderlini P, Ueno N, Champlin R. Preliminary results of fludarabine/melphalan or 2CDA/melphalan as preparative regimens for allogeneic progenitor cell transplantation in poor candidates for conventional myeloablative conditioning. Blood 1997; 90(suppl 1):417a.
46. Slavin S, Nagler A, Naparstek E, Ackerstein A, Kapelushnik Y, Varadi G, Kirschbaum M, Ben-Yosef R, Samuel S, Or R. Successful replacement of conventional allogeneic bone marrow or blood stem cell transplantation with well-tolerated non-myeloablative conditioning for the treatment of malignant and non-malignant diseases. Blood 1997; 90(suppl 1):534a.
47. Singhal S, Mehta J, Hood S, Mattox S, Siegel D, Fassas A, Desikan K, Anaissie E, Tricot G, Jagannath S, Barlogie B. Third transplants for myeloma relapsing after two prior autografts. Blood 1997; 90(suppl 1):547a.
48. Porter DL, Connors JM, Doyle B, McGarigle C, Saidman S, VanDeerlin V, Leonard D, Antin JH. Donor leukocyte infusions as primary allogeneic adoptive immunotherapy for patients with malignancies. Blood 1997; 90(suppl 1):549a.
49. Mehta J, Powles R, Singhal S, Horton C, Treleaven J. Outcome of autologous rescue after failed engraftment of allogeneic marrow. Bone Marrow Transplant 1996; 17:213–217.
50. Mehta J, Singhal S. Graft failure: diagnosis and management. In: Barrett AJ, Treleaven J, eds. The Clinical Practice of Stem Cell Transplantation. London: Isis, 1998.
51. Singhal S, Vourka-Karussis U, Mehta J, Slavin S, Weiss L. Failure of cyclosporine to induce graft-vs-host disease or graft-vs-leukemia after syngeneic bone marrow transplantation in mice. Leuk Res 1996; 20:941–946.
52. Geller RB, Esa AH, Beschorner WE, Frondoza CG, Santos GW, Hess AD. Successful in vitro graft-versus-tumor effect against an Ia-bearing tumor using cyclosporine-induced syngeneic graft-versus-host disease in the rat. Blood 1989; 74:1165–1171.
53. Giralt S, Weber D, Colome M, Dimopoulos M, Mehra R, van Besien K, Gajewski J, Andersson B, Khouri I, Przepiorka D, von Wolff B, Delasalle K, Korbling M, Seong D, Alexanian R, Champlin R. Phase I trial of cyclosporine-induced autologous graft-versus-host disease in patients with multiple myeloma undergoing high-dose chemotherapy with autologous stem-cell rescue. J Clin Oncol 1997; 15:667–673.
54. Byrne JL, Carter GI, Ellis I, Haynes AP, Russell NH. Autologous GVHD following PBSCT, with evidence for a graft-versus-myeloma effect. Bone Marrow Transplant 1997; 20:517–520.
55. Kwak LW, Sternas LA, Jagannath S, Siegel D, Munshi NC, Barlogie B. T cell responses elicited by immunization of multiple myeloma patients with idiotypic M-protein plus GM-CSF in remission after autologous transplantation. Blood 1997; 90(suppl 1):579a.

11
The Graft-Versus-Tumor Effect

Richard W. Childs and John Barrett
National Institutes of Health
Bethesda, Maryland

I. INTRODUCTION

Given justified concerns of high treatment-related mortality in a setting of unproven efficacy, few have attempted or even considered allotransplantation in patients with nonhematological malignancies. However, the demonstration of potent antileukemia effects following allogeneic BMT for a diversity of hematological malignancies [1–4] begs the question whether similar beneficial alloresponses can be used to eradicate solid tumors. From our knowledge of the GVL response, we can define the characteristics of a tumor that should make it susceptible to a graft-versus-tumor (GVT) effect. Indeed, allograft studies in mouse tumor models described by Slavin et al. in Chapter 12 demonstrate unequivocal GVT effects. Nevertheless, human solid tumors and hematological malignancies differ in some quite fundamental ways. Assumptions about GVT made by analogy with the GVL effect may not always be valid. In Table 1 the arguments for and against a GVT effect are set out.

Support for an alloimmune response to tumors comes from the demonstration of an autologous antitumor response, notably in malignant melanoma and renal cell carcinoma. The occurrence of T cells, which can in some circumstances recognize and efficiently lyse tumor, supports the possibility of a therapeutic effect from a T-cell allograft. In favor of a GVT effect is the fact that many tumors arise from the same tissues that are the direct target of GVHD damage. In theory therefore, all carcinomas arising from epithelial and endothelial surfaces and specialized organs derived from these tissues (e.g., keratinocytes, fibroblasts, exocrine glands, hepatobiliary tree, gastrointestinal tract, and lungs) should be susceptible to GVT effects [5,6]. Tumors arising in other tissues that are notably

Table 1 Arguments for and Against a GVT Effect

In favor of GVT
Tumors arising in tissues that are targets of cytotoxic damage in GVHD could also be susceptible to immune-mediated damage and control.
Tumors posessing MHC class I and II, ICAM-1, B7.1, and Fas should be targets of T-cell attack.
There is evidence of autologous antitiumor immune responses in some malignancies. Alloresponses are likely to be at least as powerful.
Alloreacting T cells can recognize a wide range of antigens on the recipient's malignant cells (minor histocompatibility antigens, alleles of tumor specific antigens [TSA]).
Clinical graft-versus-malignancy effects are being demonstrated in a widening range of diseases (leukemias, lymphomas, myeloma and some solid tumors).
Against GVT
Tumors arising in tissues not involved in GVHD are less likely to be suitable targets of alloreacting T cells. Tumors are notoriously adapted to escape from immune control.
Posttransplant immune deficiency may favor tumor progression.
GVT effects may be abrogated following the establishment of tolerance posttransplant.
Large tumor masses may limit complete infiltration by tumor infiltrating lymphocytes (TIL).
Delayed second malignancies may develop following bone marrow transplants.

uninvolved in GVHD reactions (e.g., muscle, nervous system, and renal tract) may, by the same argument, be immune to GVT effects. Tumor lysis by allogeneic CTL or NK/LAK cells, or proliferation inhibition by cytokines, are prerequisites for a GVT effect. From our understanding of GVL, the tumor-cell characteristics necessary to generate a successful GVT response would include slow proliferation (matching the relatively slow pace of the T-cell response), presence on the cell surface of MHC class I and II molecules, costimulatory molecules (CD80, CD86), adhesion molecules such as the ICAMs, and Fas expression [7,8]. Many malignancies possess some or all of these characteristics. However, it should also be noted that solid tumors may often be well adapted to escape immune-mediated killing. Locus- or allele-specific down-regulation of MHC molecules is a common mechanism whereby tumor cells escape T-cell attack [9,10]. In addition, aberrations in the number of MHC molecules on the surface of tumor cells such as melanoma have been shown to quantitatively affect their lysis by cytotoxic T lymphocytes. Increased concentrations of membrane-bound Fas ligand [12] as well as tumor-cell secretion of soluble inhibitory factors such as IL-10 [13] or transforming growth factor beta (TGF-β) [14] may all lead to immune escape from tumor infiltrating lymphocytes (TIL). Additional concerns related to transplanting patients with solid tumors include the fact that bone marrow allografts actually predispose to secondary malignancies. Malignancies particularly appearing as late effects of marrow allografting include malignant melanoma; non-Hodgkin's lymphomas; cancers of the buccal cavity, liver, brain, central nervous system, thyroid, bone, and connective tissue. The occurrence of these second cancers relates in part to the mutagenic effect of high-dose chemotherapy/radiation and in part to the immunodeficiency of chronic GVHD. After total body irradiation, second malignancies are being increasingly reported as long-term effects become better defined [15,16].

In designing allogeneic transplantation protocols for patients with solid tumors, it would be an advantage to minimize these risks by reducing the intensity of the preparative regimen and by attempting to ensure rapid immune reconstitution so as to maintain immune regulation of the tumor. T cell–replete, nonmyeloablative regimens that incorporate early cyclosporine withdrawal with delayed donor lymphocyte infusions (described later in this chapter) go some way to achieving these aims. Preliminary data suggest a significant reduction in treatment related mortality versus conventional marrow cell transplantation [17,18].

II. STRATEGIES FOR INDUCING GVT EFFECTS WITH ALLOGENEIC STEM-CELL TRANSPLANT (SCT)

The reasons for exploiting possible alloimmune responses to solid tumors are several: First, the allograft provides the opportunity to attack the tumor with the donor immune system, which is intact and unsuppressed by chemotherapy and has yet to develop tolerance to the malignancy. In addition, patients with growing tumors may lack the T-cell repetoire necessary to recognize and destroy the tumor, analogous to what is sometimes seen in patients with leukemia [19]. Finally, over and above the presentation of known tumor-specific antigens, the malignant cells may present a diversity of alloantigens to the donor immune system, which could induce powerful immunodominant responses [6,20,21].

A. The Donor-Antitumor Response

From what is already known about GVL, the response by donor T cells to the tumor is likely to be greatest when unmanipulated transplants are performed. There is a theoretical risk that the immunosuppression given to establish engraftment of the donor cells may accelerate disease progression in a tumor that has hitherto been held in check by the recipient's immunity. For this reason, a prudent approach to the allografting of tumors would be to use a T cell–replete allograft that would initiate immune competence as rapidly as possible. While GVHD inevitably requires control and suppression, it would be important to attempt to avoid the establishment of tolerance of the donor to recipient malignant tissues. In the absence of severe GVHD, therefore, withdrawal of immunosuppressive agents such as cyclosporine followed by the administration of donor lymphocyte transfusions posttransplant to amplify GVT effects should also be considered. In tumors where dose intensification is not effective in controlling disease or prolonging survival, low-intensity nonmyeloablative protocols similar to those described by Slavin et al. for hematological disorders are likely to find increasing application [17]. Such regimens may be associated with less severe GVHD, allowing larger numbers of donor lymphocytes to be safely transferred for a greater antitumor effect. Other treatment modalities that might enhance GVT could be brought to bear posttransplant. These include the use of interferons to upregulate MHC and costimulatory molecules on the tumor and interleukin-2 (IL-2) to enhance T-cell cytotoxicity [8,18]. Donor antigen-presenting cells such as dendritic cells could be pulsed with tumor-specific peptide and used for the ex vivo expansion of tumor-specific donor T cells. These tumor-specific cells could then be infused posttransplant to provide a specific GVT effect. In addition, vaccine strategies to induce donor T-cell responses to known tumor proteins and peptides could also be used to stimulate a GVT effect.

B. Tumor Antigens

There are a number of tumor-associated antigens (TAA) that might serve as targets for T cells, including nonmutated self peptides derived from tissue-specific proteins (e.g., MART-1, gp100), tumor-specific shared antigens (e.g., MAGE, BAGE, CAGE family) and tumor-specific unique antigens resulting from mutated epitopes expressed in tumors (e.g., β-catenin, MUM-1, CDK4, Her-2neu) [45]. Table 2 lists these and other classes of antigens that might be targets of donor immune cells. It will be of importance to determine whether TAA exist in allelic forms, since this would open up the exciting possibility that novel and powerful allo responses to these proteins could be induced in donors not possessing the recipient's alleles. In addition to T cell interactions with TAA, allo responses could be directed against tissue minor histocompatibility antigens (mHA) which are restricted to tumor tissue or ubiquitously expressed [6]. These latter antigens would be likely to induce both GVT and GVH responses.

1. Stem-Cell Transplants for Solid Tumors in Humans

The clinical experience with stem-cell allografts in solid tumors is scanty and at best anecdotal. To date, there are only a few case reports where allogeneic bone marrow or lymphocytes have been clearly implicated to induce a GVT effect in nonhematologic malignancies [22,23]. We are currently at the stage where more proof is needed to show that clinically measurable GVT effects occur. Inevitably in the evaluation of an experimental technique, patients with advanced disease who have failed conventional treatment options are the first to be selected. As a

Table 2 Possible Tumor Antigen Targets of GVT

1. Overexpressed normal tissue-restricted proteins
   MART-1 (Melan-A), BAGE, gp75, gp100, tyrosinase, TRP-1, TRP-2, Her2neu
2. Tumor-specific shared antigens (expressed in tumors, testis, and pancreas)
   MAGE, BAGE, CAGE family
3. Tumor-specific unique antigens
   Beta catenin, MUM-1, CDK-4
4. Oncofetal proteins
   CEA (carcinoembryonic antigen)
5. Allelic variants of any of the above
6. Protein products of chromosome translocation/mutation
   Such as *t(3;8) adenomas, t(19;20) ovarian cancer t(3;5) renal cell cancer, t(X;18) synovial sarcoma etc.*
7. Minor histocompatibility antigens
   Ubiquitously expressed, tissue-restricted
8. Major histocompatibility antigens
   Classes I and II

consequence, survival is invariably low. However, the following accounts provide the first proof of principle that GVT effects could be used to treat cancers of nonhematological origin.

III. BREAST CANCER

Slavin's group reported attempts to induce GVT effects against solid tumors, using a murine model of mammary adenocarcinoma [44] (see Chapter 12). A cell line isolated from this tumor model was highly tumorigenic in syngeneic or haploidentical mice but was nontumorigenic in a major histocompatibility complex (MHC)–unrelated strain of mice. Twenty-four hours following lethal total-body irradiation, female mice were reconstituted with minor (MiHC) or MHC-mismatched donor bone marrow cells. Some 2 to 3 months following the transplant, recipient mice carrying MiHC- or MHC-mismatched donor cells were inoculated with the breast carcinoma cell line. Chimeras reconstituted with allogeneic donor cells that were MiHC- or MHC-incompatible with tumor cells were able to suppress the development of the primary tumor, which expressed host-type MHC alloantigens, indicating an allogeneic antitumor effect in this model. Slavin's group then went on to investigate whether allogeneic cytokine-activated donor lymphocytes could induce GVT after autologous stem-cell transplants for metastatic breast cancer [23]. Six patients with metastatic breast cancer were studied. After receiving high-dose chemotherapy and peripheral-blood stem-cell transplant (PBSCT), they were treated by adoptive transfer of HLA-matched donor lymphocytes, activated in vivo with human recombinant IL-2. If no GVHD developed, donor lymphocytes preactivated in vitro with rIL-2 were also given. Two patients developed GVHD grade I–II, one of whom showed no evidence of metastatic breast cancer more than 3 years after transplant. The other five patients showed no clear evidence of benefit, with progression-free survival between 7 and 13 months.

In 1996 Eibl et al. were the first to report the use of an allogeneic BMT to induce a GVT effect in breast cancer [22]. A woman with inflammatory breast cancer received an experimental BMT from her HLA-identical sibling. Resolution of liver metastases occurred simultaneously with the onset of GVHD in the first few weeks after transplant. T lymphocytes obtained at the time of GVHD showed MHC class I–restricted cytotoxicity against several breast carcinoma cell lines, suggesting the presence of mHA on the breast tumor cells. The clinical course and the in vitro results suggested that a GVT effect could exist after allogeneic BMT for breast cancer. To evaluate the feasibility of allogeneic peripheral-blood progenitor-cell (PBPC) transplantation and to assess GVT effects in patients with metastatic breast cancer, a group of investigators at the MD Anderson Cancer Center evaluated allogeneic PBPC transplantation in 10 women (median age, 42 years) with chemoresponsive metastatic breast cancer [24]. The patients were prepared with a myeloablative regimen of cyclophosphamide, carmustine, and thiotepa (CBT regimen). GVHD prophylaxis was achieved with cyclosporine or tacrolimus. All patients engrafted with full hematological recovery; 3 developed grade ≥ II acute GVHD and 4 had chronic GVHD. After transplantation, 1 patient was in complete remission (CR), 5 achieved a partial remission (PR), and 4 had stable disease (SD). In 2 patients, metastatic liver lesions regressed in association with skin GVHD after withdrawal of immunosuppression, suggesting a GVT effect. At a median follow-up of 408 days, the median progression-free survival was 238 days. These results showed that allogeneic PBPC transplantation is feasible in patients with poor-risk metastatic breast cancer. Furthermore, the regression of tumor associated with GVHD provides some evidence for a possible GVT effect. However, because of the slow progression of some patients with metastatic breast cancer, longer follow-up and larger studies would be required to properly evaluate a beneficial effect of allografting in this disease.

A. Neuroblastoma

Philip's group investigated allogeneic BMT in children with advanced neuroblastoma in hopes of demonstrating a GVT effect analogous to that seen in patients undergoing allotransplantation for lymphoma [25]. Seventeen children with stage IV neuroblastoma underwent allogeneic BMT following dose-intensive combination chemotherapy. The outcome of these patients was compared retrospectively with that of 34 autologously transplanted patients matched for risk factors. Although there was no difference in response rates, disease-free survival, or overall survival between groups, the relapse rate at 2 years in patients who received an allograft and who developed acute GVHD was lower than that in patients without GVHD (57 versus 78%) suggesting a possible GVT effect.

IV. MALIGNANT MELANOMA

Few tumors carry a worse prognosis than metastatic melanoma, which has a median survival of about 6 months and 5-year survivals of 2–6% [26]. A recent study of over 1500 patients with metastatic melanoma showed no improvement in survival over a 22-year period despite the introduction of a variety of innovative treatments [27]. However, melanoma is exceptional among solid tumors in that abundant data indicate that T-cell immune responses to tumor occur [28]. It has been known for a long time that melanomas can undergo spontaneous regression; biopsies of regressing melanomas contain tumor-infiltrating lymphocytes (TIL) [29]; TIL isolated from melanoma tissue are predominantly CD8+ exhibiting cytotoxicity against both autologous and allogeneic melanoma targets [30]; and adoptive immunotherapy with ex vivo expanded TILs induces tumor regression in some patients [31]. The response to TIL is occasionally accompanied by the appearance of vitiligo, suggesting that there is immune attack against differentiation antigens present on both normal and malignant melanocytes [32]. Approximately 90% of human melanoma lines express HLA alleles necessary for tumor recognition by alloreacting T cells.

Furthermore a number of melanocyte-specific melanosomal antigens have been defined at the peptide level [13]. These peptides are products of melanoma self proteins often found in the normal melanocyte counterpart but overexpressed in the tumor. Such tumor associated antigens (TAAs) are capable of inducing CTL activity against the tumor. There is therefore some justification in exploring the possibility of an allogeneic GVT effect following marrow stem-cell allografts for melanoma. For reasons stated above, the alloimmune GVT effect might be more powerful than the autologous effect because of the ability of the allograft to recognize alloantigenic targets in addition to the known TAA. Furthermore, the transplant opens up the opportunity to overcome tumor tolerance by repeated treatments with lymphocytes from a healthy donor. These lymphocytes have the additional advantage over autologous lymphocytes of being chemotherapy-native and may contain the defective or absent T-cell repertoire necessary to target and destroy tumor cells.

We initiated an experimental protocol at the National Institutes of Health in Bethesda to evaluate a potential GVT effect in malignant melanoma. Eligible patients are those who have failed all standard treatment approaches and have tumor progression despite IL-2 treatment. Dose intensification has proven to be of little value in metastatic melanoma [33], therefore patients were prepared for transplant with a nonmyeloablative but highly immunosuppressive conditioning regimen consisting of fludarabine and cyclophosphamide. To ensure rapid immune recovery, patients received unmanipulated G-CSF–mobilized PBPC transplants containing a high lymphocyte dose (1–4 $\times$ 10^8CD3$^+$ cells/kg) and cyclosporine alone as GVHD prophylaxis. At 30, 60, and 100 days posttransplant, patients were reassessed for lineage-specific chimerism and tumor status by computed tomography scans. On day 30, cyclosporine was tapered and stopped in patients without grade $\geq$ II GVHD. If no GVHD developed, patients then received incremental doses of donor lymphocytes as further adoptive antitumor immunotherapy. Four patients have so far received nonmyeloablative transplants from HLA-identical siblings. One partial response and one mixed response have been seen. A definite GVT has yet to be established in this disease.

A. Renal Cell Cancer

Few advances have been made in the treatment of metastatic renal cell carcinoma (RCC). The disease is largely resistant to hormonal and cytotoxic chemotherapy [34,35], but about 20% of patients respond to IL-2 or interferons [36]. However, treatment-related toxicity can be substantial, and there is no evidence that such immunomodulators prolong survival [37,38]. In RCC, there is some evidence that autologous T lymphocytes exert an immune antitumor response: tumor-infiltrating lymphocytes can be readily isolated from some renal-cell carcinomas and have been shown in vitro to have HLA-restricted specific cytotoxicity against tumor cells [39]. Since RCC has been shown in vitro to be a target for T-cell cytotoxicity and potential renal tissue restricted minor histocompatibility antigens have been described [40], we postulated that a GVT effect might be generated following transplantation of alloreacting lymphocytes recognizing tumor or recipient-specific alloantigens. We therefore initiated an experimental protocol for patients with metastatic RCC resistant to other, more standard treatments. The same approach to transplantation for melanoma was used, namely, a nonmyeloablative immunosuppressive preparative regimen, a T-replete G-CSF mobilized PBPC allograft and posttransplant immune modulation with early discontinuation of cyclosporine, and donor lymphocyte transfusions. The clinical course of the first evaluable patient is described below.

A 50-year-old man developed progressive pulmonary metastasis resistant to IFN-α treatment 7 months after left nephrectomy for stage III renal cell carcinoma. To exploit a possible GVT effect from alloreactive lymphocytes, the patient underwent a nonmyeloablative peripheral blood stem-cell allograft. Conditioning consisted of fludarabine and cyclophosphamide, followed by a T cell–replete granulocyte colony-stimulating factor (G-CSF)–mobilized (PBSCT) from his HLA-identical brother. Cyclosporine was given from days −4 to +45 to prevent acute GVHD. Serial PCR analysis of hematopoietic lineage-specific minisatellites [41] initially showed mixed chimerism in CD15+ myeloid cells, CD3+ T cells, and CD34+ progenitor cells, with rapid conversion to 100% donor T-cell chimerism by day +60 and 100% myeloid cells by day 100. Serial computed tomography scans of the chest showed stable disease at day +30, slight regression of pulmonary lesions at day +63, and complete disappearance of all pulmonary metastatic disease by day +110 (Figure 1). Mild, transient acute GVHD disease of the skin occurred on day +60, not requiring treatment. The regression of metastatic disease, which has now been maintained for 18 months, is compatible with a GVT effect. The patient's course together with chimerism data is illustrated in Figure 2. We attribute the complete regression of biopsy-proven and radiographically progressive pulmonary renal metastasis in this pa-

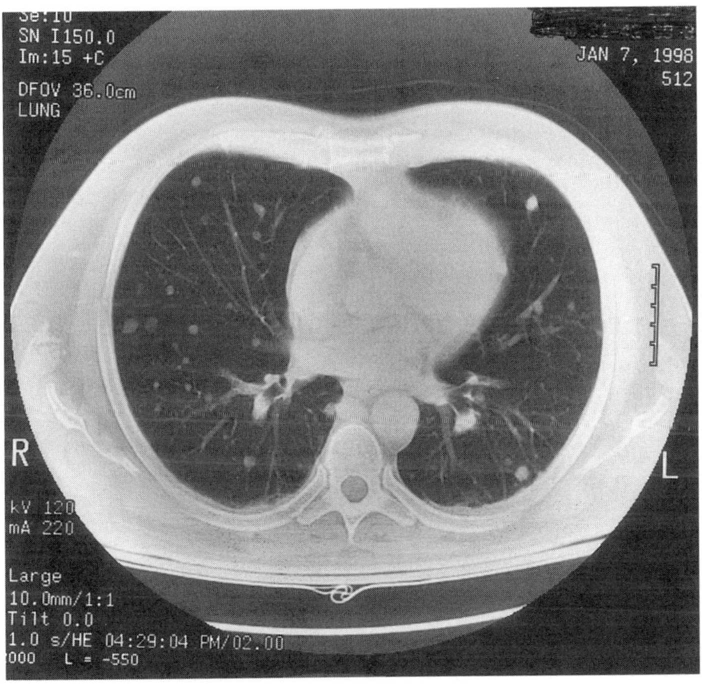

(A)

Figure 1 Serial CT scan images of the same thoracic cut showing extensive pulmonary metastases pretransplant and unchanged day 30 posttransplant (A, B), followed by rapid regression between days 60 (C), 86 (D), and 120 (E).

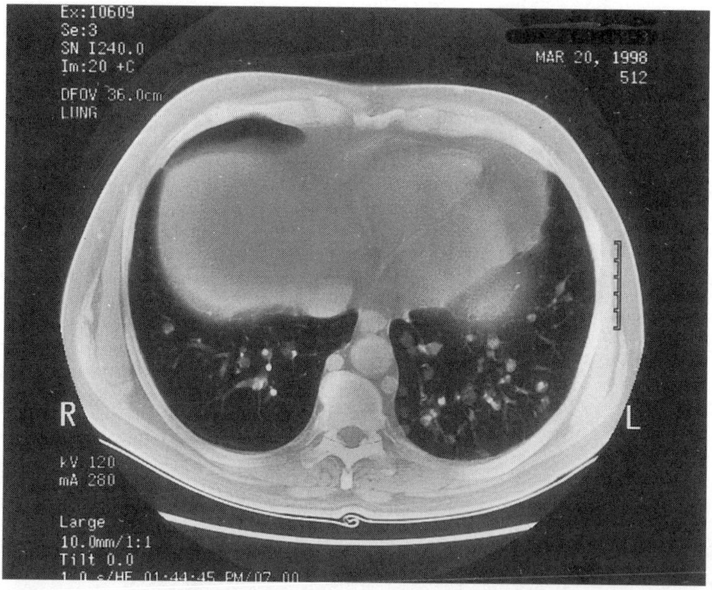

(B)

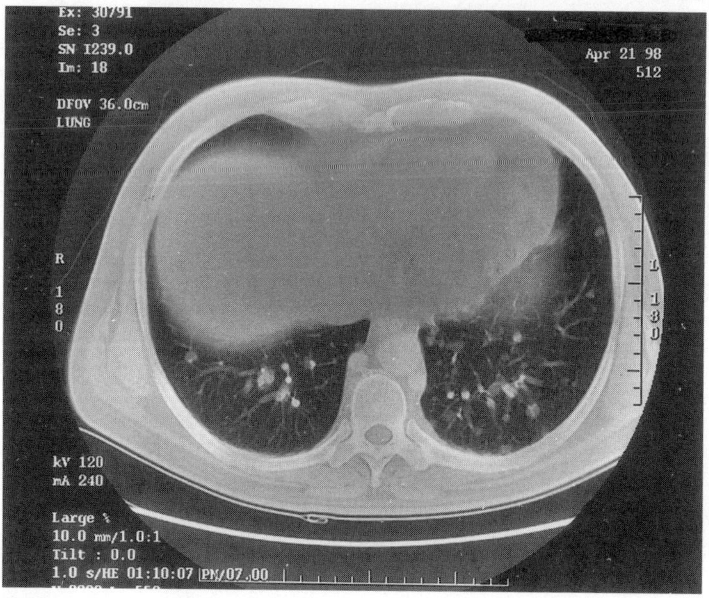

(C)

Figure 1 Continued

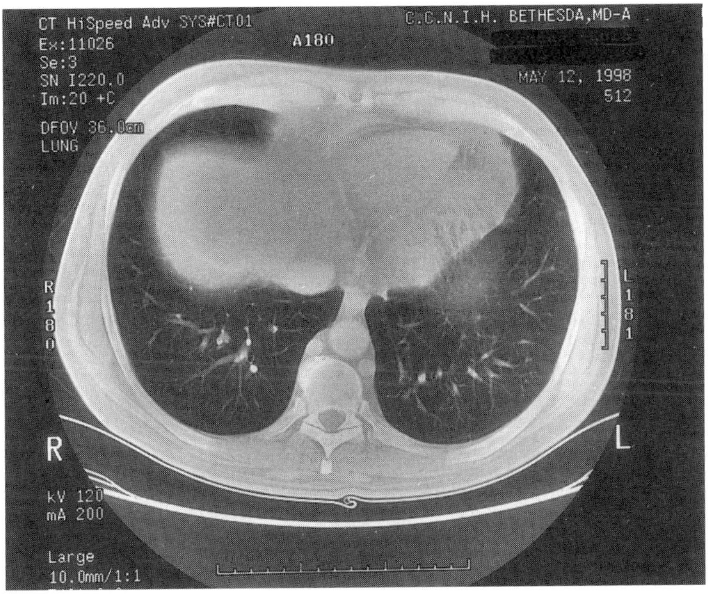
CT HiSpeed Adv SYS#CT01
Ex:11026
Se:3
SN I220.0
Im:20 +C
DFOV 36.0cm
LUNG
A180
C.C.N.I.H. BETHESDA,MD-A
MAY 12, 1998
512
R 180
L 181
R
L
kV 120
mA 200
Large
10.0mm/1:1

(D)

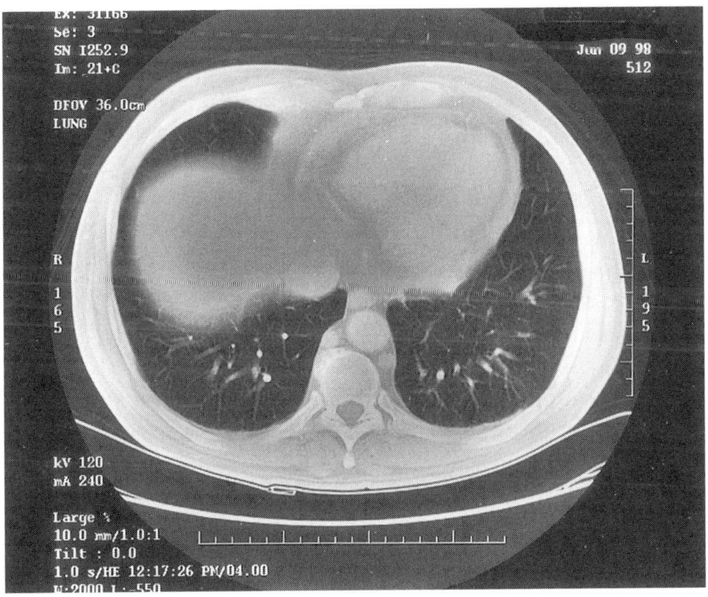
Se: 3
SN I252.9
Im: 21+C
DFOV 36.0cm
LUNG
Jun 09 98
512
R 165
L 195
kV 120
mA 240
Large
10.0 mm/1.0:1
Tilt : 0.0
1.0 s/HE 12:17:26 PM/04.00

(E)

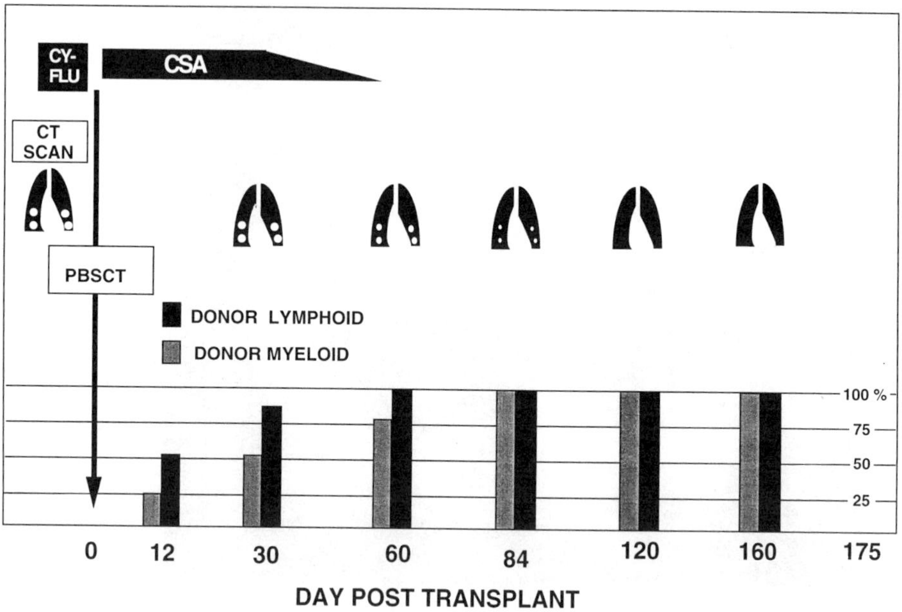

Figure 2 Clinical course of a 50-year-old man with pulmonary metastatic renal cell carcinoma receiving an HLA-identical peripheral blood stem-cell allograft (PBSCT). Cy-Flu + preparative regimen of cycloposphamide 120 mg/kg and fludarabine 125 mg/m^2. CSA = cyclosporine. CT scans show diagramatically the resolution of pulmonary metastases on successive scans. The degree of donor lymphocyte or myeloid cell chimerism is shown as a percentage.

tient to a GVT effect for the following reasons: First, the chemotherapeutic agents used have no known activity in metastatic RCC. Second, the 2-month interval between the transplant chemotherapy and the first signs of tumor regression is more compatible with an immune-mediated GVT effect. (A 2 to 6-month time period is usually required for a GVL effect from donor lymphocyte transfusions used to treat relapsed leukemia following allogenic marrow transplantation [42].) Furthermore, tumor regression did not begin until full donor T-cell chimerism was established. Although RCC can occasionally show spontaneous regression, the presence of 100% donor lymphoid chimerism indicates that if regression were immunologically induced, the principal effector cells were of donor origin. Finally, tumor regression occurred shortly following the withdrawal of cyclosporine and with the occurrence of mild acute GVHD of the skin. GVL effects have also been observed in conjunction with cyclosporine reduction and the occurrence of acute GVHD [43].

Although this patient had a dramatic and complete response, further allogeneic transplants in similar patients will be required to determine the place of nonmyeloablative allogeneic stem-cell transplantation in the treatment of metastatic RCC.

V. FUTURE PROSPECTS

These very preliminary results provide the first evidence that GVT effects can reverse or contain some advanced malignancies. Future clinical trials will be greatly helped by the adoption of low-intensity "minitransplants" that have an acceptably low toxicity. Furthermore, the use of nonmyeloablative preparative regimens is more logical in situations where the tumor has proven to be resistant to dose intensification. It is therefore likely that increasing numbers of investigators will attempt allogeneic stem-cell transplants in a widening variety of tumors. Since tumors show a wide diversity of etiology, it will be necessary to evaluate the allograft approach in each disease individually. The low mortality associated with nonmyeloablative allotransplantation will likely lead to trials in which it is studied as adjuvant therapy in patients achieving complete responses in diseases at high risk for relapse (i.e., stage III RCC and melanoma, relapsed NHL, etc). After heart disease, cancer is the single most common cause of death in the adult population. If it emerges that at least 10% of otherwise untreatable cancers respond to allogeneic stem-cell transplants, the exercise will have proved worthwhile for thousands of individuals.

REFERENCES

1. Weiden P, Flournoy N, Thomas E, et al. Antileukemic effects of graft-versus-host disease in human recipients of allogenic marrow grafts. N Engl J Med 1979; 300: 1068–1073.
2. Horowitz M, Gale RP, Sondel P, et al. Graft-versus-leukemia reactions after bone marrow transplantation. Blood, 1991; 78:2120–2130.
3. van Biesen KW, de Lima M, Giralt SA, et al. Management of lymphoma recurrence after allogeneic transplantation: the relevance of graft-versus-lymphoma effect. Bone Marrow Transplant 1997; 19:977–982.
4. Verdonck L, Lokhorst H, Dekker A, et al. Graft-versus myeloma effect in two cases. Lancet 1996; 347:800–801.
5. Leon MP, Bassendine MF, Gibbs P, et al. Immunogenicity of bilary epithelium: Study of the adhesive interaction with lymphocytes. Gastroenterology 1997, 112: 968–977.
6. De Bueger M, Bakker A, Van Rood JJ, et al. Tissue distribution of human minor histocompatibility antigens: Ubiquitous versus restricted tissue distribution indicates

heterogeneity among human cytotoxic T lymphocyte-defined non-MHC antigens. J Immunol 1992, 149:1788–1796.

7. Rivoltini L, Barracchini K, Viggiano V, et al. Quantitative correlation between HLA class I expression and recognition of melanoma cells by antigen-specific T lymphocytes. Cancer Res 1995, 55:3149–3157.
8. Webb DS, Mostowski HS, Gerrard T. Cytokine induced enhancement of ICAM-1 expression results in increased vulnerability of tumor cells to monocyte mediated lysis. J of Immunol 1991, 146:3682–3686.
9. Ruiz-Cabello F, Perz-Ayala M, Gomez O, et al. Molecular analysis of MHC-Class-I-alterations in human tumor cell lines. Cancer 1991; 6(suppl):123–130.
10. Gattoni-Celli S, Kirsh K, Timpane R, et al. Beta 2 microglobulin is mutated in human colon cancer cell line (HCT) deficient in the expression of HLA class I antigens ion the cell surface. Cancer Res 1992; 52:1201–1204.
11. Ferrone S and Marincola FM. Loss of HLA class I antigens by melanoma cells: molecular mechanisms, functional significance and clinical relevance. Immunol Today 1995; 16:487–494.
12. Hahne M, Rimoldi D, Schroter M, et al. Melanoma cell expression of Fas(apo-1/CD95) ligand: Implications for tumor immune escape. Science 1996; 274:1363–1366.
13. Mukherji B, Chakraborty NG. Immunobiology and immunotherapy of melanoma. Curr Opin Oncol 1995; 7:175–184.
14. Huber D, Phillipp J, Fontana A, et al. Protease inhibitors interfere with transforming growth factor beta-dependent but not transforming growth factor independent pathway of tumor cell mediated immunosuppression. J Immunol 1992; 148:277–284.
15. Bhatia S, Ramsay NKC, Steinbuch M, et al. Malignant neoplasms following bone marrow transplantation. Blood 1996; 87:3633–3639.
16. Curtis RE, Rowlings PA, Deeg HJ, et al. Solid cancers after bone marrow transplantation. N Engl J Med 1997; 336:897–904.
17. Slavin S, Nagler A, Naparstek E, et al. Nonmyeloablative stem cell transplantation and cell therapy as an alternative to conventional bone marrow transplantation with lethal cytoreduction for the treatment of malignant and nonmalignant hematologic diseases. Rapid Commun Blood 1998; 91:756–763.
18. Khouri IF, Keating M, Korbling M, et al. Transplant-Lite: induction of graft-versus-malignancy using fludarabine based nonablative chemotherapy and allogeneic blood progenitor-cell transplantation as treatment for lymphoid malignancies. J Clin Oncol 1998; 16:2817–2824.
19. Lewalle P, Hensel N, Guimaraes A, et al. Helper and cytotoxic lymphocyte responses to chronic myeloid leukaemia: implications for adoptive immunotherapy with T cells. Br J Haematol 1996; 92:587–594.
20. Warren EH, Greenberg PD, Riddell SR. Cytotoxic T-lymphocyte–defined human minor histocompatibility antigens with a restricted tissue distribution. Blood 1998; 91:2197–2207.
21. van der Harst D, Goulmy E, Falkenburg F, et al. Recognition of minor histocompatibility antigens on lymphocytic and myeloid leukemic cells by cytotoxic T-cell clones. Blood 1994; 83:1060–1066.
22. Eibl B, Schwaighofer H, Nachbaur D, et al. Evidence for a graft-versus-tumor effect

in a patient treated with marrow ablative chemotherapy and allogeneic bone marrow transplantation for breast cancer. Blood 1996; 88:1501–1508.
23. Or R, Ackerstein A, Nagler A, Kapelushnik J, Naparstek E, Samuel S, Amar A, Bruatbar C, Slavin S. Allogeneic cell-mediated immunotherapy for breast cancer after autologous stem cell transplantation: a clinical pilot study Cytokines Cell Mol Ther 1998; 4:1–6.
24. Ueno NT; Rondon G; Mirza NQ, et al. Allogeneic peripheral-blood progenitor-cell transplantation for poor-risk patients with metastatic breast cancer. J Clin Oncol 1998; 16:986–993.
25. Ladenstein R, Lasset C, Hartmann O, et al. Comparison of auto versus allografting as consolidation of primary treatments in advanced neuroblastoma over one year of age at diagnosis: report from the European Group for Bone Marrow Transplantation. Bone Marrow Transplant 1994; 14:37–46.
26. Houghton AN, Meyers ML, Chapman PB et al. Medical treatment of metastatic melanoma. Surg Clin North Am 1996; 76:1343–1353.
27. Barth A, Wanek LA, Morton D. Prognostic factors in 1,521 melanoma patients with distant metastases. J Am Coll Surg 1995; 6:181–193.
28. Rosenburg SA, Yang JC, Topalian SL, et al. Treatment of 283 consecutive patients with metastatic melanoma or renal cell cancer using high-dose bolus interleukin 2. JAMA 1994; 271:907–913.
29. Halliday GM, Patel A, Hunt M, et al. Spontaneous regression of human melanoma/nonmelanoma skin cancer: association with infiltrating CD4+ T cells. World J Surg 1995; 19:352–358.
30. Melioli G, Guastella M, Semino C et al. Proliferative, phenotypic and functional and molecular characteristics of tumor-infiltrating lymphocytes obtained from unselected patients with malignant melanomas and expanded in vitro in the presence of recombinant interleukin-2. Melanoma Res 1994; 4:127–133.
31. Topalian SL, Solomon D, Avis FP, et al. Immunotherapy of patients with advanced cancer using tunor-infiltrating lymphocytes and recombinant interleukin-2: a pilot study. J Clin Oncol 1988, 6:839–853.
32. Kradin RL, Kurnick JT, Lazarus DS et al. Tumor-infiltrating lymphocytes and interleukein-2 in treatment of advanced cancer. Lancet 1989; 1:577–580.
33. Thatcher N, Lind M, Morgenstern G et al. High dose double alkylating agent chemotherapy with DTIC, melphalan, or ifosphamide and marrow rescue for metastatic malignant melanoma. Cancer 1989; 63:1296–1302.
34. Savage PD. Renal cell carcinoma. Curr Opin Oncol 1996; 8:247–251.
35. Yagoda A, Abi-Rached B, Petrylak D, et al. Chemotherapy for advanced renal cell carcinoma: 1983–1993. Semin Oncol 1995; 22:42–60.
36. Negrier S, Escudier B, Lassett C, et al. Recombinant human interleukin-2, recombinant human interferon alfa-2a, or both in metastatic renal cell carcinoma. N Engl J Med 1998; 338:1272–1278.
37. Elson PJ, Witte RS, Trump DI. Prognostic factors for survival in patients with recurrent or metastatic renal cell carcinoma. Cancer Res 1988; 48:7310–7313.
38. Gleave ME, Elhilali M, Fradet Y, et al. Interferon gamma-1b compared with placebo in metastatic renal-cell carcinoma. N Engl J Med 1998; 338:1265–1271.

39. Caignard A, Guillard M, Gaudin C, et al. In situ demonstration of renal cell carcinoma specific T-cell clones. Int J Cancer 1996; 66:564–570.
40. Poindexter N, Shenoy S, Howard T, et al. Allograft infiltrating cytotoxic T lymphocytes recognize kidney-specific human minor histocompatibility antigens. Clin Transplant 1997; 11:174–177.
41. Mackinnon S, Barnett L, Bourhis JH, et al. Myeloid and lymphoid chimerism after T-cell depleted bone marrow transplantation: evaluation of conditioning regimens using the polymerase chain reaction to amplify human minisatellite regions of genomic DNA. Blood 1992; 180:3235–3241.
42. Barrett AJ, Malkovska V. Graft-versus-leukemia: understanding and using the alloimmune response to treat haematological malignancies. Br J Haematol 1996; 93: 754–761.
43. Collins RH, Rogers ZR, Bennett M, et al. Hematologic relapse of chronic myelogenous leukemia following allogeneic bone marrow transplantation: apparent graft-versus-leukemia effect following abrupt discontinuation of immunosuppression. Bone Marrow Transplant 1992; 10:391–395.
44. Morecki S, Moshel Y, Gelfend Y, et al. Induction of graft vs tumor effect in a murine mammary adenocarcinoma. Int J Cancer 1997; 71:59–63.
45. Kawakami Y, Robbins PF, Wang RF, et al. Tumor antigens recognized by T cells: the use of melanosomal proteins in the immunotherapy of melanoma. J Immunother 1998; 21:237–246.

12

Adoptive Allogeneic Cell-Mediated Immunotherapy and Nonmyeloablative Stem-Cell Transplantation

Shimon Slavin, Shoshana Morecki, Elizabeth Naparstek, Arnon Nagler, Gabor Varadi, Rami Ben-Yosef, and Reuven Or
Hadassah University Hospital
Jerusalem, Israel

I. INTRODUCTION

Allogeneic blood or marrow transplantation (alloBMT) is currently the most effective modality for the eradication of hematologic malignancies in patients at high risk for relapse or resistant to conventional chemoradiotherapeutic approaches. High-dose myeloablative chemoradiotherapy may also be supported by autologous stem-cell transplantation. However, the risk of relapse is higher in the absence of an allogeneic graft-versus-leukemia (GVL) effect [1]. A number of approaches to improve antitumor effects induced by donor T cells have been developed, including reduction or avoidance of posttransplant immunosuppression [2–5]. However, this approach is hazardous since recipients of fully or partially matched allografts may develop lethal GVHD. Allogeneic cell-mediated immunotherapy (alloCT) using donor lymphocyte transfusion (DLT) in graded increments is safer because it permits some control of GVHD [6,7]. We and others have shown that the risk of GVHD decreases with increasing intervals between the transplant and DLT [7–10]. Because of the time-interval effect, it is sometimes possible to provoke a marked GVL response with a large number of lymphocytes without causing severe GVHD. Furthermore, we have recently shown that host-type tumor cells resistant to DLT may still respond to unstimulated or in vitro activated lymphocytes in conjunction with a short course of intermediate-dose IL-2 [6]. The therapeutic action of DLT with or without IL-2 may not require durable engraftment of donor lymphocytes. In mice inoculated with 6×10^6 B-cell leukemia/lymphoma cells of BALB/c origin, eradication of host-type leukemia cells occurs within 2–3 weeks following DLT with T cells fully tolerant to host antigens. In vivo activation of the same effector cells with rIL-2 can eradicate the leukemia in 3–5 days [11]. As previously mentioned, the same strategy has been applied in a cohort of patients with a variety of hematologic malignancies relapsing after allogeneic BMT [6]. It therefore appears that alloCT in conjunction with rIL-2 activation of T cells can be an effective method of treating or preventing relapse [7,12].

In this chapter we review data in support of DLT as immunotherapy and the contribution of IL-2 in the treatment and prevention of relapse after alloBMT in experimental animals, which led to our first clinical trials. Our results have been confirmed in prospective studies in Europe and the United States (see Chapter 9). We also describe recent results where a GVL-like effect has been induced to treat recurrent disease in recipients of alloBMT with malignant and nonmalignant diseases [13]. Finally, we present preliminary data supporting the idea that alloCT could be used to eradicate minimal residual disease in the context of metastatic solid tumors.

II. GVL EFFECTS CONTROL RELAPSE IN EXPERIMENTAL ANIMALS

The possibility that allogeneic BMT eliminates leukemia through an immune-mediated action can be deduced from a large literature of experimental [14–22] and clinical data [23–25]. The unique therapeutic potential of allogeneic BMT to cure leukemia (in contrast to autologous or syngeneic BMT) relates as much to the reactivity of immunocompetent donor-derived T lymphocytes against residual host-derived cells as to the high dose chemoradiotherapy given in preparation for BMT [6,23–31]. Experiments with chimeric mice showed that by increasing the time interval between BMT and cell infusion, resistance to GVHD increases with or without T-cell depletion [14,26,28]. Recent data in murine models imply that GVL effects can also be induced by posttransplant administration of graded increments of immunocompetent allogeneic lymphocytes with rIL-2 [9,11,31–33]. The murine data show that delayed infusion of donor-derived peripheral blood lymphocytes (PBLs) is associated with a lower incidence of

GVHD even in recipients not protected by prophylaxis with cyclosporine [6,26,28,32].

III. GVL IN CLINICAL PRACTICE—TREATMENT OF RELAPSE

Preliminary data from pilot clinical trials detailed below suggest that a similar rationale for the treatment of relapse may be applicable in clinical practice. As early as 1987, we successfully induced a GVL effect by alloCT using donor PBLs in a patient who relapsed after BMT with acute lymphoblastic leukemia (ALL) with resistant bulky intra- and extramedullary disease. We thus demonstrated that alloCT could successfully eradicate leukemia, possibly through minor histocompatibility antigen differences on the leukemia cell. Our most recent data show that patients with tumor cells resistant to alloCT may still respond to donor PBLs in vivo with or without in vitro activation with IL-2. This suggests that the alloreactive potential of donor PBLs may be further exploited using IL-2. Interestingly, in a number of patients, remission was observed without clinical evidence of GVHD, suggesting that operational cure of leukemia can occasionally be achieved independently of GVHD [26]. These data imply either that tumor cells present antigens that differ from self antigens or that tumor target cells are recognized by specific effector T-cell clones. Alternatively, tumor cells may occasionally represent better targets for alloresponses than normal tissues. The occurrence of GVL without GVHD may also reflect qualitative rather than quantitative differences, with GVL occurring at the same time as low levels of subclinical GVHD. For reasons not well defined, chronic myclogenous leukemia (CML) represents the leukemia most susceptible to the GVL effect of DLT. The use of DLT to treat relapse of leukemia, CML in particular, is reviewed in Chapter 9.

IV. GVL IN CLINICAL PRACTICE—PREVENTION OF RELAPSE

Clinical experience in the treatment of relapsed leukemia using DLT indicates that patients with minimal or less advanced disease respond more frequently. We have shown that alloCT can prevent relapse even after a T cell–depleted transplant and posttransplant immunosuppression with cyclosporine, which is known to suppress the GVL response [3,4,7,34–36]. In a series of 314 patients transplanted for leukemia, including 70 patients with CML, we have shown that alloCT can prevent relapse even in patients at high risk for relapse after T cell–depleted transplants. Our results appear to be equal or superior to those currently obtained using conventional unmanipulated transplants [37]. These results need to be confirmed in a prospective study.

V. GVL FOLLOWING NONMYELOABLATIVE STEM CELL TRANSPLANTATION

We have recently studied a new approach to the treatment of bone marrow disorders, focusing on the potential of donor T cells to eradicate host malignant and non-malignant cells following nonmyeloablative chemotherapy. Our protocol uses an immunosuppressive conditioning regimen of low-dose oral busulfan, ATG and fludarabine followed by infusion of leukapheresis-collected, unmanipulated G-CSF–mobilized peripheral blood stem cells that have a high T-cell content. We anticipated that the large number of donor-derived T cells together with the stem cells would provide a GVL effect that could be augmented after transplant by DLT. To prevent GVHD, cyclosporine was used as a standard regimen.

We treated 26 patients with standard indications for BMT, 22 with hematologic malignancies and 4 with genetic disorders. The conditioning regimen produced no severe toxicity. The neutrophil count never fell below $0.1 \times 10^9/L$ in 9 patients and below $0.5 \times 10^9/L$ in two patients. Neutrophil recovery to $0.5 \times 10^9/L$ was achieved within 10–32 (median 15) days. Platelet counts did not decrease below $20 \times 10^9/L$ in 4 patients who required no platelet transfusions, and a platelet count of greater than $20 \times 10^9/L$ was reached between 0–35 (median 12) days. Stable donor chimerism was achieved, which was complete in 17 and partial in 9 patients. The single major complication was fatal grade III–IV GVHD in 4 patients following early discontinuation of cyclosporine. Relapse occurred in 3 patients but was reversed by alloCT in 2. With a follow-up of greater than 1 year (median 8 months), 22 (85%) patients were alive and 21 (81%) were disease-free. The actuarial probability of disease-free survival at 14 months was 77.5% (95% confidence intervals 53–90%). Four patients with nonmalignant disorders received this transplant regimen. All are alive and well with a Karnofsky score of 100% and no evidence of the original disorder. No residual host cells could be detected by either male-specific PCR [38] or variable nonrandom tandem repeat PCR.

These preliminary results suggest that nonmyeloablative transplants could confer major advantages over the conventional high-dose chemoradiotherapy approach. An important feature is that the state of stable mixed chimerism resulting from the nonmyeloablative preparative regimen may facilitate a new strategy of controlling GVH. The mechanism of the apparent tolerance seen in mixed chimeras is not known. However, in mice, it has been shown that host hematopoietic cells can veto donor-antihost reactivity, while donor hematopoietic cells veto residual alloreactive host cells. The result is a two-way tolerance of donor and host [39–42]. The nonmyeloablative preparative regimen also circumvents complications resulting from intensive chemoradiotherapy. This is of particular importance in older patients, who have a high transplant-related mortality. In preadolescent patients, the low-intensity regimen should reduce the problems of growth retardation and infertility caused by damage to the gonads and endocrine organs due to high-dose treatment. It remains to be seen whether the non-myeloablative regimen can also be applied to transplants from unrelated donors and to patients with nonhematopoietic malignancies.

VI. GVT EFFECTS IN EXPERIMENTAL ANIMALS

An important question is whether or not effects similar to GVL can be induced against solid tumors. Some time ago we tested the ability of allogeneic BMT to prevent spontaneously occurring lymphosarcoma in (NZB × NZW)F1 mice [43]. Interestingly, a GVT effect similar to GVL was observed despite complete absence of GVHD and host-versus-graft responsiveness. GVT effects were effective only when tumor-susceptible hosts were reconstituted with non T cell–depleted allogeneic BM at an early age. Subsequently we induced GVT effects in a murine model of a transplantable metastasizing mammary tumor (4T1) resembling the human counterpart. The tumor was subcloned from a spontaneous mammary tumor developing in a BALB/cfC3H mouse [44]. The 4T1 cells are highly tumorigenic in BALB/c mice. Following injection into the mammary fat pad, 4T1 cells metastasize to the lungs and, less frequently, to the liver and lymph nodes. To characterize GVT effects in this model, a phenotypic analysis of cell-surface alloantigen expression and tumorigenicity assays was carried out in different strains of mice, which differed at both major and minor MHC loci. We then carried out transplants in different strains of mice using major or minor MHC–incompatible marrow. When tumor cells were inoculated into fully competent BM chimeras, donor lymphocytes were barely reactive against the host but recognized tumor cells bearing host MHC molecules. The 4T1 cells were highly tumorigenic in syngeneic BALB/c (H-2^{d}) or haploidentical (BALB/c × C57BL/6) F1 (H-$2^{d/b}$), but they were only slightly tumorigenic in an H-2^{d} congenic strain (DBA/2) (H-2^{d}) and non-tumorigenic in MHC-unrelated (C57BL/6) (H-2^{b}) mice. The 4T1 cells express MHC class I antigen adhesion molecules and CD44 homing-associated adhesion molecules, but they do not express MHC class II or costimulatory molecules such as B7. Twenty-four hours after total-body irradiation (TBI), female BALB/c (H-2d) or F1 (H-2d/b) mice were reconstituted with 10^7 male BM cells derived from MiHC-mismatched DBA (H-2d) donors or with MHC mismatched C57BL/6 (H-2b) BM cells. A dose of 9 Gy TBI was given before MiHC mismatched (BALB/c-DBA) transplants and 11 Gy before MHC mismatched (BALB/c × C57BL/6 F1-C57BL/6) transplants. Donor chimerism was detected using a Y chromosome–specific PCR assay. Stable hematopoietic chimerism was established with mild features of chronic GVHD (roughened fur and weight loss) across MiHC barriers and with no overt GVHD across the MHC barrier. Median survival of 9 DBA/2 into BALB/c chimeras was 261 (range 147–341) days and >300 days in 14 C57BL/6 into F1 chimeras. Recipient mice carrying MiHc or MHC mismatched donor cells were inoculated with 4T1 cells 2–3 months after BM reconstitution. Chimeras reconstituted with donor cells mismatched by MiHC or MHC with the tumor were able to suppress the development of the primary tumor expressing the host MHC antigens. Tumor size in chimeras was significantly smaller ($p < 0.05$) when either MiHC- or MHC-mismatched donor cells were present when compared with BALB/c or F1 controls. In a subsequent study using the same tumor model, we used intravenously inoculated tumor cells to induce pulmonary metastases that caused death from widespread disease in untreated BALB/c or F1 recipients. The pulmonary metastases were completely preventable when tumor cells were inoculated into both MiHC- and MHC-mismatched chimeras. Elimination of all metastases was confirmed by adoptive transfer of single-cell suspensions of lung cells obtained from inoculated chimeras and controls. Only cell suspensions from syngeneic controls caused death in 100% secondary recipients.

These studies demonstrate the existence of a GVT effect in a murine mammary adenocarcinoma model and the ability of alloreacting donor T cells to prevent breast cancer metastasis. The results suggest a possible benefit for the treatment or prevention of metastatic disease by alloimmunotherapy in patients with breast cancer and possibly in those with other solid tumors. However, it is possible that GVT may be less effective than GVL for several reasons: epithelial tumors may be more difficult for T cells to home to; also, tumor cells (unlike hematopoietic cells) may not express MHC class II and therefore fail to present some tumor-specific, tissue-specific or tumor-associated antigens. Essential costimulatory molecules may be down-regulated, and, furthermore, epithelial tumor cells may be resistant to lysis or apoptosis. We detected MHC class I and several adhesion molecules but not MHC class II and B7 on 4T1 cells. For T-cell activation, MHC class I and II and B7 costimulatory molecules must be present. MHC class I (H-2^d) expression of 4T1 cells permitted their growth in syngeneic and semiallogeneic recipients, but they appear to have been the target of MiHC- and MHC-mismatched hosts. Loss of MHC expression on these tumor cells would therefore allow them to escape from immune recognition.

Unfortunately, in both experimental and clinical situations, GVL effects in hematologic malignancies are accompanied by GVHD [15,22,25,31]. However, this is not always the case [11,17,45,46]. In our study, BM chimeras across MiHC antigen differences suffered only mild GVHD, and no GVHD was observed in MHC-mismatched donor-recipient pairs. Despite the absence of severe GVHD, the allograft exerted an antitumor effect that inhibited the growth of primary tumors and prevented the seeding of metastases. Separation of GVT from GVHD has important clinical implications, and efforts to control GVHD must not impair GVT effects. The finding of GVT effects independent of GVHD in the 4T1 tumor model may indicate that the two effects are mediated by different T-cell populations or that tumor cells have a greater sensitivity to allogeneic effector cells. Alternatively, anti-tumor effects may be induced in parallel with subclinical GVHD. These possibilities require further investigation by experiments using well-defined T-cell and other effector-cell subsets, including MHC-unrestricted T and NK cells.

VII. GVT IN CLINICAL PRACTICE

We describe here a possible GVT effect in a 37-year-old woman with recurrent breast cancer [47]. This patient presented for evaluation of an undefined upper- and medial-quadrant mass in the left breast and a 4- by 3-cm mass in the axilla. Excision biopsy confirmed a grade II multifocal infiltrating ductal carcinoma invading lymphatic vessels and present at the surgical margin. She was treated with seven cycles of cyclophosphamide, adriamycin, and 5-fluorouracil (CAF) followed by left upper quadrantectomy axillary node dissection (3 of 17 nodes positive) and 56 Gy of irradiation to the left breast with a 14-Gy boost to the tumor area. Twenty-three months later, a small, irregular mass was noted in the medial aspect of the surgical scar, adherent to the chest wall and histologically identical to the original tumor. At that time she was found to be anemic and neutropenic; a bone marrow aspirate showed blast cells. A diagnosis of acute myelogenous leukemia (AML-M2) was made. Remission was achieved with a single course of amsacrine and high-dose cytosine arabinoside. The chest-wall mass appeared to have diminished a little in size, but no further decrease in size was observed following a consolidation course of etoposide and mitoxantrone. Four months after the diagnosis of recurrent breast cancer, she underwent an uneventful bone marrow transplant from her HLA-identical brother. She was given donor lymphocyte transfusions of 1×10^5 T cells per kilogram at 10 weeks and 6×10^5 T cells per kilogram at 20 weeks posttransplant, which induced grade I skin GVHD. Twelve months after transplant, no evidence of breast cancer or AML was detected. Although the approach in treating this patient was directed primarily to the leukemia, a beneficial effect was also seen against the breast cancer, at least in the period of follow-up. It thus appears that a GVT effect similar to a GVL effect may have played a role in achieving a complete response in recurrent breast cancer.

We have also demonstrated possible antitumor responses in six further patients given HLA-matched sibling donor lymphocyte transfusions to treat metastatic breast cancer who relapsed after autologous blood stem-cell transplantation.

Donor lymphocytes were activated with rIL-2 in vitro and in vivo. One patient treated with no evidence of disease at the time of alloCT is still alive and disease-free 5 years following DLT.

Although there is, as yet, no conclusive evidence for a clinical GVT effect, these results should encourage further attempts to evaluate this treatment.

VIII. NEW DEVELOPMENTS

The ability of nonmyeloablative transplants and DLT to prevent or treat recurrence of malignant disease suggests that the same approach could be of benefit in the treatment of genetic diseases. A full discussion of the role of nonmyeloablative transplants in nonmalignant disorders is outside the context of this book. However, the preliminary results reported here encourage further studies to evaluate the role of such transplants in disorders such as thalassemia and sickle cell anemia.

Because the therapeutic benefit of DLT is frequently offset by GVHD with an incidence and severity that is unpredictable, new approaches to limit the life span of donor lymphocytes are under development. The most promising modality for controlling GVHD and its occurrence after discontinuation of immunosuppression prophylaxis is the use of donor T cells transduced with the herpes simplex virus thymidine kinase gene. Genetically modified T cells of donor origin still retain their GVL capacity. Hence in the event of uncontrolled GVHD, these antitumor effector cells can be successfully eliminated by administering conventional doses of ganciclovir [48]. The feasibility of eliminating GVHD induced intentionally by DLT to enhance GVL effects may extend the use of DLT to treat hematological malignancies and possibly metastatic solid tumors not curable by current treatment.

REFERENCES

1. Horowitz MM, Gale RP, Sondel PM, Goldman JM, Kersey J, Kolb H-J, Rimm AA, Ringden O, Rozman C, Speck B, Truitt RL, Zwaan FE, Bortin MM. Graft-versus-leukemia reactions after bone marrow transplantation. Blood 1990; 75:555–562.
2. Sullivan KM, Storb R, Buckner CD, et al. Graft-versus-host disease as adoptive immunotherapy in patients with advanced hematologic neoplasms. N Engl J Med 1989; 320:828–834.
3. Stockschlaeder M, Storb R, Pepe M, et al. A pilot study of low-dose cyclosporin for graft-versus-host prophylaxis in marrow transplantation. Br J Haematol 1992; 80:49–54.

4. Bacigalupo A, van Lint MT, Occhini D, et al. Increased risk of leukemia relapse with high-dose cyclosporine A after allogeneic marrow transplantation for acute leukemia. Blood 1991; 77:1423–1428.
5. Collins RH, Rogers ZR, Bennett M, Kurser V, Nikein A, Fay JW. Hematologic relapse of chronic myelogenous leukemia following allogeneic bone marrow transplantation: apparent graft-versus-leukemia effect following abrupt discontinuation of immunosuppression. Bone Marrow Transplant 1992; 10:391–395.
6. Slavin S, Naparstek E, Nagler A, Ackerstein A, Samuel S, Kapelushnik J, Brautbar C, Or R. Allogeneic cell therapy with donor peripheral blood cells and recombinant human interleukin-2 to treat leukemia relapse post allogeneic bone marrow transplantation. Blood 1996; 87:2195–2204.
7. Naparstek E, Or R, Nagler A, et al. T-cell depleted allogeneic bone marrow transplantation for acute leukemia using Campath-1 antibodies and post transplant administration of donor's peripheral blood lymphocytes for prevention of relapse. Br J Haematol 1995; 89:506–515.
8. Slavin S, Fuks Z, Kaplan HS, Strober S. Transplantation of allogeneic bone marrow without graft vs host disease using total lymphoid irradiation. J Exp Med 1978; 147: 963–972.
9. Weiss L, Reich S, Slavin S. Use of recombinant human interleukin-2 in conjunction with bone marrow transplantation as a model for control of minimal residual disease in malignant hematological disorders: I. Treatment of murine leukemia in conjunction with allogeneic bone marrow transplantation and IL2-activated cell-mediated immunotherapy. Cancer Invest 1992; 10:19–26.
10. Johnson BD, Drobyski WR, Truitt RL. Delayed infusion of normal donor cells after MHC-matched bone marrow transplantation provides an antileukemia reaction without graft-versus-host disease. Bone Marrow Transplant 1993; 11:329–336.
11. Weiss L, Lubin I, Factorowich Y, Lapidot Z, Reich S, Reisner Y, Slavin S. Effective graft vs leukemia effects independent of graft vs host disease after T-cell depleted allogeneic bone marrow transplantation in a murine model of B cell leukemia/lymphoma: role of cell therapy and rIL-2. J Immunol 1994; 153:2562–2567.
12. Naparstek E, Nagler A, Or R, Slavin S. Allogeneic cell mediated immunotherapy using donor lymphocytes for prevention of relapse in patients treated with allogeneic BMT for hematological malignancies. Clin Transplant 1996; 281–290.
13. Slavin S, Nagler A, Naparstek E, Kapelushnik Y, Aker M, Cividalli G, Varadi G, Kirschbaum M, Ackerstein A, Samuel S, Ben-Tal O, Eldor A, Or R. Non-myeloablative stem cell transplantation and cell therapy as an alternative to conventional bone marrow transplantation with lethal cytoreduction for the treatment of malignant and non-malignant hematologic diseases. Blood 1998; 91:756–763.
14. Sinkovics JG, Shullenberger CC. Effect of hematopoietic chimerism on the course of Rauscher's viral mouse leukemia. Proc Am Assoc Cancer Res 1963; 4:62–72.
15. Boranic M, Tonkovic I. Time pattern of the antileukemia effect of graft-versus-host reaction in mice: I. Cellular events. Cancer Res 1971; 31:1140–1147.
16. Bortin MM, Truitt RL, Rimm AA, Bach FH. Graft-versus-leukaemia reactivity induced by alloimmunization without augmentation of graft-versus-host reactivity. Nature 1979; 281:490–491.

17. Slavin S, Weiss L, Morecki S, Weigensberg M. Eradication of murine leukemia with histoincompatible marrow grafts in mice conditioned with total lymphoid irradiation (TLI). Cancer Immunol Immunother 1981; 11:155–161.
18. Truitt RL, Shih F-H, LeFever AV, et al. Characterization of alloimmunization-induced T lymphocytes reactivated against AKR leukemia in vitro and correlation with graft-vs-leukemia activity in vivo. J Immunol 1983; 131:2050–2058.
19. Slavin S, Weiss L, Morecki S, Weingensberg M. Eradication of murine leukemia with histoincompatible marrow grafts in mice conditioned with total lymphoid irradiation (TLI). Cancer Immunol Immunother 1981; 11:155–158.
20. Meredith RF, O'Kunewick JP. Possibility of graft-vs-leukemia determinants independent of the major histocompatibility complex in allogeneic marrow transplantation. Transplantation 1983; 35:378–385.
21. Weiss L, Weigensberg M, Morecki S, et al. Characterization of effector cells of graft vs leukemia (GVL) following allogeneic bone marrow transplantation in mice inoculated with murine B-cell leukemia (BCL1). Cancer Immunol Immunother 1990; 31:236–242.
22. Truitt RL, Atasoylu AA. Impact of pretransplant conditioning and donor T cells on chimerism, graft-versus-host disease, graft-vs-leukemia reactivity, and tolerance after bone marrow transplantation. Blood 1991; 77:2515–2523.
23. Weiden PL, Sullivan KM, Fluornoy N, et al. Antileukemic effect of chronic graft-versus-host disease: contribution to improved survival after allogeneic marrow transplantation. N Engl J Med 1981; 304:1529–1533.
24. Weiden PL, Fluornoy N, Sanders JE, Sullivan KM, Thomas ED. Antileukemic effect of graft-versus-host disease contributes to improved survival after allogeneic marrow transplantation. Transplantation 1981; 13:248–251.
25. Sullivan KM, Weiden PL, Storb R, et al. Influence of acute and chronic graft-versus-host disease on relapse and survival after bone marrow transplantation from HLA-identical siblings as treatment of acute and chronic leukemia. Blood 1989; 73:1720–1726.
26. Slavin S, Naparstek E, Nagler A, Ackerstein A, Kapelushnik Y, Or R. Allogeneic cell therapy for relapsed leukemia following bone marrow transplantation with donor peripheral blood lymphocytes. Exp Hematol 1995; 23:1553–1562.
27. Kolb HJ, Mittermueller J, Clemm CH, et al. Donor leukocyte transfusions for treatment of recurrent chronic myelogenous leukemia in marrow transplant patients. Blood 1990; 76:2462–2465.
28. Slavin S, Ackerstein A, Weiss L, Nagler A, Or R, Naparstek E. Immunotherapy of minimal residual disease by immunocompetent lymphocytes and their activation by cytokines. Cancer Invest 1992; 10:221–227.
29. Horowitz M, Gale RP, Sondel PM, et al. Graft-versus-leukemia reactions after bone marrow transplantation. Blood 1990; 75:555–562.
30. Slavin S, Or R, Kapelushnik Y, Drakos P, Ackerstein A, Vourka-Karussis U, Weiss L, Nagler A. Immunotherapy of minimal residual disease in conjunction with autologous and allogeneic bone marrow transplantation (BMT). Leukemia 1992; 6:164–166.
31. Vourka-Karussis U, Karussis D, Ackerstein A, Slavin S. Enhancement of graft versus leukemia effect (GVL) with recombinant human interleukin 2 (rIL-2) following

bone marrow transplantation in a murine model for acute myeloid leukemia in SJL/J mice. Exp Hematol 1995; 23:196–201.
32. Soiffer RJ, Murray C, Cochran K, et al. Clinical and immunologic effects of prolonged infusion of low-dose recombinant interleukin-2 after autologous and T-cell-depleted allogeneic bone barrow transplantation. Blood 1992; 79:517–526.
33. Soiffer RJ, Murray C, Gonin R, et al. Effect of low-dose interleukin-2 on disease relapse after T-cell-depleted allogeneic bone marrow transplantation. Blood 1994; 84:964–971.
34. Weiss L, Reich S, Slavin S. Effect of cyclosporine A and methylprednisolone on the GVL effect across major histocompatibility barriers in mice following allogeneic bone marrow transplantation. Bone Marrow Transplant 1990; 6:229–233.
35. Odom LF, August CS, Githens JH, et al. Remission of relapsed leukaemia during a graft-versus-host reaction: a "graft-versus-leukaemia reaction" in man? Lancet 1978; 2:537–538.
36. Higano CS, Brixey M, Bryant EM, et al. Durable complete remission of acute non-lymphocytic leukemia associated with discontinuation of immunosuppression following relapse after allogeneic bone marrow tranplantation: a case report of a probable graft-versus-leukemia effect. Transfusion 1990; 50:175–178.
37. Naparstek E, Nagler A, Or R, Kapelushnik J, Slavin S. Allogeneic cell mediated immunotherapy using donor lymphocytes for prevention of relapse in patients treated with allogeneic BMT for hematological malignancies. Clin Transpl 1996; 281–290.
38. Pugatsch T, Oppenheim A, Slavin S. Improved single step PCR assay for sex identification post allogeneic sex-mismatched BMT. Bone Marrow Transplant 1996; 17: 273–275.
39. Slavin S, Strober S, Fuks Z, Kaplan HS. Induction of specific tissue transplantation tolerance using fractionated total lymphoid irradiation in adult mice: long-term survival of allogeneic bone marrow and skin grafts. J Exp Med 1977; 146:34–48.
40. Slavin S. Total lymphoid irradiation (TLI). Immunol Today 1987; 8:88–92.
41. Ildstad ST, Sachs DH. Reconstitution with syngeneic plus allogeneic or xenogeneic bone marrow leads to specific acceptance of allografts and xenografts. Nature 1984; 307:168.
42. Sykes M, Sachs DH. Mixed allogeneic chimerism as an approach to transplantation tolerance. Immunol Today 1988; 9:23.
43. Moscovitch M, Slavin S. Anti-tumor effects of allogeneic bone marrow transplantation in (NZB × NZW) F1 hybrids with spontaneous lymphosarcoma. J Immunol 1984; 132:997–1000.
44. Dexter DL, Kowalski HM, Blazar BA, Fligiel Z, Vogel R, Heppner G. Heterogeneity of tumor cells from a single mouse mammary tumor. Cancer Res 1978; 38:3174–3181.
45. Abraham VS, Sykes M. Mechanism of the anti-GVHD effect of IL-2: I. Protective host-type cell populations are not induced by IL-2 treatment alone. Bone Marrow Transplant 1991; 7(suppl 1):29–32.
46. Slavin S, Ackerstein A, Naparstek E, Or R, Weiss L. The graft-versus-leukemia (GVL) phenomenon: is GVL separable from GVHD? Bone Marrow Transplant 1990; 6:155–161.
47. Ben-Yosef R, Or R, Nagler A, Slavin S. Graft vs tumor and graft vs leukemia in

patients with concurrent breast cancer and acute myelocytic leukemia. Lancet 1996; 348:1242–1243.

48. Bonini C, Ferrari G, Verzeletti S, Srvida P, Zappone E, Ruggieri L, Ponzoni M, Rossini S, Mavilio F, Traversari C, Bordignon C. HSV-TK gene transfer into donor lymphocytes for control of allogeneic graft versus leukemia. Science 1997; 276: 1719–1724.

13

Clinical and Basic Science Studies of Human Umbilical Cord Blood

Implications for the GVL Effect Following Cord Blood Transplantation

Jay Gaddy, Pierluigi Porcu, and Hal E. Broxmeyer
Indiana University School of Medicine and the Walther Cancer Institute
Indianapolis, Indiana

I. INTRODUCTION

Human umbilical cord blood (CB) is a readily available source of stem cells and naive or ontogenically immature leukocytes [1–7]. Increasingly, CB is being utilized as an alternative to bone marrow (BM) for stem-cell transplants. The first CB transplant was performed in 1988 as a treatment for Fanconi's anemia [8]. Numerous CB transplants have since been performed to treat a variety of malignant and nonmalignant hematopoietic diseases as well as metabolic disorders [9,10]. Umbilical cord blood presents multiple advantages over bone marrow as a source of stem cells: harvesting presents no donor risk or discomfort, the product carries less likelihood of infectious disease transmission, and collection can be targeted to include minority groups underrepresented in BM donor registries [11–13]. Clinical results worldwide of CB transplantation performed in settings—ranging from matched sibling to mismatched unrelated—are encouraging. In general, the time to neutrophil engraftment is similar to that for bone marrow transplant (BMT) [10]. Importantly, there is less likelihood of severe acute graft-versus-host disease (aGVHD) following CB transplants even when unrelated mismatched grafts are used [9,12,14–17]. Potential downsides to CB transplantation are delayed time to platelet independence and questions regarding the ability to engraft adults [13]. However, there are reports in the literature of adult-size patients being successfully engrafted by CB [17–19].

It is now well accepted that there is a graft-versus-leukemia (GVL) effect following allogeneic BMT [20], although the mechanisms for such an effect are not completely known and probably differ according to the type of malignancy being treated [21]. Of great interest, especially given the reduced incidence of aGVHD following CB transplantation, is whether CB is effective in mediating a GVL effect. However, because CB transplants have only recently begun to be performed, reported CB transplants are still too few in number and the time of follow-up too short to determine if a GVL effect is mediated by CB.

In this chapter, we will discuss relevant clinical and laboratory data that may give insight into the capacity of CB transplantation to mediate a GVL effect.

II. CLINICAL RESULTS

Recently published or internationally presented results relating to GVHD and GVL effects for both related and unrelated CB transplants are presented below. Results for other parameters regarding the overall efficacy of CB transplants are given in detail in summaries by Wagner and Kurtzberg [17] and Gluckman et al. [22].

A. Related CB Transplantation

Most of the data regarding related CB transplants performed worldwide have been compiled and reported by two major organizations; the International Cord Blood Transplant Registry (ICBTR) and the Eurocord Transplant Group. The results of 74 transplants (56 HLA-matched or mismatched for one HLA antigen, 18 mismatched for two or three HLA antigens) reported by the ICBTR, demonstrated a relatively low incidence of aGVHD for related CB transplants [17]. In patients receiving HLA-matched or one-antigen-mismatched CB transplants, the actuarial probabilities of grade II–IV and grades III–IV aGVHD at day 100 were 0.03 ± 0.02 and 0.03 ± 0.02, respectively. In 15 evaluable recipients of two or three HLA-antigen-mismatched GB transplants, 11 developed grade 0–I aGVHD and 4 developed Grade II–IV aGVHD. Very few patients receiving CB transplants had evidence of chronic GVHD (cGVHD), with none having extensive disease. At a median follow-up of 2 years the actuarial probability of survival for patients receiving HLA-matched and one-antigen-mismatched CB grafts was

0.61 ± 0.12. Only one patient, who received a three-antigen-mismatched graft, died of GVHD. For patients who received CB transplants to treat malignancy, the actuarial probability of disease-free survival was 0.41 ± 0.11.

The results of 78 transplants reported by Eurocord (60 HLA-matched, 3 mismatched for one HLA antigen, 5 mismatched for two HLA antigens, 9 mismatched for three HLA antigens and 1 mismatched for four HLA antigens) were fairly similar [22]. The incidence of aGVHD in recipients of HLA-matched CB transplants was 9%; in recipients of HLA-mismatched CB transplants, it was 50%. HLA-mismatching was the only factor associated with an increased risk of aGVHD. Relapse of leukemia occurred in 10 of 38 patients receiving transplants to treat malignant disease. The overall 1-year survival rate was 73% for recipients of HLA-matched and 33% for recipients of HLA-mismatched CB grafts, with only 1 person dying of GVHD.

B. Unrelated Cord Blood Transplantation

The promising early results regarding related CB transplants, as well as the limited number of suitable HLA-compatible BM donors available at any one time, led investigators to attempt to expand the potential stem-cell donor pool by utilizing banked CB units for unrelated transplants. Extensive analysis of unrelated CB transplants performed to date has been encouraging. Wagner et al. have reported on 111 evaluable unrelated CB transplants performed at the University of Minnesota and Duke University between August 1993 and August 1997 [23]. A total of 51 recipients received CB grafts mismatched at 0–1 HLA antigens, 58 at 2–3 HLA antigens, and 2 at 4 HLA antigens. The probabilities of grade II–IV and grade III–IV aGVHD were 0.35 ± 0.14 and 0.12 ± 0.06, respectively. For recipients of 0–1 HLA antigen and 2–3 HLA antigen-mismatched CB grafts, the probabilities of grade II–IV aGVHD were 0.31 ± 0.13 and 0.39 ± 0.15, while the probabilities of 2-year survival were 0.41 ± 0.18 and 0.49 ± 0.14, respectively. Extensive cGVHD was only rarely demonstrated. In this study, no risk factor predicted higher incidence of aGVHD, while the only factor that correlated with improved survival was cell dose. No report of relapse rates was given.

The Eurocord Transplant Registry has reported somewhat similar results for unrelated CB transplants regarding GVHD and survival. Acute GVHD was observed in 21 of 65 recipients of unrelated CB transplants with 8 having grade II, 9 having grade III, and 4 having grade IV disease. Chronic GVHD was not observed. Recipient cytomegalovirus-positive serologic status was the only risk factor associated with a higher risk of GVHD. The overall survival rate at 1 year was 29%, with recipient cytomegalovirus-negative serologic status associated with longer median survival. Of 49 patients receiving CB transplants to treat malignant disease, 7 suffered leukemic relapse.

C. Analysis of Immune Recovery Following CB Transplantation

Few studies have been reported regarding the recovery of the immune system following CB transplantation. Laughlin et al. have reported on phenotypic and functional analyses of lymphocyte populations present in 9 adult patients following unrelated CB transplantation for hematologic malignancies [24]. One patient developed grade III aGVHD, while the remaining 8 patients had grade 0–II aGVHD. Immune recovery in these patients post–CB transplant was marked by increased B and natural killer (NK) cell populations, while T-cell recovery demonstrated early emergence of CD4+ T cells with mature T-cell receptor repertoire but diminished cytokine production and response to recall antigens. Another report demonstrated the immune recovery following matched related CB transplantation in three children with ALL, none experiencing aGVHD or cGVHD [25]. The pattern and kinetics of recovery mimicked those of BMT with an early recovery of NK cells and rapid increase in CD8+ T cells with the characteristic inversion of the CD4/CD8 ratio. As with the unrelated CB transplants reported above, there was also a marked increase in the percentage and absolute number of B cells. Many more and expanded studies of immune recovery following CB transplant need to be performed before conclusions can be drawn regarding this important subject.

In general, the clinical studies suggest that there is a reduced incidence and/or severity of GVHD following related or unrelated CB transplantation as compared with age-matched BMT transplants. It has been postulated that the reduced incidence and/or severity of GVHD is simply due to a relative T-cell depletion during CB transplantation. However, the reduction in the absolute number of CD3+ cells infused during CB transplantation is modest, and such a T-cell depletion would not be expected to reduce the incidence of aGVHD during BMT [26]. Clinical trials currently under way should help determine conclusively whether CB transplantation is marked by a lessened incidence and/or severity of GVHD as compared to BMT performed under comparable conditions.

Whether a reduced incidence and/or severity of GVHD will have a negative impact on the GVL effect of CB transplants needs to be determined. Many more CB transplants need to be performed and followed for a longer time period to determine the relapse rate of malignant disease and whether CB can indeed mount an effective GVL response—and, if so, against which cancers. In this regard, a recent case report has demonstrated that even if a CB transplantation is ineffective in eliminating all minimal residual disease, the possibility exists to utilize donor-derived peripheral blood leukocyte infusions to increase the GVL effect [27].

III. CHARACTERIZATION OF CB IMMUNE CELLS

The results of CB transplantation regarding the lessened incidence and/or severity of GVHD—as compared with BMT performed in similar patients—suggest that there are quantitative and/or qualitative differences in the cells involved in GVHD. Such differences may affect the ability of CB immune cells to mount an effective GVL response. Interest in the mechanisms of reduced GVHD of CB transplantation and the possible effects on GVL responses has resulted in a great expansion in knowledge regarding the basic biology of CB immune cells, including T cells, NK cells, B cells, monocytes and macrophages, and dendritic cells. Both similarities and important differences have been noted.

A. Cord-Blood T Cells

1. Surface Antigen Phenotype of CB T Cells

While some results are conflicting, most reports demonstrate that the percentage of CD3+ T cells in CB is slightly but significantly lower than in adult peripheral blood (PB) [6,28–30]. We have found similar results even when contaminating granulocytes and nucleated erythroblasts are eliminated by antibody and complement prior to immunological staining [31]. Although the frequency of CD3+ T cells in CB is less than in PB, the absolute number is higher per unit volume owing to a general leukocytosis in CB [6,29]. Importantly, CB $\alpha\beta$ T cells have a fully formed, polyclonal T-cell receptor β-chain repertoire, suggesting that CB T cells have not been previously exposed to or responded to antigenic stimulation [32]. That CB T cells are naive is supported by the nearly uniform expression of CD45RA, a marker of previously unstimulated cells, and lack of expression of CD45RO, a marker for memory cells that can respond to recall antigens and provide help for B-cell antibody synthesis [6,33–40]. CB T cells also express CD26 and CD38 [33,41], antigens typically expressed on naive T cells or recent thymic emigrants. However, CB T cells do not express CD56 [42,43], CD57 [41,43], or inhibitory receptors for HLA class I molecules [44], which are typically found on a significant proportion of previously activated T cells. Important functional molecules such as CD28 and LFA-1 are expressed at normal levels on comparable numbers of freshly isolated CB and PB T cells [36,39], while anti-CD3 activated CB T cells express fully functional CD40L [45].

A significantly lower percentage of gamma-delta ($\gamma\delta$) T cells are found in CB than in PB [37,46]. Only a small proportion of those $\gamma\delta$ T cells present in CB express the cytotoxicity-associated marker serine esterase [46].

2. Functional Responses of CB T Cells

We and others have found that purified CB T cells demonstrate normal proliferative responses to alloantigens [38,39] or anti-CD3 plus anti-CD28 [47]. However, we have found that such primary stimulation induces a state of proliferative unresponsiveness upon secondary alloantigen or anti-CD3 plus anti-CD28 stimulation [47,48]. This state of unresponsiveness is marked by an inability to activate Ras upon secondary stimulation [47]. Stimulation of tolerized CB T cells with phorbol-12-myristate-13-acetate (PMA) and the calcium ionophore ionomycin, which bypasses the T-cell receptor (TcR) and CD3 complex by inducing calcium flux and stimulating protein kinase C (PKC) directly, can induce activation of Ras and subsequent proliferation [47]. This suggests that unresponsive CB T cells are viable and capable of proliferation and that any block in normal signaling is upstream of Ras. Tolerized CB T cells respond to interleukin-2 (IL-2) with vigorous proliferation, but the inclusion of IL-2 during primary stimulation does not prevent CB T-cell unresponsiveness to secondary TCR-dependent stimulation. Similar results were seen by Takahishi et al. in that primary stimulation with the bacterial superantigen toxic shock syndrome toxin-1 (TSST-1) induced proliferation and blastogenesis followed by a state of secondary unresponsiveness [40].

Differences in cytotoxic T-cell responses to alloantigen also exist between CB and bone marrow (BM) or peripheral blood (PB) T cells. Using CB mononuclear cells (MNCs) as responders in mixed lymphocyte culture (MLC), others have reported reduced cytotoxicity against stimulator cells [36,38]. We have observed similar results, even following secondary or tertiary stimulation, using purified CB T cells as responders [39]. In our assays, the percentage of CD8+ T cells was comparable between the CB and PB or BM samples. In contrast, a study by Roncarolo et al. found significant cytotoxic responses by CB when purified CD5+ T cells were used as responders and purified PB monocytes as stimulators. The reason for the conflicting results in these studies is not known, but they may be due to differences in the isolation procedures and the presence of different populations of cells that affected activation of the CB T cells.

Although most studies agree that CB T-cell cytotoxicity is reduced in comparison to that of BM or PB and that CB T cells can be rendered unresponsive to secondary TCR-dependent stimulation, CB contains normal frequencies of alloantigen-directed helper T-lymphocyte precursors (HTLp) and cytotoxic T-lymphocyte precursors (CTLp) [49,50]. While data regarding HTLp and CTLp frequencies and the data above regarding reduced cytotoxic activity and secondary proliferative responses seem contradictory, this may be due to the different readouts employed and the different conditions used in the assays. HTLp and CTLp assays determine only the frequencies of cells capable of mediating even very small responses, while other assays measure quantitative differences in the strengths of such responses.

Cytokine production by CB T cells differs both quantitatively and qualitatively with respect to that of PB T cells. Depending upon the stimulus provided, CB T cells either produce less [30,39] or comparable [49,51,52] amounts of IL-2 as similarly stimulated PB T cells. However, interferon-gamma (IFN-γ) production by CB T cells is uniformly low, with almost none produced [30,39,49,51–53]. Tumor necrosis factor-alpha (TNF-α) and IL-4 production by CB T cells is also low or nonexistent [39,52]. The provision of cytokines such as IL-4 or IL-12 during stimulation can modulate the types and amounts of cytokines produced by CB T cells, skewing them toward a T-helper 2 (Th2) or Th1 phenotype respectively [54–56].

Overall the data regarding CB T-cell phenotype and function suggest that they are very different from BM or PB T cells. Potentially relevant to the ability to mediate an effective GVL response is the lower cytotoxic activity, secondary unresponsiveness, and unusual cytokine production profile of CB T cells. It is important to determine the mechanisms behind these phenomena so that it will be possible to selectively counteract them and possibly improve the GVL capabilities of CB T cells.

B. Natural Killer Cells in CB

Human NK cells are a distinct lineage of lymphoid cells defined as being membrane CD3−, CD16+, and/or CD56+ [57,58]. The majority of adult PB NK cells are CD16+56+ with a minor population of CD16−56+ cells present [59]. NK cells typically have a large granular lymphocyte morphology and can lyse certain target cells without prior sensitization and without major histocompatibility (MHC) restriction [58]. A number of in vivo functions have been ascribed to NK cells including destruction of tumor cells, resistance to viral and bacterial infections, regulation of hematopoiesis, and resistance to allogeneic blood cell grafts [58]. These activities may be the result of direct lytic functions of NK cells, production of cytokines, or direct interactions with other leukocytes [58].

1. Surface Antigen Phenotype of CB NK Cells

In studying CB and PB, different investigators find either a comparable [60–64] or lesser [65] frequency of CD16-expressing lymphocytes and either a comparable [63,64] or lesser [62,65] frequency of CD56-expressing lymphocytes in CB. To address these discrepancies, we performed surface marker analysis on CB and PB samples and determined that in comparison to PB nonadherent MNC (naMNCs), CB naMNCs contain on average a comparable percentage of CD16-expressing lymphocytes but a lesser percentage of CD56-expressing lymphocytes [5]. In further comparing the phenotype of CB and PB NK cells we find the existence of a unique and large population of CD16+56− cell in CB as determined by two-color flow-cytometric analysis [5]. Other groups have also reported the existence of this unique population in CB [43,66], while one group failed to identify these cells [67]. We find that such CD16+56− cells typically comprise 10–30% of the CD16+ lymphocyte population in CB. NK cells with a

CD16+56− phenotype are very rare or nonexistent in blood cell compartments of healthy individuals [57,58]. However, such cells have been found in the peripheral blood of HIV-infected patients with or without AIDS [68], in the blood of children who received IL-2 following autologous bone marrow transplant for adjunct treatment of solid tumors [69], and in cancer patients receiving bolus high-dose IL-2 [70]. The relationship of the CD16+56− NK cells in these studies to CB CD16+56− NK cells is unknown and their relationship to CD56+ NK cells was not investigated. Another difference is that CB mCD3− CD56+ NK cells do not express the CD57 antigen [43,60,65], which is found on 50–60% of PB NK cells, but do express CD69 [43], which is characterized as an inducible lymphocyte antigen. We find that similar percentages of CB and PB NK cells express the T and NK cell–associated markers CD2, CD7, and CD8 [71].

2. Functional Activity of CB NK Cells

Most studies of CB NK activity have reported reduced lytic activity against K562 cells in comparison to adult PB [60–62,64,66,72–76], while a few have reported similar lytic activity [43,77]. Our studies to confirm the NK lytic abilities of CB using naMNCs agree with the majority of previous reports that CB NK lytic activity is on average significantly reduced in comparison to PB NK activity [5]. However, approximately 10% of individual CB samples have lytic activity comparable to that of PB. The reason for this heterogeneity of activity is unknown. These results suggest that previous reports of NK activity may not be as contradictory as first thought but rather may reflect the present but limited diversity of NK lytic activity of CB samples. Further functional studies performed in our laboratory using sorted CB and PB NK-cell subsets reveal distinct differences [5,78]. CB CD16+56− NK cells display little or no lytic activity against K562 cells, consistent with the findings using CD16+56− NK cells from HIV infected patients and cancer patients receiving IL-2 discussed above [68,70]. CB CD16+56+ NK cells have lytic activities ranging from little or none to adult-like levels; while PB CD16+56+ NK cells had high adult levels of activity. These results suggest a hierarchy of lytic activity CB CD16+56− $\leq$ CB CD16+56+ $\leq$ PB CD 16+56+. The mechanism for the reduced lytic activity of CB NK-cell subsets is unclear. CB NK cells are able to bind target cells and express the lytic moieties perforin and granzyme-B [5,71]. In addition, CB NK-cell subsets demonstrate high lytic activity when induced by PMA and ionomycin treatment during lytic assays to undergo efficient granule exocytosis [71]. These results suggest that the mechanism of reduced lytic activity of CB NK-cell subsets include absent or reduced expression of triggering receptor(s) and/or deficient stimulus-dependent granule exocytosis due to inefficient signalling.

Whatever mechanism is responsible for the defects in CB NK lytic activity, we and others have demonstrated that overnight incubation of CB MNCs or CB

CD16+56− and CD16+56+ cell populations with IL-2 [5,43,60–63,66,75], IL-12 [5,63], or IL-15 [71,79], but not IL-7 [63,78], IFN-γ [61,63,78], or tumor necrosis factor-α (TNF-α) [63,78], increases the lytic activity of CB NK cells against K562 targets. Also, 5- to 7-day culture with IL-2 [5,63,80,81], IL-12 [5,63], and IL-15 [79] but not IL-7, IFN-γ or TNF-α [63], induces lymphokine activated killer (LAK) activity against NK-resistant target cell lines or fresh leukemic cells.

In addition to increasing the lytic activity of CB NK cells, IL-2, IL-12, and IL-15 induce the phenotypic maturation of CB CD16+56− NK cells. Five- to seven-day culture of CB CD16+56− cells with IL-2 or IL-15 generates CD16+56+ NK cells, while culture with IL-12 generates both CD16+56+ and CD16−56+ NK cells. Studies utilizing the membrane-staining dye PKH2 demonstrate that IL-2 and IL-15 cause significant proliferation, that IL-12 causes little if any proliferation, and that proliferation is not necessary for phenotypic change induced by IL-2, IL-12, or IL-15.

Together, the data suggest that CB NK cells are functionally and phenotypically immature. However, proper cytokine stimulation induces the maturation of CB NK cells. The ability of cytokines possibly encountered in vivo following transplantation—such as IL-2, IL-12, and IL-15—to increase the lytic activity of CB NK cells and generate CB LAK activity suggests that CB NK cells will mediate GVL effects in vivo. This may compensate for the possible reduced ability of CB T cells to mediate such an effect. While other effector functions, such as the ability to produce cytokines, may be important in NK-cell GVL effects, they have not been well studied in CB NK cells.

C. Biology of CB B Cells

1. Surface Antigen Phenotype of CB B Cells

Similar percentages of B cells are present in CB and adult PB [6,37]. However, CB B cells have unique phenotypic characteristics. The antigens CD1c, CD38, CD5, and CD23, although normally expressed on only a small percentage of circulating B cells in adults, are highly expressed on CB B cells and suggest an immature phenotype [4,6,37,42]. Conversely, CB B cells do not express CD27, which is associated with high immunoglobulin production, nor surface immunoglobulin G (IgG) or IgA [82,83]. Expression of HLA class II molecules on CB B cells is normal [36], although antigen-presentation functions have not been tested.

2. Functional Activity of CB B Cells

Although CB B cells have unique phenotypic characteristics and there are no significant levels of endogenously produced IgG, IgA, or IgE in CB serum, they do not seem to be functionally immature. Culture of CB B cells in the presence of cytokines such as IL-2, IL-4, or IL-6 induces the secretion of all Ig isotypes [84], whereas incubation with IL-4 and anti-CD40 antibodies induces secretion of IgM, IgG, IgG4, and IgE antibodies [49]. Activation of CB T cells with anti-CD3 antibodies induces the expression of functional CD40L and allows CB T cells to provide proper helper functions and induce CB B cell Ig production and CD86 expression [45]. These results suggest that CB B-cell deficits in Ig isotype production are probably secondary to deficient T-cell help.

Whether CB B cells would contribute to a GVL effect following transplantation via either antibody production or antigen presentation is unknown.

D. Biology of CB Monocytes

Human monocytes mediate potent phagocytic and antigen-presenting functions and typically express the CD14 surface antigen. Phenotypic analysis reveals that significantly reduced amounts of Fc-receptor-gamma III (Fc_γRIII or CD16) are present on CB CD14dim monocytes relative to adult CD14dim monocytes, but that Fc_γRI (CD64) and Fc_γRII (CD32) are expressed at normal levels [85,86]. HLA class II antigens, CD28, and ICAM-1 are also expressed at lower levels and in lower percentages of CB monocytes [49,85]. Direct assays of the antigen-presenting abilities of CB monocytes have not been reported. The relevance of these data to the GVL capabilities of CB is unknown.

E. Biology of CB Dendritic Cells

A single study of freshly isolated CB dendritic cells reveals evidence for phenotypic and functional immaturity [87]. Flow cytometric analysis showed that ICAM-1, HLA class I, and HLA class II antigens are expressed at significantly lower levels those observed on adult PB dendritic cells. More importantly, CB dendritic cells were poor stimulators of mixed leukocyte reactions when adult MNCs or T cells were used as responders. The role that functionally immature dendritic cells play in the reduced functionality of CB T cells is unknown. It is likely that a reduced ability to present antigen in a stimulatory manner would reduce the GVL capabilities of CB T cells.

Although freshly isolated CB dendritic cells have decreased functional capability, fully functional dendritic cells can be generated from CB progenitor cells. In response to GM-CSF+TNF-α, CD34+ hematopoietic progenitors from human cord blood differentiate along two independent dendritic cell pathways to become either CD1a Langerhans-like cells or CD14+ dendritic cells [88]. Dendritic cells can also be generated from CB CD34+ progenitors upon culture with IL-3 plus TNF-α [89], or upon cross-linking CD40 independent of exogenous cytokine addition [90]. Overall, these data suggest that dendritic cells could be generated from CB progenitors for the purpose of presenting exogenously added or vector-encoded leukemia-specific antigens or to provide other moieties necessary to develop competent CB T-cell responses.

IV. GENE THERAPY POTENTIAL

Various populations of CB progenitor cells can be transduced at high efficiency by either retrovirus [91,92] or adeno-associated virus [93]. This raises the possibility of using gene transduction technology to enhance the GVL potential of CB. Of interest, fully functional retrovirally transduced dendritic cells can be generated during culture of CB progenitors [91–93]. In addition, T cells expressing novel genes can be generated from retrovirally transduced CB CD34+ cells [91–93]. Obviously, before gene transduction technology can be used to increase the GVL capabilities of CB, GVL-enhancing gene products must be identified and characterized.

V. SUMMARY

Human CB has only recently begun to be used as a source of stem cells for transplant purposes. While there are as yet no indications that CB transplantation is associated with enhanced relapse rates compared with those noted with BMT, not enough CB transplants have been performed and not enough time has elapsed to determine whether CB can mediate an effective GVL effect. Initial clinical and laboratory results regarding the reduced incidence and/or severity of GVHD and the reduced functions of many immune cell types in CB suggest that CB would potentially have a reduced capacity to mediate GVL effects. It is therefore important to continue to study immune reconstitution; rates and severity of GVHD, relapse rates of leukemias, lymphomas, or tumors; and—most importantly—overall survival rates following CB transplantation. It is also important to continue to study the basic biology of CB immune cells, especially the mechanisms of induction of T-cell unresponsiveness and the antigen-presenting capabilities of cells such as dendritic cells, B cells, and monocytes. Only with more extensive combined clinical and laboratory investigation will it be determined whether CB is capable of mediating an effective GVL response, and if not, how to enhance its ability to do so.

ACKNOWLEDGMENT

J.G. and P.P. were supported by Public Health Service Training Grant T32DK07519 from the NIH to H.E.B.

REFERENCES

1. Broxmeyer HE, Douglas GW, Hangoc G, Cooper S, Bard J, English D, Arny M, Thomas L, Boyse EA. Human umbilical cord blood as a potential source of transplantable hematopoietic stem/progenitor cells. Proc Natl Acad Sci USA 1989; 86: 3828.
2. Broxmeyer HE, Kurtzberg J, Gluckman E, Auerbach AD, Douglas G, Cooper S, Falkenburg JH, Bard J, Boyse EA. Umbilical cord blood hematopoietic stem and repopulating cells in human clinical transplantation. Blood Cells 1991; 17:313.
3. Broxmeyer HE, Hangoc G, Cooper S, Ribeiro RC, Graves V, Yoder M, Wagner J, Vadhan-Raj S, Benninger L, Rubinstein P, Brown ER. Growth characteristics and expansion of human umbilical cord blood and estimation of its potential for transplantation in adults. Proc Natl Acad Sci USA 1992; 89:4109.
4. Cicuttini FM, Boyd AW. Hemopoietic and lymphoid progenitor cells in human umbilical cord blood. Dev Immunol 1994; 4:1.
5. Gaddy J, Risdon G, Broxmeyer HE. Cord blood natural killer cells are functionally and phenotypically immature but readily respond to interleukin-2 and interleukin-12. J Interferon Cytokine Res 1995; 15:527.
6. Hannet I, Erkeller-Yuksel F, Lydyard P, Deneys V, DeBruyere M. Developmental and maturational changes in human blood lymphocyte subpopulations (see comments). Immunol Today 1992; 13:215.
7. Miller ME. Phagocyte function in the neonate: selected aspects. Pediatrics 1979; 64: 709.
8. Gluckman E, Broxmeyer HE, Auerbach AD, Friedman HS, Douglas GW, Devergie A, Esperou H, Thierry D, Socie G, Lehn P, Cooper S, English D, Kurtzberg J, Bard J, Boyse EA. Hematopoietic reconstitution in a patient with Fanconi's anemia by means of umbilical cord blood from an HLA-identical sibling. N Engl J Med 1989; 321:1174.
9. Gluckman E. Umbilical cord blood transplant in human. Bone Marrow Transplant 1996; 18:166.
10. Wagner JE. Umbilical cord blood transplantation: overview of the clinical experience [see comments]. Blood Cells 1994; 20:227.
11. Kogler G, Callejas J, Hakenberg P, Enczmann J, Adams O, Daubener W, Krempe C, Gobel U, Somville T, Wernet P. Hematopoietic transplant potential of unrelated cord blood: critical issues. J Hematother 1996; 5:105.
12. Kurtzberg J. Umbilical cord blood: a novel alternative source of hematopoietic stem cells for bone marrow transplantation (editorial). J Hematother 1996; 5:95.
13. Newburger PE, Quesenberry PJ. Umbilical cord blood as a new and promising source of unrelated-donor hematopoietic stem cells for transplantation. Curr Opin Pediatr 1996; 8:29.
14. Kurtzberg J, Laughlin M, Graham ML, Smith C, Olson JF, Halperin EC, Ciocci G, Carrier C, Stevens CE, Rubinstein P. Placental blood as a source of hematopoietic stem cells for transplantation into unrelated recipients (see comments). N Engl J Med 1996; 335:157.
15. Wagner JE, Kernan NA, Steinbuch M, Broxmeyer HE, Gluckman E. Allogeneic

sibling umbilical-cord-blood transplantation in children with malignant and non-malignant disease (see comments). Lancet 1995; 346:214.
16. Wagner JE, Rosenthal J, Sweetman R, Shu XO, Davies SM, Ramsay NK, McGlave PB, Sender L, Cairo MS. Successful transplantation of HLA-matched and HLA-mismatched umbilical cord blood from unrelated donors: analysis of engraftment and acute graft versus host disease. Blood 1996; 88:795.
17. Wagner JE, Kurtzberg J. Allogeneic Umbilical Cord Blood Transplantation. Bethesda, MD: AABB Press, 1998.
18. Lambertengh Delliers, G, Soligo D, Della Volpe A, Bertolini F, Poli F, Romitti L, Tagliaferri E, Ibatici A, Onida F, Annaloro C, Gattinoni L, Sirchia G. Unrelated mismatched cord blood transplantation in an adult with secondary AML. Bone Marrow Transplant 1996; 18:469.
19. Fernandez MN, Regidor C, Diez JL, Fores R, Sanjuan I, Briz M, Cabrera R. HLA haploidentical cord blood cell transplantin a 15-year-old, 50 kg weight patient: successful treatment for chronic myeloid leukemia after myeloid blastic transformation. Bone Marrow Transplant 1996; 17:1175.
20. Horowitz MM, Gale RP, Sondel PM, Goldman JM, Kersey J, Kolb HJ, Rimm AA, Ringden O, Rozman C, Speck B, Truitt RL, Zwaan FE, Burtin MM. Graft versus-leukemia reactions after bone marrow transplantation. Blood 1990; 75:555.
21. Nash RA, Storb R. Graft-versus-host effect after allogeneic hematopoietic stem cell transplantation: GVHD and GVL. Curr Opin Immunol 1996; 8:674.
22. Gluckman E, Rocha V, Boyer-Chammard A, Locatelli F, Arcese W, Pasquini R, Ortega J, Souillet G, Ferreira E, Laporte JP, Fernandez M, Chastang C. Outcome of cord-blood transplantation from related and unrelated donors: Eurocord Transplant Group and the European Blood and Marrow Transplantation Group. N Engl J Med 1997; 337:373.
23. Wagner JE, DeFor T, Rubinstein P, Kurtzberg J. Transplantation of unrelated donor umbilical cord blood: outcomes and analysis of risk factors. Blood 1997; 90:1767a.
24. Laughlin MJ, McKinnon K, Demarest J, Buckley R, Weinhold K, Kaufman R, Koropchak CM, DeSombre K, Iaobucci M, Cook JM, Martinek L, DeOliveira D, Kurtzberg J. Immune recovery post-unrelated allogeneic umbilical cord blood transplantation in adult recipients. Blood 1997, 90:1868a.
25. Locatelli F, Maccario R, Comoli P, Bertolini F, Giorgiani G, Montagna D, Bonetti F, De Stefano P, Rondini G, Sirchia G, Severi F. Hematopoietic and immune recovery after transplantation of cord blood progenitor cells in children. Bone Marrow Transplant 1996; 18:1095.
26. Kernan NA. T-cell depletion for the prevention of graft-versus-host disease. In: Forman SJ, Blume KG, Thomas ED, eds. Bone Marrow Transplantation. Cambridge, England: Blackwell, 1994, p. 124.
27. Locatelli F, Comoli P, Giorgiani G, Carra AM, Di Giulio G, Di Maggio EM, Pellegrini N, Maccario R. Infusion of donor-derived peripheral blood leukocytes after transplantation of cord blood progenitor cells can increase the graft-versus-leukaemia effect. Leukemia 1997; 11:729.
28. Griffiths-Chu S, Patterson JA, Berger CL, Edelson RL, Chu AC. Characterization of immature T cell subpopulations in neonatal blood. Blood 1984; 64:296.

29. Lim FT, van Winsen L, Willemze R, Kanhai HH, Falkenburg JH. Influence of delivery on numbers of leukocytes, leukocyte subpopulations, and hematopoietic progenitor cells in human umbilical cord blood. Blood Cells 1994; 20:547.
30. Milosevits J, Pocsik E, Schmidt B, Remenyi P, Intodi ZS, Reti M, Batai A, Illes P, Mihalik R, Petranyi GG, Paloczi K. Immunophenotypic and functional characteristics of haemopoietic cells from human cord blood. Scand J Immunol 1995; 42:493.
31. Risdon G, Gaddy J, Broxmeyer HE. Allogeneic responses of human umbilical cord blood. Blood Cells 1994; 20:566.
32. Garderet L, Dulphy N, Douay C, Chalumeau N, Schaeffer V, Zilber M, Lim A, Even N, Mooney N, Gelin C, Gluckman E, Charron D, Toubert A. The umbilical cord blood αβ T-cell repertoire: characteristic of a polyclonal and naive but completely formed repertoire. Blood 1998; 91:340.
33. Amlot PL, Tahami F, Chinn D, Rawlings E. Activation antigen expression on human T cells: I. Analysis by two-colour flow cytometry of umbilical cord blood, adult blood and lymphoid tissue. Clin Exp Immunol 1996; 105:176.
34. Beck R, and Lam-Po-Tang PR. Comparison of cord blood and adult blood lymphocyte normal ranges: a possible explanation for decreased severity of graft versus host disease after cord blood transplantation. Immunol Cell Biol 1994; 72:440.
35. Han P, Hodge G, Story C, Xu X. Phenotypic analysis of functional T-lymphocyte subtypes and natural killer cells in human cord blood: relevance to umbilical cord blood transplantation. Br J Haematol 1995; 89:733.
36. Keever CA. Characterization of cord blood lymphocyte subpopulations. J Hematother 1993; 2:203.
37. Osugi Y, Hara J, Kurahashi H, Sakata N, Inoue M, Yumura-Yagi K, Kawa-Ha K, Okada S, Tawa A. Age-related changes in surface antigens on peripheral lymphocytes of healthy children. Clin Exp Immunol 1995; 100:543.
38. Roncarolo MG, Bigler M, Martino S, Ciuti E, Tovo PA, Wagner J. Immune functions of cord blood cells before and after transplantation. J Hematother 1996; 5:157.
39. Risdon G, Gaddy J, Stehman FB, Broxmeyer HE. Proliferative and cytotoxic responses of human cord blood T lymphocytes following allogeneic stimulation. Cell Immunol 1994; 154:14.
40. Takahishi N, Imanishi K, Nishida H, Uchiyama T. Evidence for immunologic immaturity of cord blood T cells. J Immunol 1995; 155:5213.
41. Lucivero G, Dalla Mora L, Bresciano E, Loria MP, Pezone L, Mancino D. Functional characteristics of cord blood T lymphocytes after lectin and anti-CD3 stimulation: differences in the way T cells express activation molecules and proliferate. Int J Clin Lab Res 1996; 26:255.
42. Motley D, Meyer MP, King RA, Naus GJ. Determination of lymphocyte immunophenotypic values for normal full-term cord blood. Am J Clin Pathol 1996; 105: 38.
43. Phillips JH, Hori T, Nagler A, Bhat N, Spits H, Lanier LL. Ontogeny of human natural killer (NK) cells: fetal NK cells mediate cytolytic function and express cytoplasmic CD3 epsilon, delta proteins. J Exp Med 1992; 175:1055.
44. Mingari MC, Ponte M, Vitale C, Schiavetti F, Bertone S, Moretta L. Inhibitory receptors for HLA class I molecules on cytolytic T lymphocytes. Functional rele-

vance and implications for anti-tumor immune responses. Int J Clin Lab Res 1997; 27:87.
45. Splawski JB, Nishioka J, Nishioka Y, Lipsky PE. CD40 ligand is expressed and functional on activated neonatal T cells. J Immunol 1996; 156:119.
46. Smith MD, Worman C, Yuksel F, Yuksel B, Moretta L, Ciccone E, Grossi CE, MacKenzie L, Lydyard PM. T gamma delta-cell subsets in cord and adult blood. Scand J Immunol 1990; 32:491.
47. Porcu P, Gaddy J, Broxmeyer HE. Alloantigen-induced unresponsiveness in cord blood T-lymphocytes is associated with defective activation of Ras. Proc Natl Acad Sci USA 1998; 95(8):4538.
48. Risdon G, Gaddy J, Horie M, Broxmeyer HE. Alloantigen priming induces a state of unresponsiveness in human umbilical cord blood T cells. Proc Natl Acad Sci USA 1995; 92:2413.
49. Roncarolo MG, Bigler M, Ciuti E, Martino S, Tovo PA. Immune responses by cord blood cells. Blood Cells 1994; 20:573.
50. Falkenburg JH, van Luxemburg-Heijs SA, Lim FT, Kanhai HH, Willemze R. Umbilical cord blood contains normal frequencies of cytotoxic T-lymphocyte precursors (ctlp) and helper T-lymphocyte precursors against noninherited maternal antigens and noninherited paternal antigens. Ann Hematol 1996; 72:260.
51. Miyawaki T, Seki H, Taga K, Sato H, Taniguchi N. Dissociated production of interleukin-2 and immune (gamma) interferon by phytohaemagglutinin stimulated lymphocytes in healthy infants. Clin Exp Immunol 1985; 59:505.
52. Sautois B, Fillet G, Beguin Y. Comparative cytokine production by in vitro stimulated mononucleated cells from cord blood and adult blood. Exp Hematol 1997; 25: 103.
53. von Freeden U, Zessack N, van Valen F, Burdach S. Defective interferon gamma production in neonatal T cells is independent of interleukin-2 receptor binding. Pediatr Res 1991; 30:270.
54. Wu CY, Demeure C, Gately M, Podlaski F, Yssel H, Kiniwa M, Delespesse G. In vitro maturation of human neonatal CD4 T lymphocytes: induction of IL-4-producing cells after long-term culture in the presence of IL-4 plus either IL-2 or IL-12. J Immunol 1994; 152:1141.
55. Sornasse T, Larenas PV, Davis KA, de Vries JE, Yssel H. Differentiation and stability of T helper 1 and 2 cells derived from naive human neonatal CD4+ T cells, analyzed at the single-cell level. J Exp Med 1996; 184:473.
56. Ehlers S, Smith KA. Differentiation of T cell lymphokine gene expression: the in vitro acquisition of T cell memory. J Exp Med 1991; 173:25.
57. Lanier LL, Phillips JH, Hackett J, Jr, Tutt M, Kumar V. Natural killer cells: definition of a cell type rather than a function [published errata appear in J Immunol 1987; 138:996 and 1987; 138:2745] J Immunol 1986; 137:2735.
58. Robertson MJ, Ritz J. Biology and clinical relevance of human natural killer cells. Blood 1990; 76:2421.
59. Lanier LL, Le AM, Civin CI, Loken MR, Phillips JH. The relationship of CD16 (Leu-11) and Leu-19 (NKH-1) antigen expression on human peripheral blood NK cells and cytotoxic T lymphocytes. J Immunol 1986; 136:4480.

60. Seki H, Ueno Y, Taga K, Matsuda A, Miyawaki T, Taniguchi N. Mode of in vitro augmentation of natural killer cell activity by recombinant human interleukin 2: a comparative study of Leu-11+ and Leu-11-cell populations in cord blood and adult peripheral blood. J Immunol 1985; 135:2351.
61. Ueno Y, Miyawaki T, Seki H, Matsuda A, Taga K, Sato H, Taniguchi N. Differential effects of recombinant human interferon-gamma and interleukin 2 on natural killer cell activity of peripheral blood in early human development. J Immunol 1985; 135: 180.
62. Yabuhara A, Kawai H, Komiyama A. Development of natural killer cytotoxicity during childhood: marked increases in number of natural killer cells with adequate cytotoxic abilities during infancy to early childhood. Pediatr Res 1990; 28:316.
63. Webb BJ, Bochan MR, Montel A, Padilla LM, Brahmi Z. The lack of NK cytotoxicity associated with fresh HUCB may be due to the presence of soluble HLA in the serum. Cell Immunol 1994; 159:246.
64. McDonald T, Sneed J, Valenski WR, Dockter M, Cooke R, Herrod HG. Natural killer cell activity in very low birth weight infants. Pediatr Res 1992; 31:376.
65. Slukvin II, Chemishov VP. Two-color flow cytometric analysis of natural killer and cytotoxic T-lymphocyte subsets in peripheral blood of normal human neonates. Biol Neonate 1992; 61:156.
66. Bradstock KF, Luxford C, Grimsley PG. Functional and phenotypic assessment of neonatal human leucocytes expressing natural killer cell-associated antigens. Immunol Cell Biol 1993; 71:535.
67. Cicuttini FM, Martin M, Petrie HT, Boyd AW. A novel population of natural killer progenitor cells isolated from human umbilical cord blood. J Immunol 1993; 151: 29.
68. Hu PF, Hultin LE, Hultin P, Hausner MA, Hirji K, Jewett A, Bonavida B, Detels R, Giorgi JV. Natural killer cell immunodeficiency in HIV disease is manifest by profoundly decreased numbers of CD16+CD56+ cells and expansion of a population of CD16dim CD56− cells with low lytic activity. J Acquir Immune Defic Syndr Human Retrovirol 1995; 10:331.
69. Dilloo D, Laws HJ, Hanenberg H, Korholz D, Nurnberger W, Burdach SE. Induction of two distinct natural killer cell populations, activated T cells and antineoplastic cytokines, by interleukin-2 therapy in children with solid tumors. Exp Hematol 1994; 22:1081.
70. McKenzie RS, Simms PE, Helfrich BA, Fisher RI, Ellis TM. Identification of a novel CD56− lymphokine-activated killer cell precursor in cancer patients receiving recombinant interleukin 2. Cancer Res 1992; 52:6318.
71. Gaddy J, Broxmeyer HE. Cord blood CD15+56− cells with low lytic activity are possible precursors of mature natural killer cells. Cell Immunol 1997; 180:132.
72. Baley JE, Schacter BZ. Mechanisms of diminished natural killer cell activity in pregnant women and neonates. J Immunol 1985; 134:3042.
73. Kaplan J, Shope TC, Bollinger RO, Smith J. Human newborns are deficient in natural killer activity. J Clin Immunol 1982; 2:350.
74. Lubens RG, Gard SE, Soderberg-Warner M, Stiehm ER. Lectin-dependent T-lymphocyte and natural killer cytotoxic deficiencies in human newborns. Cell Immunol 1982; 74:40.

75. Nair MP, Schwartz SA, Menon M. Association of decreased natural and antibody-dependent cellular cytotoxicity and production of natural killer cytotoxic factor and interferon in neonates. Cell Immunol 1985; 94:159.
76. Toder V, Durdana A, Elrad H, Gleicher N. Natural killing (NK) potential of cord blood lymphocytes. J Clin Lab Immunol 1985; 17:29.
77. Poros A, Klein E. Distinction of anti-K562 and anti-allocytotoxicity in in vitro stimulated populations of human lymphocytes. Cell Immunol 1979; 46:57.
78. Gaddy J, Broxmeyer HE. Cord blood CD16+56− cells with low lytic activity are possible precursors of mature natural killer cells. Cell Immunology 1997; 180(2): 132.
79. Qian JX, Lee SM, Suen Y, Knoppel E, van de Ven C, Cairo MS. Decreased interleukin-15 from activated cord versus adult peripheral blood mononuclear cells and the effect of interleukin-15 in upregulating antitumor immune activity and cytokine production in cord blood. Blood 1997; 90:3106.
80. Malygin AM, Timonen T. Non-major histocompatibility complex-restricted killer cells in human cord blood: generation and cytotoxic activity in recombinant interleukin-2-supplemented cultures. Immunology 1993; 79:506.
81. Ghin TW, Ank BJ, Murakami D, Gill M, Spina C, Strom S, Stiehm ER. Cytotoxic studies in human newborns: lessened allogeneic cell-induced (augmented) cytotoxicity but strong lymphokine-activated cytotoxicity of cord mononuclear cells. Cell Immunol 1986; 103:241.
82. Agematsu K, Nagumo H, Yang FC, Nakazawa T, Fukushima K, Ito S, Sugita K, Mori T, Kobata T, Morimoto C, Komiyama A. B cell subpopulations separated by CD27 and crucial collaboration of CD27+ B cells and helper T cells in immunoglob ulin production. Eur J Immunol 1997; 27:2073.
83. Wedgwood JF, Weinberger BI, Hatam L, Palmer R. Umbilical cord blood lacks circulating B lymphocytes expressing surface IgG or IgA. Clin Immunol Immunopathol 1997; 84:276.
84. Splawski JB, Lipskey PE. Cytokine regulation of immunoglobulin secretion by neonatal lymphocytes. J Clin Invest 1991; 88:967.
85. Murphy FJ, Reen DJ. Differential expression of function-related antigens on newborn and adult monocyte subpopulations. Immunology 1996; 89:587.
86. Maeda M, van Schie RC, Yuksel B, Greenough A, Fanger MW, Guyre PM, Lydyard PM. Differential expression of Fc receptors for IgG by monocytes and granulocytes from neonates and adults. Clin Exp Immunol 1996; 103:343.
87. Hunt DW, Huppertz HI, Jiang HJ, Petty RE. Studies of human cord blood dendritic cells: evidence for functional immaturity. Blood 1994; 84:4333.
88. Caux C, Vanbervliet B, Massacrier C, Dezutter-Dambuyant C, de Saint-Vis B, Jacquet C, Yoneda K, Imamura S, Schmitt D, Banchereau J. CD34+ hematopoietic progenitors from human cord blood differentiate along two independent dendritic cell pathways in response to GM-CSF+TNF alpha. J Exp Med 1996; 184:695.
89. Caux C, Vanbervliet B, Massacrier C, Durand I, Banchereau J. Interleukin-3 cooperates with tumor necrosis factor alpha for the development of human dendritic/Langerhans cells from cord blood CD34+ hematopoietic progenitor cells. Blood 1996; 87:2376.
90. Flores Romo L, Bjorck P, Duvert V, van Kooten C, Saeland S, Banchereau J. CD40

ligation on human cord blood CD34+ hematopoietic progenitors induces their proliferation and differentiation into functional dendritic cells. J Exp Med 1997; 185: 341.

91. Bello-Fernandez C, Matyash M, Strobl H, Pickl WF, Majdic O, Lyman SD, Knapp W. Efficient retrovirus-mediated gene transfer of dendritic cells generated from CD34+ cord blood cells under serum-free conditions. Hum Gene Ther 1997; 8: 1651.
92. Szabolcs P, Gallardo HF, Ciocon DH, Sadelain M, Young JW. Retrovirally transduced human dendritic cells express a normal phenotype and potent T-cell stimulatory capacity. Blood 1997; 90:2160.
93. Broxmeyer HE, Cooper S, Etienne-Julan M, Wang XS, Ponnazhagan S, Braun S, Lu L, Srivastava A. Cord blood transplantation and the potential for gene therapy. Gene transduction using a recombinant adeno-associated viral vector. Ann NY Acad Sci 1995; 770:105.

14
Separating GVHD and GVL Reactions

Dimitrios Mavroudis
University General Hospital
Heraklion, Crete, Greece

John Barrett
National Institutes of Health
Bethesda, Maryland

I. INTRODUCTION

When the phenomenon of the graft-versus-leukemia (GVL) effect was first described by Barnes and Loutit [1], there was no indication that it was anything other than a particular aspect of a graft-versus-host disease (GVHD) reaction. This perception persisted into the era of clinical transplantation, along with the assumption that GVL and GVHD were inseparable. While it is correct to state that GVL and GVH reactions share common mechanisms and that GVL reactions typically accompany GVHD, there is good clinical evidence indicating that the two phenomena can be separated. These data are summarized in Table 1.

II. EXPERIMENTAL BASIS FOR SEPARATION OF GVH AND GVL

Besides the clinical data, there is a large body of evidence supporting the separability of T-cell responses to leukemia and other tissues. In the fully allogeneic setting, it is possible to identify T-cell lines with reactivity against leukemia blasts and nonreactivity against normal hematological cells from the same individual

Table 1 Clinical Situations Where GVHD and GVL Reactions Are Separated

Leukemia patients not developing GVHD and receiving T cell–replete BMT have a lower risk of relapse than patients receiving T cell–depleted transplants demonstrating a "pure" GVL effect of donor T cells [2].
Leukemia patients given DLT to treat relapse after allogeneic BMT can achieve further remissions without developing GVHD [3].
Leukemic relapse after BMT can be reversed by prompt cessation of cyclosporine immunosuppression without onset of GVHD (Chapter 14).

[4]. In HLA-identical siblings, cytotoxic T lymphocytes (CTLs) specifically lysing leukemic or nonleukemic targets have also been isolated [5]. Furthermore, murine experiments confirm the presence of GVL reactivity independent of GVHD [6]. In another study, CTL lines were generated from patients at different time points during the course of acute GVHD after an HLA-identical sibling bone marrow transplant (BMT). Clones with three different reactivities were identified: clones reacting only against normal peripheral blood lymphocytes (PBLs), clones reacting only against leukemic cells, and clones reacting with both [7]. This was also confirmed in another in vitro model, where allogeneic T-cell clones able to selectively destroy Philadelphia chromosome–bearing human leukemia lines were also able to recognize Ph-cells from the same patient [8]. Similar results have been announced using minor histocompatibility antigen (mHA)-specific CTLs from patients with GVHD. The targeted mHAs were simultaneously expressed on several host cell lines, including lymphoblastoid cell lines, PHA blasts, leukemic cells, and keratinocytes [9].

The challenge now is to devise clinical techniques to control immune recovery after allogeneic stem-cell transplantation so as to exploit the GVL reaction without causing GVHD. However, before the clinical separation of GVL from GVHD can become a clinical reality, those factors that positively or negatively influence the separability of GVHD from GVL must be considered. These are outlined in Table 2 and discussed below.

III. FACTORS INFLUENCING SEPARABILITY OF GVL FROM GVHD

A. Tissue-Restricted Minor Histocompatibility Antigens (mHA)

The major argument favoring the separability of GVL from GVHD rests on the diversity of the antigens presented to alloreacting T cells and the corresponding diversity of the T-cell repertoire. Although sharing many common protein constit-

Table 2 Factors For and Against the Separability of GVL from GVHD

	GVL Without GVHD	GVL with GVHD
Antigens	Leukemia-specific or hematopoietic cell lineage–restricted antigens eliciting tissue-restricted T cell responses.	Ubiquitously expressed mHA direct T-cell attack to both leukemia and other host tissues.
Antigen presentation	Myeloid leukemia cells expressing MHC class I and II are better APC than cells from nonhematopoietic tissues.	All cells expressing MHC class I and II are subject to allogeneic T-cell recognition and cytotoxicity.
Effector cells	In vitro evidence of CTLs specific for leukemia. In vivo evidence of expanded CTL populations with Vβ restriction and antileukemic specificity.	In vitro and in vivo evidence of T cells with indiscriminate cytotoxicity to leukemia and nonleukemic recipient tissues.
	CD4 cells have greater GVL reactivity than GVHD reactivity. Th2 subsets have greater GVL reactivity than GVHD reactivity.	Some leukemias may only be responsive to CD8 and Th1 T cell–mediated GVL effects.
Cytokines and effector pathways	Leukemia cells with greater sensitivity than normal cells to proliferation inhibition and cytotoxicity from cytokines.	GVHD and GVL responses end in a final common pathway of nonspecific cytokine-mediated tissue damage.
Timing	Delayed infusion of T cells conserves GVL reactivity but confers low GVHD reactivity.	GVHD still occurs following delayed infusion of T cells.
	Time to achieve leukemia reduction more rapid than time for major organ damage from GVHD (rationale for suicide gene strategy).	Molecular cures of CML after DLT takes many months.
T-cell homing	T cells with different specificities home to different tissues.	Homing not discriminative for GVH and GVL reactions.
Tolerance	Tolerance is established after GVL effect is complete. Tolerance can be broken by DLT.	Tolerance is an early feature of immune reconstitution without GVHD. Tolerance is associated with mixed chimerism, absence of GVHD, and lack of GVL effect.

uents, cells from different tissues also have distinct patterns of protein expression that define their lineage. Cells from different tissues could therefore induce alloresponses in different T-cell responder clones by presenting lineage-restricted self peptides through their MHC molecules. However, in most clinical situations, where steps are not taken to select leukemia-specific T cells, the recognition of ubiquitously expressed immunodominant mHA results in a strong nonspecific GVL/GVHD alloresponse. The fine specificity of the T-cell repertoire can only be exploited by selecting T-cell lines or clones with specific reactivity to defined leukemia-restricted antigens. Such leukemia-restricted antigens may be either mHAs expressed on lymphoid and myeloid cells (Chapter 5), normal proteins overexpressed in leukemia cells (Chapter 6), or antigens unique to the leukemia cell (Chapter 7). The occurrence of these antigens is the basis for strategies to create leukemia-specific CTL clones for adoptive immunotherapy. Hitherto this approach has been limited by our almost complete ignorance of the antigens involved. This is beginning to change: apart from the 8 mHAs identified by Goulmy's group (see Chapter 5), other mHAs are beginning to be identified. Riddell has described over 50 new mHA T-cell clones, derived from posttransplant donor T cells, defined by their characteristic profile of activity with a panel of cells from different tissues of the same individual [10]. Dolstra et al. have recently identified a B cell–specific mHA [11]. An alternative approach to finding new antigens has been to study known myeloid or lymphoid-restricted proteins for peptide sequences that bind to common HLA molecules: synthetic peptides are then tested for their ability to induce CTL with antileukemic or tissue-restricted specificity. Additionally, well-expressed proteins such as CD33 have been studied to identify alleles that could function as mHAs [12]. A similar approach has been taken with leukemia-specific fusion proteins, where peptide sequences spanning the fusion region have been used to induce CTLs with antileukemic specificity (see Chapters 6 and 19). Table 3 lists the defined protein antigens so far characterized.

B. Antigen Presentation

Malignancies arising from the lymphohematopoietic system retain some of the characteristics of the unique antigen-presenting capacity that characterizes their normal B-cell, monocyte-macrophage, or dendritic cell counterparts. It is thus possible that leukemias are better antigen-presenting cells (APCs) than nonhematopoietic tissues and could induce stronger alloresponses against hematopoietic cells than tissues involved in GVHD. However not all leukemias are efficient antigen presenting cells [13]. Furthermore against a potential GVL selection mechanism is the fact that both host and donor APCs may capture and present host antigens from many tissue sources, thereby inducing indiscriminate alloge-

Table 3 Candidate Target Antigens for the Generation of GVL Specific T Cells

Tissue-restricted minor histocompatibility antigens HA-1, HA-2 (Chapter 5) others [10]
Lineage-restricted markers (= known polymorphisms)* panleukocyte: CD45*
  Myeloid: CD33* [12]
  B cell: CD19, CD20, CD21, CD22 [11]
Overexpressed normal myeloid or lymphoid proteins (Chapter 6) e.g., Primary granule
  proteins—proteinase-3, myeloperoxidase MDR-1
  BCL-1, BCL-2
Leukemia-specific proteins (Chapter 7)
  Fusion proteins: e.g., BCR-ABL, PML-RARα
  Mutations: RAS, p53

neic responses in donor T cells. Currently the relative contribution that host and donor APCs make to the alloresponse is not known.

C. Effector Cells

Both CD4+ and CD8+ cytotoxic T cells as well as NK cells with antileukemic function have been implicated for the GVL effect of allogeneic BMT or donor lymphocyte transfusions [14–17]. There is good evidence that while not causing GVHD in HLA-identical donor-recipient pairs, CD4+ T cells are effectors of cytotoxicity in some myeloid leukemias [18]. This has led to several studies using CD8+-depleted donor lymphocyte transfusions to prevent or treat relapse of chronic myeloid leukemia (CML) (see below). A potential difference between GVL and GVHD resides in the distinct behaviors of T-helper Th1 and Th2 lymphocyte subsets. In murine studies, the administration of donor cells with Th2 cytokine phenotype reduces the severity and lethality of experimental GVHD. Such cells have been generated by treating the mice with a combination of IL-2 and IL-4 [19,20] or granulocyte colony-stimulating factor (G-CSF) [21]. Furthermore the Th2 cells in this model had a GVL effect in a transplantable murine leukemia. The relevance of this observation in humans is that G-CSF mobilization of peripheral blood progenitor cells for transplant can induce a skewing of the T-cell profile to a Th2 phenotype. Whether this may induce a favorable bias in favor of GVL responses to human leukemias is not known. Another T-cell subset that has been claimed to be associated with a GVL effect after mismatched transplants are T cells expressing the gamma-delta T-cell receptor [22]. Patients who remain in remission have a significantly higher number of circulating gamma-delta T cells but a comparable incidence of acute GVHD. Finally, T-cell responses can be characterized by the T-cell receptor (TCR) Vβ family usage. Jiang et al. raised alloreacting T-cell clones using CML stimulators from an HLA

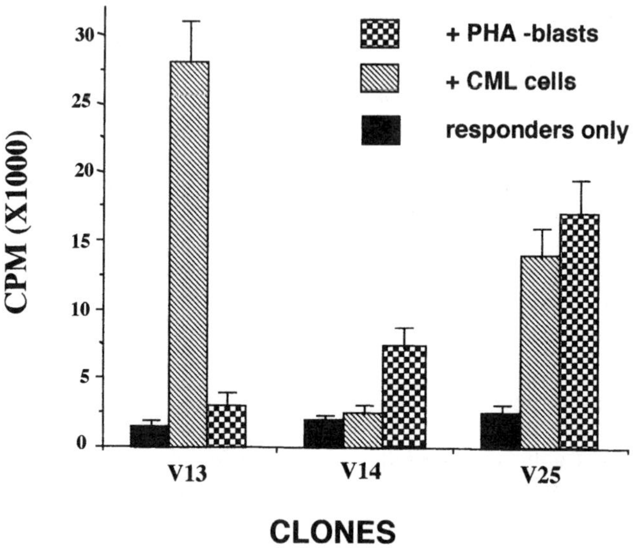

Figure 1 Examples of donor-derived clones with distinct reactivities against patient's leukemic and nonleukemic cells. Clone V13 reacts against patient's CML leukemia cells, clone V14 reacts against patient's PHA-blasts, and clone V25 reacts with both. (From Ref. 23.)

partially matched relative [23]. Of 18 clones studied in depth, 10 reacted exclusively with leukemic cells, 3 only with nonleukemic cells (PHA-blasts), and 4 with both. Clones recognizing leukemia cells had a different Vβ TCRs than clones recognizing nonleukemic cells from the same individual (Figure 1). These results indicate that antigens on leukemia cells may elicit responses in specific Vβ TCR families that distinguish these responders from T cells recognizing other tissues. Analysis of the Vβ repertoire after BMT frequently reveals oligoclonal expansion of a small number of Vβ families [24–27]. In mice, mHA-specific donor T cells show Vβ TCR restriction [26]. These expansions have been correlated with GVHD and GVL responses. Furthermore, the prompt disappearance of the leukemia after donor lymphocyte transfusion (DLT) has sometimes been observed to correspond temporally with the clonal dominance distinct Vβ family, suggesting a possible GVL specificity [28]. This observation makes possible a new approach to reconstituting the recipient with T cells with GVL but not GVHD reactivity. First, the Vβ restriction of the donor T cells responding uniquely to recipient leukemia would be identified by in vitro culture. Then the recipient would be transfused posttransplant with the appropriate Vβ subsets selected from a leukapheresis donation using Vβ antibody–coated magnetic beads [23].

D. Effector Pathways of GVL/GVHD

In vivo, the effector phase of the alloresponse involves more than the interaction of a cytotoxic T cell with its target. Activation of nonspecific accessory cells and local production of cytokines may ultimately reduce the fine specificity of a T-cell response to an antigen-bearing cell. Natural killer (NK) cells have been implicated in GVHD, but the evidence for a GVL effect of NK cells in clinical transplantation remains to be clearly established [29]. It is unlikely that GVL and GVHD would be easily separable if NK cells were the main effectors of these responses. The contribution of tumor necrosis factor alpha (TNF-α) and interferon gamma (IFN-γ) in particular to the tissue damage seen in acute GVHD has been studied in animal and human in vitro models [30]. The nonspecific action of cytokines released during a GVHD or a GVL alloresponse could transform a specific effector–target cell interaction into a nonspecific immune reaction. Of relevance to this discussion is the clinical outcome of treating posttransplant Epstein-Barr virus (EBV) lymphoproliferative disease with DLT. Using very low doses of donor lymphocytes (around 10^6 CD3+ cells per kilogram), Papadopoulos observed temporary enlargement of the tumor with local inflammation before rapid reduction in tumor size associated with a dense infiltrate of donor lymphocytes [31]. No acute GVHD was observed in these patients. It therefore appears that nonspecific mechanisms of effector cells can remain localized in effective GVL responses. Whether GVHD reactions also have an antimalignant effect through indirect cytokine and accessory cell activation is not known. In this regard we found that granulocyte-macrophage colony-forming units (GM-CFU) in CML were more susceptible to growth inhibition by TNF-α and IFN-γ produced by alloreacting CTL clones than normal marrow GM-CFU [32]. This suggests that some leukemias may be particularly susceptible to cytokines released during GVHD reactions.

E. Time Scale of GVL and GVHD Responses

There are fundamental differences in the nature of the GVHD reaction, which causes extensive tissue damage, and the GVL effect, which results in permanent suppression and possibly eradication of a malignant clone. Given the robustness of malignant cells, it is all the more surprising that GVL can achieve such complete and durable eradication of disease, while normal tissues survive the same onslaught from alloreactive cells. The time required for GVL to reduce the leukemia clone to undetectable levels is not known in detail. However, the unique observation of a DLT effect from leukemia clones reported by Falkenburg suggests that permanent eradication of leukemia (once clonal expansion has occurred) is extremely rapid [33]. This observation provides the rationale for strategies to treat patients with suicide gene–transfected T cells, which can be destroyed before the recipient develops serious complications from GVHD but after a GVL effect has been produced [34].

F. Lymphocyte Homing

It has been known for some time that T cells have different patterns of tissue distribution. Numerous studies of V_B type of T cells infiltrating different tissues indicate that repertoires differ widely in different tissues. Most of these analyses concern autoimmune disease states and tumor-infiltrating lymphocytes [35]. Tissue distribution of T cells may be determined by addressins—the growing family of integrins or ‘‘addressins’’ that retain T cells in certain tissues in a specific manner [36].

G. Tolerance

While an essential goal for restoring normal immune competence after allo-BMT is the induction of donor-recipient tolerance, the process may also terminate a GVL response. The mechanism of tolerance is still incompletely understood. However, two important events after bone marrow stem cell transplant (BMSCT) may be instrumental: (1) conversion of the host dendritic cell APC system to that of the donor and (2) emergence of naive T cells derived from prethymic donor stem cells processed through the host thymus (‘‘central tolerance’’) or through peripheral pathways (‘‘peripheral tolerance’’) (see Chapter 1). The presentation of recipient leukemia antigens through recipient APCs may uniquely stimulate alloresponses because of allogeneic differences or different processing of antigens by the recipient versus the donor APCs. The substitution of donor APCs could reduce the chance of generating mHA-specific T cells, resulting in a state of tolerance. This event probably occurs in the first few months after BMT and may be responsible for the observation in a mouse model that it is possible to transfuse mature donor T cells into the recipient without causing GVHD provided that 3 weeks elapse after a T cell–depleted transplant. In this model a GVL response is conserved when experimental leukemias are transfused into recipient mice [37]. The protective effect of delayed T-cell add-back on GVHD is strictly dose-related, but higher doses can be given without causing GVHD the longer the time interval from the transplant [38]. A state of mixed donor-recipient chimerism is also conducive to tolerance. Patients with mixed lymphoid chimerism have a higher relapse risk and have a very low risk of developing acute GVHD [39].

Table 4 Clinical Strategies to Separate the GVL Response from GVHD

Delayed add-back of donor T cells following T-depleted transplant
Incremental add-back of donor lymphocytes without cyclosporine [42]
Scheduled add-back of large T cell doses under cyclosporine cover [43]
Add-back of "suicide gene"–transfected T cells to T-depleted transplant [34,50]
Add-back of non–specifically expanded T cells
Add-back of specifically expanded T cells
CD8-depleted T cells [46–49]
After allogeneic BMT to prevent relapse in CML
Treatment of relapsed leukemia
Selectively depleted donor T cells [51–61]
Add-back of donor T cells depleted in vitro of antihost reactivity
Immunotoxin against CD25
Selection of CD25+ donor cells using antibody-coated magnetic beads
Selection of TCR Vβ T-cell subsets that contain antileukemic reacting clones [23]
Selection of appropriate Vβ family using antibody-coated immunomagnetic beads
Generation of leukemia-reactive T-cell clones ([33] chapters 6 and 18)
In vitro culture with recipient leukemia to generate leukemia-specific T cell lines
In vitro culture of donor lymphocytes with leukemia-specific peptides
Vaccination with leukemia-specific proteins [71]
Donor pretransplant
Recipient posttransplant

Thymic tolerance develops slowly in the first 6–12 months after BMT. This may allow sufficient time for the alloreaction against the residual leukemia to be completed.

IV. STRATEGIES FOR SEPARATING GVHD AND GVL RESPONSES

Based on the above data and assumptions, a number of approaches to conferring GVL without GVHD are being explored in clinical trials or are currently at a preclinical stage of development. Table 4 categorizes these strategies.

A. Delayed Add-Back of Donor Cells

Based on new understanding of the importance of cytokines in the process of acute GVHD, Johnson and Truitt elegantly showed in murine MHC matched and haplotype mismatched BMT models that infusion of immunocompetent donor cells delayed until 21 days after transplantation conferred a long-lasting antileukemic effect without causing severe acute GVHD [37,40]. In these experiments, alloreactive donor cells behaved differently when infused at different time points posttransplant. The mechanism of the protective effect is not yet defined. The reduced risk from GVHD may be due to avoidance of the ''cytokine storm'' or to the emergence of tolerance accompanying the establishment of a donor-derived antigen-presenting system [41]. The concept of delayed lymphocyte add-back has now been tested clinically by Slavin's group. In a study where Campath-1 antibodies were used for T-cell depletion, donor lymphocytes were infused, either starting early after transplant with weekly 1 log increments for up to four doses (days +1, +6, +14, +21 with 10^4, 10^5, 10^6, 10^7 T cells per kilogram of recipient weight, respectively) or starting on day 28 and given only to patients without signs of acute GVHD (days +28, +56, +84 infused with 10^5, 10^6, and 10^7 T cells per kilogram, respectively) [42]. In this nonprospective, randomized, heterogeneous group of relatively young patients, delayed administration of donor lymphocytes caused clinically significant acute GVHD in 42–53% of patients and was associated with a low probability of leukemia relapse. Unfortunately, due to patient variability and study design, it is not possible from these data to determine the cell dose and timing critical for the prevention of acute GVHD. We investigated the effect of delayed T-cell add-back on the risk of acute GVHD in 38 patients with hematological malignancies receiving T cell–depleted BMTs and cyclosporine to prevent acute GVHD (a-GVHD) [43]. Donor lymphocytes were added back at varying times after transplant to prevent leukemia relapse. In 26 patients scheduled for donor T-cell add-back of 2×10^6 cells per kilogram on day 30 and 5×10^7 cells per kilogram on day 45 (schedule 1), the overall probability of grade $\geq$ II a-GVHD developing was 31.5%, with a 15.5% probability of a-GVHD occurring after T-cell add-back. In 12 patients receiving 10^7 donor T cells per kilogram on day 30 (schedule 2), the probability of grade $\geq$ II a-GVHD was 100%. The incidence of grade III–IV a-GVHD was higher in schedule 2 than in schedule 1 ($p = 0.02$). Of 24 evaluable patients, 10 (46%) developed chronic GVHD, which was limited in 8 and extensive in 2. Current disease-free survival for 18 patients at standard risk for relapse of chronic myeloid leukemia (CML) in chronic or accelerated phase, acute myeloid leukemia in remission versus 20 patients with more advanced leukemia or multiple myeloma were respectively 72% versus 12% ($p < 0.01$) with a 29% versus 69% probability of relapse ($p = 0.08$). In 12 CML patients surviving more than 3 months, PCR analysis of the BCR/ABL transcript showed that minimal residual disease after T-cell add-back was transient except in two patients, who developed hematological relapse. Results indicate that the risk of acute GVHD is low following substantial T-cell doses transfused 45 days after transplant using cyclosporine prophylaxis. Furthermore a GVL effect was conserved.

Delayed lymphocyte add-back has also been investigated in partially mismatched related transplants [44]. Twenty-seven patients with advanced hematological malignancies were transplanted with T cell–depleted bone marrow grafts from 1–3 antigen-mismatched related donors. Starting between days 26 and 74, a cumulative T-cell dose of 0.23 to 16.5 × 10^6/kg was infused to preempt leukemia relapse under low-dose cyclosporine and steroid coverage. The results were compared with a historical group of similar patients treated at the same institution with T cell–depleted BMT without the delayed addition of donor lymphocytes. A high incidence of acute GVHD was observed in the group receiving lymphocyte add-back compared with historical controls (56% versus 11%). When more than 10^6/kg donor T cells were infused, the risk of developing GVHD was higher (88%), with significant GVHD-related mortality. Moreover, development of acute GVHD did not result in more GVL reactivity, since there was no difference in relapse rate between the add-back group and historical controls at 18 months posttransplant (56% versus 58%).

Based on our current experience with delayed donor lymphocyte infusions, it thus appears that for HLA-matched sibling pairs, a T-cell dose of 10^6/kg given on day 30 or 10^7/kg given on day 45 under cyclosporine coverage is associated with a low risk of inducing severe acute GVHD and may still confer a GVL effect, especially in CML. However, in the HLA-mismatched setting, despite cyclosporine and steroid protection, administration of even low doses of unmanipulated donor lymphocytes induces severe GVHD. More studies are needed to measure the impact of cyclosporine on the GVL effect and to determine whether smaller T-cell doses without cyclosporine are preferable. Since there is significant variation in the individual recipient's susceptibility to GVHD, it will be necessary to escalate T-cell add-back, starting from a low T-cell dose and allowing sufficient time between each dose to observe development of GVHD.

B. CD8+ Subset Depletion

There have been several clinical trials using CD8+ T-cell depletion for the prevention of GVHD [45,46]. In the initial study [45], 36 patients with leukemia received bone marrow grafts from HLA-identical siblings and CD8+ T cell–depleted bone marrow combined with posttransplant cyclosporine. Twenty-eight percent of recipients developed acute GVHD > grade I, usually mild and limited to the skin. Four patients failed to engraft, confirming an important role of CD8+ cells in engraftment. The leukemia relapse rate was only 11%, and none of the 13 patients with CML relapsed, suggesting that the GVL effect was retained. In a prospective, randomized, double-blind study [46], 38 patients with leukemia received bone marrow grafts from their HLA-identical sibling donors, either unmanipulated or CD8+ depleted, with posttransplant cyclosporine. Acute GVHD > grade I developed in 20% of the CD8-depleted group versus 80% (with 5 deaths) in the control group. Leukemia relapse was the same in the two groups and graft failure occurred in two patients in the CD8-depleted group but in none of the controls. Although GVHD prophylaxis was suboptimal for the control group, it seems that CD8+ T-cell depletion in combination with cyclosporine is an effective method to reduce acute GVHD in HLA-identical sibling transplants without losing the GVL effect, but at the expense of compromising engraftment in some patients. In another study [47], CD8+ T-cell depletion with posttransplant cyclosporine effectively prevented acute GVHD in HLA-identical siblings but not in transplants from less well matched donors. More recently, CD8-depleted donor lymphocytes have been used successfully to treat CML and multiple myeloma relapsing after allogeneic BMT, with a low incidence of acute GVHD [48,49].

C. Tk Gene Transfection of Donor T Cells

Gene transfer technology has made it possible to transduce donor lymphocytes with a "suicide gene" that makes them a target for pharmacological elimination in vivo. Bonini et al. first used a retrovirus to transfect herpes simplex thymidine kinase (HS-tk) and neomycin phosphotransferase (neo) genes into proliferating T lymphocytes [34]. G418-selected T cells retained their function in allorecognition but could be killed by addition of ganciclovir (GCV). They subsequently showed that efficient transfection could also be achieved if the T cells were subjected to allogeneic stimulation prior to retrovirus-mediated gene transfer. Such an approach could be used to generate cells both strongly alloreactive and GCV-sensitive for in vivo therapeutic use. The in vitro insertion of the HS-tk gene has been developed for clinical use. This makes it possible to carry out transplants with Tk gene-transfected T cells and to deplete gene-marked T cells in vivo by treating the patient with the antiviral drug ganciclovir should GVHD occur. The approach could be useful as a "safety net" to abort GVHD reactions in experimental add-back studies to treat relapsed leukemia, EBV lymphoproliferative disease, and cytomegalovirus (CMV) reactivation. It would be particularly applicable in mismatched donor-recipient pairs, where the risk from lethal acute GVHD is high. Clinical studies have been reported by Bonini et al. and Tiberghien et al. [34,50]. Data from both groups are preliminary, but several patients have sucessfully been treated for GVHD by administration of GCV. A potential problem with highly efficient elimination of donor lymphocytes is the risk of severe immune deficiency, which could increase the chance of leukemic relapse, recurrent infection, or reactivation of viruses, leading to CMV disease and EBV lymphoproliferation. Furthermore, at least in transplants for CML, it may be necessary to maintain the GVL effect: the BCR-ABL fusion gene is sometimes detectable for several years after BMT in the absence of relapse.

D. Selective Immunodepletion of Alloreactive T Cells

This model of selective T-cell depletion eliminates T cells that react against a specific stimulator (see Figure 2). Donor peripheral blood mononuclear cells

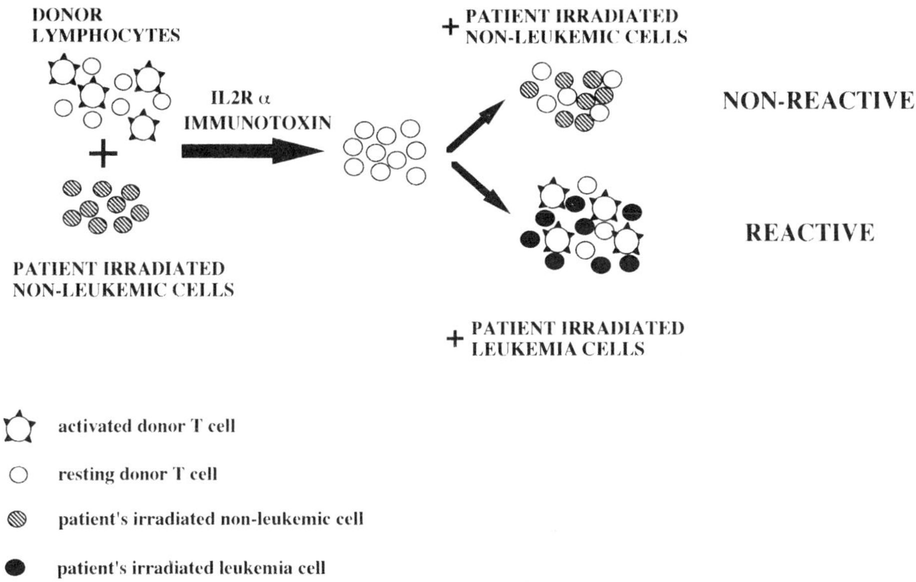

Figure 2 Selective immunodepletion method. First, donor T cells are stimulated in a mixed lymphocyte culture by patient's irradiated nonleukemic cells. Then the activated alloreactive donor T cells are eliminated by exposure to an IL-2Rα chain-specific immunotoxin. Finally, the remaining donor T cells are tested against the original nonleukemic stimulator or against leukemia cells from the patient. The method results in depletion of alloreactivity against the nonleukemic cells and preservation of alloreactivity against leukemia cells.

(PBMNCs) are stimulated by irradiated nonleukemic recipient cells in a cellular culture system to allow for activation of the alloreacting donor T cells. The activated donor T cells are then eliminated, using an immunotoxin specific for the IL-2 receptor alpha chain, which is expressed only on activated but not on resting T cells. The remaining donor T cells should be depleted of alloreactivity against the original stimulator (recipient nonleukemic cells) but may retain reactivity against recipient leukemic cells or other antigens. This model system can achieve a functional depletion by selectively destroying T cells capable of reacting against a specific stimulator while preserving T cells with other reactivities. In the transplant setting, this method could be applied to selectively deplete the donor T cells, causing GVHD while retaining donor T cells reacting against the leukemia or various infectious agents.

The selective immunodepletion method has been used successfully in preclinical studies using samples from patients and HLA-identical sibling donors undergoing BMT for CML. In chronic phase CML, T lymphocytes usually are not part of the leukemic clone and can therefore serve as normal recipient cells [51,52]. Using a ricin-conjugated anti-CD25 antibody and irradiated phytohemaglutinin (PHA) blasts as nonleukemic stimulator cells, Datta et al. have shown that the method results in selective depletion of alloreactivity against the PHA blasts, with significant preservation of reactivity against the CML cells [53]. In 10 HLA-identical sibling pairs and another 10 unrelated HLA-matched donor-recipient pairs, the mean residual reactivity against the PHA blasts after the depletion was 7.5% and 9.2% of the original value while the remaining reactivity against CML cells was 76.5% and 118% respectively (Figure 3).

Using a more sensitive measurement of alloreactivity for HLA-identical siblings by estimating the precursor frequency of alloreactive IL-2–producing helper T cells (HTLPfs), Mavroudis et al. have shown that selective immunodepletion significantly reduces the HTLPfs against host PBMNCs while preserving,

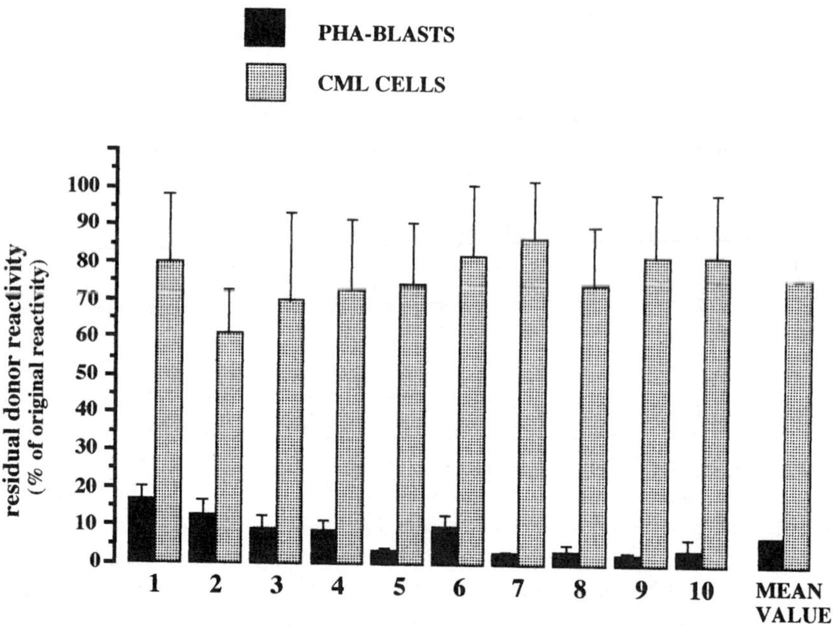

Figure 3 Depletion of alloreactivity in 10 HLA-identical sibling pairs using the selective immunodepletion method. Residual donor reactivity against the patient's PHA-blasts and CML cells after the depletion is shown as a percentage of the original donor response against the same stimulators. The original response against each stimulator has been normalized to 100%. After the depletion, reactivity against PHA-blasts is severely diminished while reactivity against CML cells is largely preserved. (From Ref. 53.)

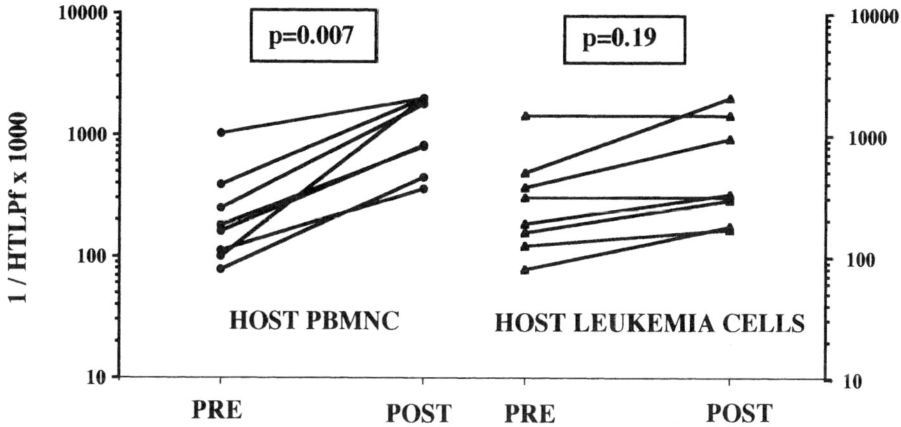

Figure 4 Donor HTLPf against host PBMNC or host leukemia cells before and after selective immunodepletion in eight HLA-identical sibling pairs. Following initial stimulation of donor PBMNC by irradiated OKT3-IL-2-expanded lymphocytes of the patient, the activated T cells were depleted using a recombinant IL-2Rα chain-specific immunotoxin [anti-Tac(Fv)PE38]. The method resulted in significant reduction of donor-versus-host PBMNC HTLPf ($p = 0.007$) but not significant reduction of donor-versus-host leukemia HTLPf ($p = 0.19$). (From Ref. 54.)

to a large extent, the HTLPfs against host leukemia cells (Figure 4) [54]. The donor-antirecipient HTLPfs have been shown to predict the risk of acute and chronic GVHD in HLA-identical siblings [55,56]. Given the important role of CD4+ T cells in the eradication of CML [57,58], the preserved donor-antileukemia HTLPfs may mediate a strong GVL effect. Therefore selective immunodepletion can separate GVHD and GVL effectors at the precursor T-cell level.

The same method can be used to deplete alloreactivity against a haplotype mismatch. In 10 parent-child pairs, selective immunodepletion reduced the alloreactivity against the haploidentical stimulator to a mean of 7.6% of the original reactivity while the third-party response was retained (Figure 5) [59].

Using a similar approach in a haploidentical murine BMT model, Cavazzano-Calvo et al. have shown that this depletion induces donor-specific tolerance by preventing the development of severe GVHD and graft rejection [60]. Other investigators, using the same principle with cell-sorting techniques instead of immunotoxins to remove the activated alloreactive T cells, have produced similar results [61].

This ex vivo stimulation of donor T cells, followed by the selective removal or elimination of activated cells, provides a crude method for separating reactivities conferred by different effector cells. Whether the residual alloreactivity, after

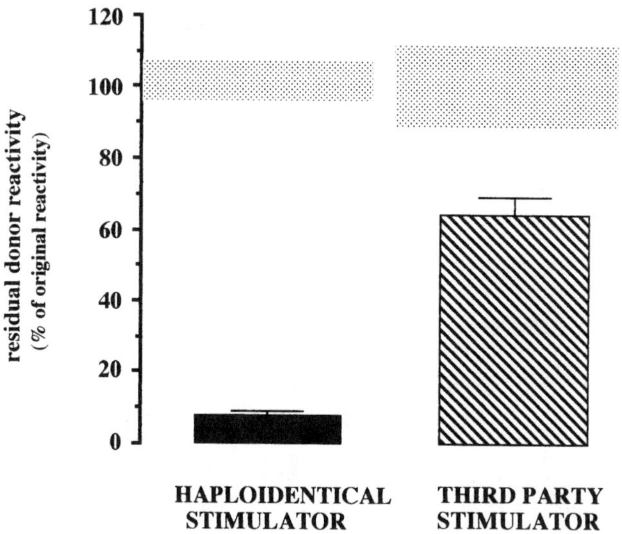

Figure 5 Specific depletion of alloreactivity in 10 haploidentical pairs. The original response to the haploidentical and third-party stimulators has been normalized to 100% ± SD; it is shown as a shaded bar. After the depletion, the alloreactivity against the haploidentical stimulator is reduced, but not against the third party. (From Ref. 59.)

the depletion, is enough to cause severe GVHD, especially in the mismatched setting, or whether the remaining GVL reactivity is enough to eradicate the leukemia can be answered only by the clinical application of the method. However, the preclinical results are encouraging and promising.

Taking advantage of recent technological advances, it is now feasible and easy to collect a large number of allogeneic CD34+ progenitor cells for transplantation by putting the donor through repeated leukaphereses procedures. These megagrafts have been shown to achieve stable donor engraftment even after extensive T-cell depletion in haploidentical BMT [62,63]. Furthermore, the beneficial effect of GVH-reacting donor lymphocytes on allogeneic engraftment has been questioned in animal T cell–depleted BMT models, where the cell dose and the immunosuppressive properties of the preparative regimen were most important [64]. Additionally, the immunotoxins used in the selective immunodepletion experiments have been shown to have no adverse effect on GM-CFU growth of bone marrow cells from normal donors [59]. It is therefore expected that engraftment will not be compromised by the application of the method.

The anticipated retained GVL effect of this method is more than with nonselective T-cell depletion but probably less than that of an unmanipulated graft.

Donor effector cells that react against both the normal and leukemic cells of the patient can be eliminated by the immunotoxin. This is the reason why the retained HTLPfs against leukemic cells are slightly reduced after selective immunodepletion [54]. However, the method preserves the donor T cells with ''pure'' antileukemic reactivity as well as other T cells with immunity against infectious agents such as EBV [54]. This may be especially important in HLA-mismatched BMT, where T-cell depletion is associated with a significant risk for the development of posttransplant EBV-related lymphoproliferations [66,67]. These potentially lethal lymphoid neoplasms are chemoresistant and susceptible only to donor lymphocyte infusions [31,67]. Selective immunodepletion by retaining the anti-EBV reactivity is expected to avoid this problem.

V. FUTURE DEVELOPMENTS

A. Amplifying and Extending the Clinical Application of GVL Responses

To improve the options for generating leukemia-specific T cells, it will be necessary to know precisely what antigenic differences exist between leukemia cells and normal tissues. This requires detailed mapping of the minor histocompatibility antigen system and the search for and identification of leukemia-specific antigens. While some advances have been made in the expansion in vitro of T-cell lines exhibiting leukemia-specific cytotoxicity, a major limitation is the inability of current culture techniques to generate sufficient numbers of T cells for therapy [68]. Furthermore, it is not known whether cultured T cells survive long enough in the recipient to exert a GVL effect [69] or whether they home to all the leukemia-containing tissues [36,70]. Vaccination of the donor with leukemia-specific peptides might be a better way of expanding leukemia specific T cells. Once a repertoire of lymphoid- and myeloid-specific antigens have been defined, the alternative approach of using peptides and proteins as vaccines would become possible. Tumor vaccine techniques are still under development—for example, following allotransplants for myeloma [71]. With the use of new specific antigens, it might ultimately be possible to stimulate strong specific GVL responses.

REFERENCES

1. Barnes DWH, Loutit JF. Treatment of murine-leukemia with x-rays and homologous bone marrow. Br Med J 1956; 2:626–627.
2. Horowitz MM, Gale RP, Sondel PM, Goldman JM, Kersey J, Kolb H-J, Rimm AA, Ringden O, Rozman C, Speck B, Truitt RL, Zwaan FE, Bortin MM. Graft-versus-leukemia reactions after bone marrow transplantation. Blood 1991; 75:555–562.

3. Kolb HJ, Schattenberg A, Goldman JM, et al. Graft-versus-leukemia effect of donor lymphocyte transfusions in marrow grafted patients. Blood 1995; 86:2041–2050.
4. Salomo M, Steinmann J, Glass B, et al. Leukemia-specific allogeneic donor T cells: quantification by limiting dilution assay. Bone Marrow Transplant 1995; 15:179 186.
5. Hoffmann T, Theobald M, Bunjes D, et al. Frequency of bone marrow T cells responding to HLA-identical non-leukemic and leukemic stimulator cells. Bone Marrow Transplant 1993; 12:1–8.
6. Glass B, Uharek L, Gassmann W, et al. Graft-versus-leukemia activity after bone marrow transplantation does not require graft-versus-host disease. Ann Hematol 1992; 64:255–259.
7. van Lochem E, de Gast B, Goulmy E. In vitro separation of host specific graft-versus-host and graft-versus-leukemia cytotoxic T cell activities. Bone Marrow Transplant 1992; 10:181–183.
8. Oettel K, Wesly O, Albertini M, et al. Allogeneic T cell clones able to selectively destroy Philadelphia chromosome–bearing human leukemia lines can also recognize Ph-cells from the same patient. Blood 1994; 83:3390–3402.
9. Niederwieser D, Grassegger A, Aubock J, et al. Correlation of minor histocompatibility antigen-specific cytotoxic T lymphocytes with graft-versus-host disease status and analyses of tissue distribution of their target antigens. Blood 1993; 81:2200–2208.
10. Warren EH, Greenberg PD, Riddell SR. Cytotoxic T-lymphocyte-defined human minor histocompatibility antigens with a restricted tissue distribution. Blood 1998; 91:2197–2207.
11. Dolstra H, Fredrix H, Preijers F, Goulmy E, Figdor CG, de Witte TM, van de Wiel-van Kemenade E. Recognition of a B cell leukemia-associated minor histocompatibility antigen by CTL. J Immunol 1997; 158:560–565.
12. Raptis A, Clave E, Mavroudis D, Molldrem J, Van Rhee F, Barrett AJ. Polymorphism in CD33 and CD34 genes: a source of minor histocompatibility antigens on hematopoietic stem cells? Br J Haematol 1998; 102:1354–1358.
13. Delain M, Tiberghien P, Racadot E, et al. Variability of the alloreactive T cell response to leukemia blasts. Leukemia 1994; 8:642–647.
14. Faber L, van Luxemburg-Heijs S, Veenhof W, et al. Generation of CD4+ cytotoxic T lymphocyte clones from a patient with severe graft-versus-host disease after allogeneic bone marrow transplantation: implications for graft-versus-leukemia reactivity. Blood 1995; 86:2821–2828.
15. Jiang YZ, Kanfer E, Macdonald D, et al. Graft-versus-leukemia following allogeneic bone marrow transplantation: emergence of cytotoxic T lymphocytes reacting to host leukemia cells. Bone Marrow Transplant 1991; 8:253–258.
16. Jiang YZ, Cullis J, Kanfer E, et al. T cell and NK cell mediated graft-versus-leukemia reactivity following donor buffy coat transfusion to treat relapse after marrow transplantation for chronic myeloid leukemia. Bone Marrow Transplant 1993; 11: 133–138.
17. Albi N, Ruggeri L, Aversa F, et al. Natural killer cell function and antileukemic activity of a large population of CD3+/CD8+ T cells expressing NK receptors for

major histocompatibility complex class I after "three-loci" HLA-incompatible bone marrow transplantation. Blood 1996; 87:3993–4000.

18. Jiang YZ, Barrett AJ. The allogeneic CD4+ T cell mediated graft-versus-leukaemia effect. Leuk Lymph 1997; 28:33–42.
19. Fowler DH, Kurasawa K, Husebekk A, et al. Cells of the Th2 cytokine phenotype prevent LPS-induced lethality during graft-versus-host reaction. J Immunol 1994; 152:1004–1013.
20. Fowler DH, Kurasawa K, Smith R, et al. Donor CD4-enriched cells of Th2 cytokine phenotype regulate graft-versus-host disease without impairing allogeneic engraftment in sublethally irradiated mice. Blood 1994; 84:3540–3554.
21. Pan L, Delmonte J, Jalonen CK, et al. Pretreatment of donor mice with granulocyte colony-stimulating factor polarizes donor T lymphocytes toward type-2 cytokine production and reduces severity of experimental graft-versus-host disease. Blood 1995; 86:4422–4429.
22. Lamb LS Jr, Henslee-Downey PJ, Parrish RS, Godder K, Thompson J, Lee C, Gee AP. Increased frequency of TCR gamma delta + T cells in disease-free survivors following T cell-depleted, partially mismatched, related donor bone marrow transplantation for leukemia. J Hematother 1996; 5:503–509.
23. Jiang YZ, Mavroudis D, Hensel N, Barrett AJ. Preferential usage of T cell receptor (TCR) Vβ by allogeneic T cells recognising myeloid leukemia cells: implications for separating GVL from GVHD. Bone Marrow Transplant 1997; 19:899–903.
24. Akatsuka Y, Cerveny C, Hansen JA. T cell receptor clonal diversity following allogeneic marrow grafting. Hum Immunol 1996; 48:125–134.
25. Liu X, Chesnokova V, Forman SJ, Diamond DJ. Molecular analysis of T-cell receptor repertoire in bone marrow transplant recipients: evidence for oligoclonal T-cell expansion in graft-versus-host disease lesions. Blood 1996; 87:3032–3044.
26. Friedman TM, Gilbert M, Briggs C, Korngold R. Repertoire analysis of CD8+ T cell responses to minor histocompatibility antigens involved in graft-versus-host disease. J Immunol 1998; 161:41–48.
27. Dietrich PY, Caignard A, Lim A, Chung V, Pico JL, Pannetier C, Kourilsky P, Hercend T. In vivo T cell clonal amplification at time of acute graft versus host disease. Blood 1994; 84:2815–2820.
28. Claret EJ, Alyea EP, Orsini E, Pickett CC, Collins H, Wang Y, Neuberg D, Soiffer RJ, Ritz J. Characterization of T cell repertoire in patients with graft-versus-leukemia after donor lymphocyte infusion. J Clin Invest 1997; 100:855–866.
29. Rhoades JL, Cibull ML, Thompson JS, et al. Role of natural killer cells in the pathogenesis of human acute graft-versus-host disease. Transplantation 1993; 56:113–120.
30. Antin JH, Ferrara JLM. Cytokine dysregulation and acute graft-versus-host disease. Blood 1992; 80:2964–2968.
31. Papadopoulos EB, Ladanyi M, Emmanuel D, Mackinnon S, Boulad F, Carabasi M, Castro-Malaspina H, Childs BH, Gillio AP, Small TN, Young JW, Kernan NA, O'Reilly RJ. Infusion of donor leukocytes to treat Epstein-Barr-virus–associated lymphoproliferative disorder after allogeneic bone marrow transplantation. N Engl J Med 1994; 330:1185–1191.

32. Jiang YZ, Barrett AJ. Cellular and cytokine mediated effects of CD4-positive lymphocyte lines generated in vitro against chronic myelogenous leukemia. Exp Hematol 1995; 23:1167–1172.
33. Falkenburg JHF, Wafelman AR, van Bergen CAM, et al. Leukemia-reactive cytotoxic T lymphocytes (CTL) induce complete remission in patients with relapsed accelerated phase chronic myeloid leukemia. Blood 1997; 90 (suppl 1):589a.
34. Bonini C, Ferrari G, Verzeletti S, Servida P, Zappone E, Ruggieri L, Ponzoni M, Rossini S, Mavilio F, Traversari C, Bordignon C. HSV-TK gene transfer into donor lymphocytes for control of allogeneic graft-versus-leukemia. Science 1997; 276: 1719–1724.
35. Silver J, Gulwani-Akolkar B, Akolkar P. The influence of genetics, environment and disease state on the human T cell receptor repertoire. Ann NY Acad Sci 1995; 756:19–28.
36. Sackstein R. Physiologic migration of lymphocytes to lymph nodes following bone marrow transplantation: role in immune recovery. Semin Oncol 1993; 20:34–39.
37. Johnson BD, Truitt RL. Delayed infusion of immunocompetent donor cells after bone marrow transplantation breaks graft-host tolerance and allows for persistent antileukemic reactivity without severe graft-versus-host disease. Blood 1995; 85: 3302–3312.
38. Slavin S, Naparstek E, Nagler A, et al. Allogeneic cell therapy with donor peripheral blood cells and recombinant human interleukin-2 to treat leukemia relapse after allogeneic bone marrow transplantation. Blood 1996; 87:2195–2204.
39. McKinnon S, Barnett L, Heller G, O'Reilly RJ. Minimal residual disease is more common in patients who have mixed T-cell chimerism after bone marrow transplantation for chronic myelogenous leukemia. Blood 1994; 83:3409–3416.
40. Johnson BD, Drobyski WR, Truitt RL. Delayed infusion of normal donor cells after MHC-matched bone marrow transplantation provides an antileukemia reaction without graft-versus-host disease. Bone Marrow Transplant 1993; 11:329–336.
41. Antin J, Ferrara J. Cytokine dysregulation and graft-versus-host disease. Blood 1992; 80:2964–2968.
42. Naparstek E, Or R, Nagler A, Cividalli G, Engelhard D, Aker M, Gimon Z, Manny N, Sacks T, Tochner Z, Weiss L, Samuel S, Brautbar C, Hale G, Waldmann H, Steinberg SM, Slavin S. T-cell-depleted allogeneic bone marrow transplantation for acute leukemia using Campath-1 antibodies and posttransplant administration of donor's peripheral blood lymphocytes for prevention of relapse. Br J Haematol 1995; 89:506–515.
43. Barrett J, Mavroudis D, Tisdale J, Molldrem J, Dunbar C, Cottler-Fox M, Phang S, Carter C, Okunnieff P, Young NS, Read EJ. T-cell depleted bone marrow transplantation followed by delayed T-cell add-back to prevent severe acute GVHD. Bone Marrow Transplant 1998; 21:543–551.
44. Pati AR, Godder K, Parrish R, et al. Pre-emptive therapy with donor leukocyte infusions to prevent relapse following partially mismatched related donor bone marrow transplantation. Blood 1996; 88(suppl 1):259a.
45. Champlin R, Giralt S, Przepiorka D, et al. Selective depletion of CD8-positive T-lymphocytes for allogeneic bone marrow transplantation: engraftment, graft-versus-host disease and graft-versus-leukemia. Prog Clin Biol Res 1995; 377:385–398.

46. Nimer SD, Giorgi J, Gajewski JL, Ku N, Schiller GJ, Lee K, Territo M, Ho W, Feig S, Selch M, Isacescu V, Reichert TA, Champlin RE. Selective depletion of CD8+ cells for prevention of graft-versus-host disease after bone marrow transplantation: A randomized controlled trial. Transplant 1994; 57:82–88.
47. Giralt S, Hester J, Huh Y, et al. CD8-depleted donor lymphocyte infusion as treatment for relapsed chronic myelogenous leukemia after allogeneic bone marrow transplantation. Blood 1995; 86:4337–4343.
48. Giralt S, Hester J, Huh Y, Hirsch-Ginsberg C, Rondon G, Guo J, Lee M, Gajewski J, Talpaz M, Kantarjian H, Fischer H, Deisseroth A, Champlin RE. CD8+-depleted donor lymphocyte infusion as treatment for relapsed chronic myelogenous leukemia after allogeneic bone marrow transplantation: graft vs. leukemia without graft vs. host disease. Blood 1995; 86:4337–4343.
49. Alyea EP, Soiffer RJ, Canning C, Neuberg D, Schlossman R, Pickett C, Collins H, Wang Y, Anderson KC, Ritz J. Toxicity and efficacy of defined doses of CD4(+) donor lymphocytes for treatment of relapse after allogeneic bone marrow transplant. Blood 1998; 91:3671–3680.
50. Thiberghien P, Reynolds CW, Keller J, Spence S, Deschaseaux M, Certoux J-M, Contassot E, Murphy WJ, Lyons R, Chiang Y, Herve P, Longo D, Ruscetti FW. Ganciclovir treatment of herpes simplex thymidine kinase-transduced primary T lymphocytes: an approach for specific in vivo donor T-cell depletion after bone marrow transplantation? Blood 1994; 84:1333–1341.
51. Bartram CR, Raghavachar A, Anger B, et al. T lymphocytes lack rearrangement of the bcr gene in Philadelphia chromosome-positive chronic myelocytic leukemia. Blood 1987; 69:1682.
52. Jonas D, Lubbert M, Kawasaki E, et al. Clonal analysis of bcr-abl rearrangement in T lymphocytes from patients with chronic myelogenous leukemia. Blood 1992; 79:1017–1023.
53. Datta AR, Barrett AJ, Jiang YZ, et al. Distinct T cell populations distinguish chronic myeloid leukemia cells from lymphocytes in the same individual: a model for separating GVHD from GVL reactions. Bone Marrow Transplant 1994; 14:517–524.
54. Mavroudis D, Dermime S, Jiang YZ, et al. Selective immunodepletion between HLA matched siblings that reduces the risk for GVHD and preserves reactivity against the leukemia and Epstein-Barr virus. Blood 1996; 88(suppl 1):245a.
55. Schwarer A, Jiang YZ, Brookes P, et al. Frequency of anti-recipient alloreactive helper T-cell precursors in donor blood and graft-versus-host disease after HLA-identical sibling bone marrow transplantation. Lancet 1993; 341:203.
56. Bunjes D, Theobald M, Nierle T, et al. Presence of host-specific interleukin 2-secreting T helper cell precursors correlates closely with active primary and secondary chronic graft-versus-host disease. Bone Marrow Transplant 1995; 15:727.
57. Jiang YZ, Barrett AJ. Cellular and cytokine-mediated effects of CD4-positive lymphocyte lines generated in vitro against chronic myelogenous leukemia. Exp Hematol 1995; 23:1167.
58. Giralt S, Hester J, Huh Y, et al. CD8-depleted donor lymphocyte infusion as treatment for relapsed chronic myelogenous leukemia after allogeneic bone marrow transplantation. Blood 1995; 86:4337.
59. Mavroudis D, Jiang YZ, Hensel N, et al. Specific depletion of alloreactivity against

haplotype mismatched related individuals by a recombinant immunotoxin: a new approach to graft-versus-host disease prophylaxis in haploidentical bone marrow transplantation. Bone Marrow Transplant 1996; 17:793–799.
60. Cavazzana-Calvo M, Stephan J, Sarnacki S, et al. Attenuation of graft-versus-host disease and graft rejection by ex vivo immunotoxin elimination of alloreactive T cells in an H-2 haplotype disparate mouse combination. Blood 1994; 83:288–298.
61. Rencher SD, Houston JA, Lockey TD, et al. Eliminating graft-versus-host potential from T cell immunotherapeutic populations. Bone Marrow Transplant 1996; 18: 415–420.
62. Martin P. The role of T cells in allogeneic marrow engraftment. Bone Marrow Transplant 1995; 15(suppl 1):S78–S81.
63. Aversa F, Tabilio A, Terenzi A, et al. Successful engraftment of T-cell depleted haploidentical "three-loci" incompatible transplants in leukemia patients by addition of recombinant human granulocyte colony-stimulating factor–mobilized peripheral blood progenitor cells to bone marrow inoculum. Blood 1994; 84:3948–3955.
64. Reisner Y, Martelli M. Bone marrow transplantation across HLA barriers by increasing the number of transplanted cells. Immunol Today 1995; 16:437–440.
65. Uharek L, Gassmann W, Glass B, et al. Influence of cell dose and graft-versus-host reactivity on rejection rates after allogeneic bone marrow transplantation. Blood 1992; 79:1612–1621.
66. Zutter M, Martin P, Sale G, et al. Epstein-Barr virus lymphoproliferation after bone marrow transplantation. Blood 1988; 72:520.
67. Shapiro R, McClain K, Frizzera G, et al. Epstein-Barr virus associated B cell lymphoproliferative disorders following bone marrow transplantation. Blood 1988; 71: 1234.
68. Falkenberg JHF, Faber LM, van der Elshout M, van Luxemburg-Heijs SAP, Hooftman den Otter A, Smit WM, Boogt PJ, Willemz R. Generation of donor-derived antileukemic cytotoxic T-lymphocyte responses for treatment of relapsed leukemia after allogeneic HLA-identical bone marrow transplantation. J Immunother 1993; 14:305–309.
69. Rooney CM, Smith CA, Ng CY, Loftin S, Li C, Krance RA, Brenner MK, Heslop HE. Use of gene-modified virus-specific T lymphocytes to control Epstein-Barr virus–related lymphoproliferation. Lancet 1995; 345:9–13.
70. Goldberg SL, Mangan KF, Klumpp TR, Cropper TM, Schnall SF, Macdonald JS. Lack of a graft-versus-leukemia effect in an immunologically privileged sanctuary site. Bone Marrow Transplant 1993; 12:180–181.
71. Kwak LW, Taib DD, Duffey PL, Bensinger WI. Bryant EM, Reynolds CW, Longo DL. Transfer of myeloma idiotype-specific immunity from an actively immunised marrow donor. Lancet 1995; 345:1016–1020.

15
T-Cell Subsets and Separation of GVL from GVHD

Sergio A. Giralt and Richard E. Champlin
M. D. Anderson Cancer Center
Houston, Texas

I. INTRODUCTION

Donor lymphocyte infusions (DLI) have rapidly become established as an important treatment for patients who relapse after an allogeneic progenitor cell transplant [1–3]. The dramatic responses seen primarily in chronic myelogenous leukemia (CML) but also on occasions in other hematologic malignancies after DLI represent the most direct evidence of a graft-versus-leukemia (GVL) effect mediated by donor lymphocytes [2,3].

Graft-versus-host disease (GVHD) is the most significant adverse side effect of DLI, and exploration of ways to mediate GVL without provoking or reducing the risk of GVHD is an active area of research. In this chapter we review current strategies to make DLI safer and more effective in the treatment and prevention of relapse after allogeneic progenitor cell transplantation.

II. LYMPHOCYTE SUBSETS AND ANTITUMOR EFFECTS

Three main types of effector cells are involved in antitumor responses: CD8+ cells recognizing MHC class I antigens, CD4+ cells recognizing MHC class II antigens, and non-MHC-restricted natural killer (NK) cells. CD4+ cells can be further subdivided into T helper (Th) cells—Th0, Th1, and Th2 subclasses—depending on their cytokine-production profile [4].

It is likely that all lymphocyte subsets contribute to the antileukemic effect; however, the relative importance of each specific lymphocyte subset may vary from disease to disease and even from patient to patient, depending on the extent and type of antigen expression, accessory cells, and costimulatory molecules on the leukemia.

The responses to donor lymphocytes has been most studied in CML, mainly because the response rate is high and the bcr-abl fusion has been the focus of considerable interest as a possible leukemia-specific target antigen [5]. However, the relevance of leukemia-specific reactions in CML is doubtful. Oettel et al. evaluated 1871 T-cell lines derived from 6 normal donors against Ph+ and Ph− targets. Sixty-three lines showed selective lysis of Ph+ cells initially, but only 3 cell lines remained specific against Ph+ cells after 3 months of culture. Two of these cell lines were CD4+, and cytotoxicity was inhibited by anti class II antibodies [6].

This observation supports the hypothesis that the response to DLI represents a non-leukemia-specific allogeneic response. However the observation that responses after DLI can be seen without concurrent GVHD suggest that the antihost response may be directed against hematopoietic-specific antigens, and thus GVL could be potentially separable from GVHD [1,2].

Characterization of the roles of different lymphocyte subsets is currently under investigation. CML and hematological progenitor cells express DR antigens on their surfaces [7]. Therefore, CD4-mediated responses may be relevant in these cases, and indeed antileukemic CD4+ lines have been generated both in vivo and in vitro [8–12]. CD8+ cells and natural killer cells with both leukemia-specific and nonspecific alloreactivity have also been described [13,14].

III. SELECTIVELY DEPLETED DONOR LYMPHOCYTE INFUSIONS

In the two largest registry reports to date, the risk of GVHD following DLI was 60% [2,3]. Conflicting data emerges from both studies in regards to risk factors for development of GVHD after DLI. In the European registry, recipients of T-cell depleted allografts during their initial transplant had a higher incidence of GVHD, interferon therapy also predicted for GVHD [2]. In the American registry, T-cell depleted allografts did not have a higher risk of GVHD, and interferon only increased the risk of GVHD if given after the DLI. Neither of the registry studies was able to show a correlation between T-cell dose and GVHD, but the doses given were relatively high for most patients. In both reports, GVHD was the most important cause of nonrelapse mortality.

Selective T-cell depletion of donor lymphocyte subsets may help dissect the roles that different lymphocyte subsets play in the antileukemic effect of donor lymphocytes in CML. Selective CD8 depletion of donor bone marrow has been associated with a lower incidence of GVHD without increases in disease relapse, suggesting that CD8+ cells may not be essential for the GVL effect [15,16]. Thus CD8-depleted donor lymphocytes may be as effective as unmanipulated donor lymphocyte infusions, but with a lower incidence of GVHD.

We treated 18 patients with CML relapses after an allogeneic transplant with CD8-depleted DLI [17,18]. Five patients had isolated cytogenetic relapses, 7 were in chronic phase, 3 were in accelerated phase, and 3 were in blast crisis. Other patient and disease characteristics are summarized in Table 1.

CD8 cells were purged using immunomagnetic or panning techniques, and adequacy of depletion was assessed by flow cytometry. After depletion, the median number of CD3+ cells infused on each occasion was 31.4×10^6/kg, with a median of 30.8×10^6 CD4+ cells and 0.3×10^6 CD8+ cells (Table 2).

Six patients developed significant cytopenias, three had neutrophil counts $<0.5 \times 10^9$/L persisting for 1–10 weeks, and four had platelet counts of $<20.0 \times 10^9$/L lasting between 1 and 26 weeks. One patient required an infusion of CD8-depleted peripheral blood stem cells from the donor due to prolonged thrombocytopenia, with subsequent recovery of a normal platelet count.

The risk of acute GVHD appeared to be lower than with unmanipulated donor lymphocytes. Two patients developed acute GVHD of grades 2 and 3, responding to steroids, and 2 developed chronic GVHD. One case was steroid-refractory and eventually fatal.

Table 1 Characteristics of Patients Receiving CD8 Depleted DLI for Treatment of CML Relapse at M.D. Anderson Cancer Center

Number of patients	18
Age in years: median (range)	39 (23–57)
Time to relapse, days: median (range)	563 (50–1852)
Donor type	
Matched sibling	13
Unrelated donor	5
Status at time of DLI	
Cytogenetic relapse	5
Clinical chronic phase	7
Clinical accelerated phase	3
Blast crisis	3
Prior treatment of relapse	
None	3
Interferon/other	15

Table 2 Infusion Characteristics of CD8 Depleted Donor Lymphocytes

	Pre–CD8 Purge (Median)	Post–CD8 Purge (Median)
MNC × 10^8/kg		0.6
CD3 × 10^6/kg	68.8	31.4
CD4 × 10^6/kg	53.8	30.8
CD8 × 10^6/kg	24.0	0.3
CD56 × 10^6/kg	9.8	4.7

MNC: mononuclear cells.

Among the 12 patients in nontransformed phases, 10 achieved complete cytogenetic remissions. Among the 6 patients with clinically transformed phases at the time of DLI, 1 achieved a complete cytogenetic and hematologic remission, 1 had a hematologic remission with no cytogenetic improvement, and the other 4 had progressive disease. Seven patients died, four from progressive disease and three in remission from chronic GVHD, pneumonia, and sepsis. Median follow-up for the surviving patients is approximately 2 years (range, 200–1282 days). These results support the hypothesis that CD8+ cells are not essential for the GVL effect in CML—also that CD8-depleted donor lymphocytes seem to be as effective and may be associated with a lower risk of acute GVHD than unmanipulated DLI [17,18].

Other groups have confirmed the efficacy of CD8 depleted DLI. The Dana Farber group reported that in patients with CML and multiple myeloma, the use of CD8-depleted DLI resulted in an overall response rate of 78% in CML [19] and 30% in myeloma [20], with 8 of 31 patients developing acute GVHD, 6 of whom had received greater than 1 × 10^8 CD4+ cells per kilogram [19,20]. A randomized trial comparing unmanipulated to CD8 depleted DLI will be needed to confirm the suggestion that CD8-depleted DLI are associated with a lower risk of GVHD at the same lymphocyte dose.

IV. LOW DOSES OR ESCALATING DOSES OF DONOR LYMPHOCYTES

Mackinnon and collaborators reported that patients with CML who received <1.0 × 10^7 CD3+ cells per kilogram for treatment of EBV lymphoma had an antiviral response without any evidence of an antileukemic effect [21]. This observation suggested that there may be a threshold lymphocyte dose that may be different for each disease. These same investigators also reported that lymphocyte doses of 0.5×10^7 CD3+ cells per kilogram could achieve remissions in patients with isolated molecular relapses, suggesting that the threshold lymphocyte dose may be dependent on disease stage at the time of infusion. Similarly, since no GVHD was seen in patients receiving the lower doses of donor lymphocytes, it was possible to separate GVL from GVHD without any form of donor-cell manipulation [22]. Earlier donor lymphocyte infusion also reduces the risk of pancytopenia, which depends primarily on the amount of residual donor cells left at the time of the lymphocyte infusion [23].

Recently there has been considerable interest in using escalated doses of donor lymphocytes as a way of obtaining a GVL effect with a lower risk of GVHD. With this strategy, patients initially receive a very low dose of donor lymphocytes, usually 1×10^6 CD3+ cells per kilogram. The Hammersmith group reported 61 patients receiving DLI for CML relapsing after an allogeneic transplant. Thirty-two patients who received unmanipulated DLI at a median dose of 1.4×10^8 CD3+ cells per kilogram had a 66% incidence of GVHD. A second group of 29 patients who received graded doses of donor lymphocytes at 12-week intervals beginning with a dose of 1×10^6 CD3+ cells per kilogram had only a 22% incidence of GVHD. This difference was even more dramatic among recipients of HLA-related transplants (57% versus 6%). Response rates were similar for both groups. These data suggest that low but escalating lymphocyte doses may permit the harnessing GVL without GVHD [24].

V. DISEASE-SPECIFIC DONOR LYMPHOCYTE INFUSIONS

The existence of leukemia-reactive cytotoxic T lymphocytes capable of inhibiting leukemic cell growth has been demonstrated by Falkenberg et al. [8,25]. This group subsequently used leukemia-reactive cytotoxic T lymphocytes to treat a patient with CML who relapsed after an allogeneic transplant and failed to respond to a standard DLI. Through exposure of donor lymphocytes to the patient's CML and incubation in IL-2, three cytotoxic T-lymphocyte lines were obtained, exhibiting 88%, 78%, and 97% growth inhibition of CML progenitor cells from the patient. The three lines were infused into the patient at 4-week intervals. Twelve weeks after the last infusion, the patient was found to be in a complete cytogenetic and hematologic remission. Although labor-intensive, this technique promises more specific anti-leukemia therapy and less risk of GVHD than the use of bulk lymphocytes (see Chapter 18) [26].

VI. SUICIDE GENE–TRANSDUCED DONOR LYMPHOCYTES

Donor lymphocytes genetically modified to carry the herpes simplex virus thymidine kinase gene have been developed. These have been used to reinduce remissions in patients relapsing after allogeneic BMT. The modified lymphocytes have been shown to exert an immune-mediated antileukemia response and can induce GVHD. In two patients developing GVHD, treatment with ganciclovir resulted in GVHD improvement without loss of the antileukemic effect. This novel approach may also be useful in harnessing and controlling the antileukemic effect of donor lymphocytes [27].

VII. SUMMARY AND FUTURE DIRECTIONS

The antileukemic potential of DLI represents a major discovery in the field of allogeneic transplantation. When initially explored by the Seattle group, donor lymphocytes given shortly after transplant as a method for relapse prevention were associated with a high incidence of GVHD [28]. However, modern immunosuppressive therapy and delayed infusion of donor lymphocytes may produce better results.

The numerous observations of GVL effects independent of a GVHD reaction demonstrate that it is possible to separate these two phenomena clinically, by using either smaller doses of cells, selective T-cell depletion of donor lymphocytes, gene-modified lymphocytes, or leukemia-reactive cytotoxic T lymphocytes. It is likely that one or more strategies may be needed and that individual patients may require different DLI strategies at different stages of the disease.

Improving the response rate in other hematological malignancies will require a deeper understanding of tumor immunology. Cytokine therapy with interferon alpha and interleukin-2 has been associated with significant toxicity and only minimal responses [29]. However, in vitro IL-2–activated donor lymphocytes have shown encouraging initial results in acute leukemia and warrant further exploration [30].

The expansion and cloning of specific lymphocyte subsets exhibiting primarily antileukemic specificity without targeting other host tissues has not yet been achieved. Current advances in our understanding of cell-mediated toxicity and techniques of lymphocyte expansion and selection will make this a feasible goal in the near future.

REFERENCES

1. Giralt S, Kolb HJ. Donor lymphocyte infusions. Curr Opin Oncol 1996; 8:96–102.
2. Kolb H, Schattenberg A, Goldman J, et al. Graft-versus-leukemia effect of donor lymphocyte transfusions in marrow grafted patients. Blood 1995; 86:2041–2050.
3. Collins R, Shpilberg O, Drobyski W, et al. Donor leukocyte infusion in 140 patients

with relapsed malignancy after allogeneic bone marrow transplantation. J Clin Oncol 1997; 15:433–444.

4. Bast R, Mills G, Gibson S, Boyer C: Tumor immunology. In: Holland J, Bast R, Morton D, Frei E, Kufe D, Weichselbaum R, eds. Cancer Medicine, 4th ed. Eds: Baltimore: Williams & Wilkins, 1997, pp. 207–242.
5. Chen W, Peace D, Rovira D, You S, Cheever M. T-cell immunity to the joining region of p210 BCR-ABL protein. Proc Natl Acad Sci USA 1992; 89:1468–1472.
6. Oettel K, Wesly O, Albertini M, et al. Allogeneic T-cell clones able to selectively destroy Philadelphia chromosome-bearing (Ph1+) human leukemia lines can also recognize Ph− cells from the same patient. Blood 1994; 83:3390–3402.
7. Verfaillie CM, Miller WJ, Boylan K, McGlave PB. Selection of benign primitive hematopoietic progenitors in chronic myelogenous leukemia on the basis of HLA-DR antigen expression. Blood 1992; 79:1003.
8. Van der Harst D, Goulmy E, Falkenburg J, et al. Recognition of minor histocompatibility antigens on lymphocytic and myeloid leukemic cells by cytotoxic T-cell clones. Blood 1994; 83:1060–1066.
9. Falkenburg J, Goselink van der Harst D, et al. Growth inhibition of clonogenic leukemic precursor cells by minor histocompatibility antigen-specific cytotoxic T-lymphocytes. J Exp Med 1991; 174:27–33.
10. Van Lochem E, De Gast B, Goulmy E. In vitro separation of host specific graft-versus-host and graft-versus-leukemia cytotoxic T cell activities. Bone Marrow Transplant 1992; 10:181–186.
11. Faber L, van Luxemburg-Heijs S, Willemze R, et al. Generation of leukemia-reactive cytotoxic T lymphocyte clones from the HLA-identical bone marrow donor of a patient with leukemia. J Exp Med 1992; 176:1283–1289.
12. Hoffmann T, Theobald M, Bunjes D, et al. Frequency of bone marrow T cells responding to HLA-identical non-leukemic and leukemic stimulator cells. Bone Marrow Transplant 1993; 12:1–9.
13. Hercend T, Takvorian T, Nowill A, et al. Characterization of natural killer cells with anti-leukemia activity following allogeneic bone marrow transplantation. Blood 1986; 67:722–730.
14. Jiang Y, Cullis J, Kanfer E, Goldman J, Barrett A. T cell and NK cell mediated graft-versus-leukemia reactivity following donor buffy coat infusion to treat relapse after marrow transplantation for chronic myeloid leukemia. Bone Marrow Transplant 1993; 11:133.
15. Champlin R, Giralt S, Przepiorka D, et al. Selective depletion of CD8-positive T-lymphocytes for allogeneic bone marrow transplantation; engraftment, graft-versus-host disease and graft-versus-leukemia. Prog Clin Biol Res 1995; 377:385–398.
16. Nimer S, Giorgi J, Gajewski J, et al. Selective depletion of CD8+ cells for prevention of graft-versus-host disease after bone marrow transplantation: a randomized controlled trial. Transplantation 1994; 57:82–87.
17. Giralt S, Hester J, Huh Y, et al. CD8-depleted donor lymphocyte infusion as treatment for relapsed chronic myelogenous leukemia after allogeneic bone marrow transplantation. Blood 1995; 86:4337–4343.
18. Hoff P, Giralt S, Huh Y, et al. Long term follow up of CD8 depleted donor lymphocyte infusions (DLI): an effective treatment for relapsed chronic myelogenous leuke-

mia (CML) after allogeneic bone marrow transplantation (BMT). Blood 1997; 90: 102a.
19. Alyea E, Chillemi A, Canning C, Soiffer R, Ritz J. Allogeneic graft-versus-leukemia is directed against host hematopoietic antigens and is not leukemia specific as determined by cytogenetic and molecular analysis in patients with CML following donor lymphocyte infusions. Blood 1997; 90:589a.
20. Alyea E, Schlossman R, Canning C, et al. CD8 depleted donot lymphocyte infusions mediate graft-versus-myeloma effect. Blood 1996; 88:258a.
21. Mackinnon S, Papadopoulos E, Carabasi M, Reich L, Collins N, O'Reilly R. Adoptive immunotherapy using donor leukocytes following bone marrow transplantation for chronic myeloid leukemia: is T cell dose important in determining biologic response? Bone Marrow Transplant 1995; 15:591–596.
22. Mackinnon S, Papadopoulos E, Carabasi M, et al. Adoptive Immunotherapy evaluating escalating doses of donor leukocytes for relapse of chronic myeloid leukemia after bone marrow transplantation: separation of graft-versus-leukemia responses from graft-versus-host disease. Blood 1995; 86:1261–1270.
23. van Rhee F, Lin F, Cullis J, et al. Relapse of chronic myeloid leukemia after allogeneic bone marrow transplant: the case for giving donor leukocyte transfusions before the onset of hematologic relapse. Blood 1994; 83:3377–3383.
24. Olavarria E, Dazzi F, Craddock C, et al. Donor lymphocyte infusion for treatment of CML in relapse after allogeneic BMT: low incidence of GVHD using an escalation dose protocol. Blood 1997; 90:589a.
25. Smit W, van Bergen C, Fibbe W, Willemze W, Falkenberg J. The antileukemic effect of donor lymphocyte transfusions (DLT) for relapsed chronic myeloid leukemia (CML) is mediated by cytotoxic T lymphocytes (CTL) recognizing leukemic CD34+ progenitor cells. Blood 1997; 90:548a.
26. Falkenberg J, Wafelman A, van Bergen C, et al. Leukemia-reactive cytotoxic T lymphocytes (CTL) induce complete remission in a patient with refractory accelerated phase chronic myeloid leukemia (CML). Blood 1997; 90:589a.
27. Bonini C, Verzeletti S, Servida P, et al. HSV-TK gene transfer into donor lymphocytes for control of allogeneic graft-versus-leukemia. Science 1997; 276:1719–1723.
28. Sullivan K, Storb R, Buckner C, et al. Graft versus host disease as adoptive immunotherapy in patients with advanced hematologic malignancies. N Engl J Med 1989; 320:828–834.
29. Giralt S, O'Brien S, Talpaz M, et al. Alpha interferon and interleukin-2 as treatment for leukemia relapse after allogeneic bone marrow transplantation. Cytokines Mol Ther, 1995; 1:115–122.
30. Slavin S, Naparstek E, Nagler A, et al. Allogeneic cell therapy with donor peripheral blood cells and recombinant human interleukin-2 to treat leukemia relapse after allogeneic bone marrow transplantation. Blood 1996; 87:2195–2204.

16

Molecular Immunological Modulation of Target Cells to Enhance the GVL Effect

Joachim L. Schultze and John G. Gribben
Harvard Medical School,
Dana-Farber Cancer Institute
Boston, Massachusetts

I. INTRODUCTION

Although there is considerable evidence to support a graft-versus-leukemia effect in allogeneic hematopoietic stem-cell transplantation (HSCT), the molecular basis for this effect remains unclear. It is likely that donor T-cell recognition of host alloantigens present on the tumor cells mediates a major component of the GVL effect. For HLA-matched sibling donors, these represent the minor histocompatibility antigens. With increasing mismatch between host and donor, this effect will potentially be increased. This type of GVL effect may be difficult to separate from GVHD, and most studies to date have demonstrated a close association between GVHD and GVL. However, the existence of immunogenic tumor antigens has now been well established [1–4]. These antigens represent targets for recognition by donor T lymphocytes. Importantly, this GVL effect will be distinct from GVHD and represents a mechanism that could be exploited for therapeutic purposes. Nevertheless, despite the documented presence of these tumor antigens, patients fail to mount clinically significant immune responses against tumor. This suggests either that tumor antigens are only very weakly immunogenic or that mechanisms exist whereby tumor cells are capable of escaping host-cell recognition. These mechanisms similarly will provide obstacles to development of a maximal GVL effect against tumor-specific antigens. Maximization of this tumor-specific GVL will require manipulation of tumor cells and host T cells and will likely be based upon an understanding of the basic molecular and immunological mechanisms required for a maximal T cell–mediated effect against antigen.

II. MOLECULAR BASIS OF IMMUNE RESPONSIVENESS AND ANERGY

A. Costimulation and the T Cell Response

For T-cell proliferation and effector function, T cells require cellular interactions with antigen presenting cells (APCs). Interactions between APCs and T cells include adhesion and recognition by MHC presentation of antigen to the T-cell receptor (TCR) and costimulation (signal 1). Although both adhesion and antigen recognition are necessary, they are not in themselves sufficient to induce a full immune response. In addition to the MHC-restricted, antigen-specific signal delivered by signal 1, there, is an absolute requirement for a second or costimulatory signal. A whole array of potentially costimulatory molecules is present on the surface of APCs, many of which also function as adhesion molecules. Among the most important costimulatory molecules are those of the B7 family. Presentation of antigen by competent APCs expressing MHC, adhesion molecules, and B7 results in productive immunity. In contrast, engagement of the TCR by antigen in the absence of costimulation fails to induce T-cell activation but rather results in the induction of long-term unresponsiveness, termed *anergy* (Figure 1).

B. B7 Family Mediated Costimulation

Recent evidence suggests that costimulation provided by members of the B7 family, CD80 (B7-1) and CD86 (B7-2), appears to be unique among costimulatory molecules. Ligation by either B7-1 or B7-2 of their counterreceptor CD28 is both necessary and sufficient to prevent the induction of anergy [5–9]. B7-1 and B7-2 have been shown to bind to and signal via CD28 on the T cell [10–13]. CD28 is constitutively expressed on 95% of resting CD4+ cells and 50% of resting CD8+ peripheral blood T cells, and its expression increases following activation [14]. In the mouse, CD28 is expressed on virtually all T cells [15]. Following a TCR-mediated signal, ligation of CD28 results in up-regulation of IL-2ra and IL-2ry receptors [16,17], increased IL-2 mRNA transcription [18], cytokine secretion, T-cell proliferation [11,12], up-regulation of CD40 ligand [19], and up-regulation of cytotoxic T-lymphocyte antigen 4 (CTLA4) mRNA [20]. CD28 signaling leads to increased expression of a number of cytokine genes, including IL-2, IFN-γ, GM-CSF, and TNF-α [21]. CD28 mediated costimulation

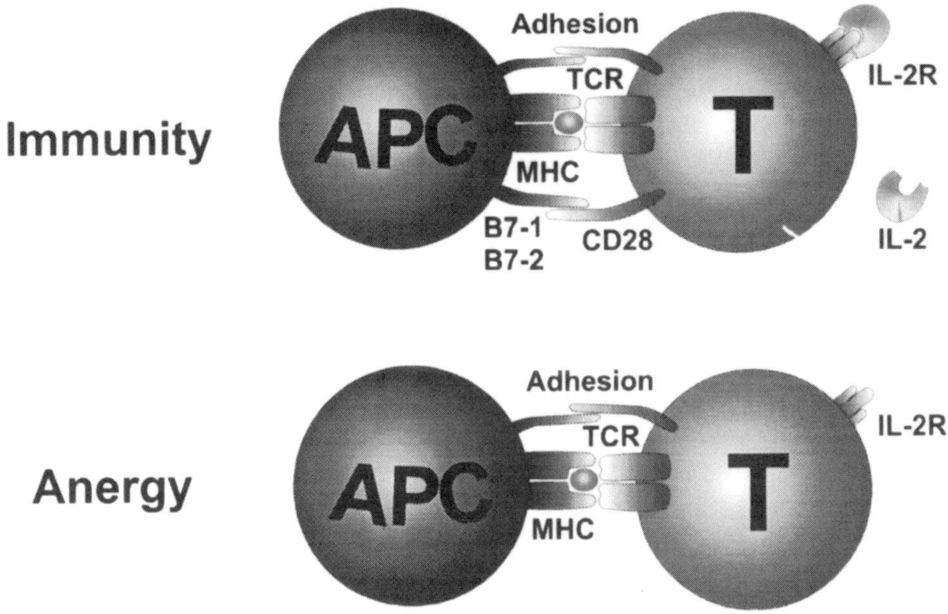

Figure 1 Requirements for T-cell proliferation following stimulation by antigen-presenting cells. (Top) Presentation by competent antigen-presenting cells leads to productive immunity. (Bottom) Presentation of antigen in the absence of costimulation results in anergy.

also enhances T-cell survival by up-regulating cell survival factors such as bcl-xL [22,23]. CTLA4 is the second high-affinity receptor for the B7 family members on T cells [11]. Unlike CD28, CTLA4 it is not expressed on resting T cells [24–26] but is induced only following T-cell activation. Since B7 family members have higher affinity for CTLA4 than for CD28, an immunoglobulin fusion protein of CTLA4 (CTLA4-lg) has proven to be an effective reagent to inhibit the costimulatory function of the B7 family both in vitro and in vivo [7,11]. Although it had been postulated that CTLA4 mediates a redundant CD28 like signal, signaling through CTLA4 in the absence of CD28 signaling results in down-regulation of T-cell responses [27]. In this model, concomitant antigen-receptor signaling and CTLA4 cross linking results in apoptosis of the previously activated T cells. Mice in whom the CTLA4 gene is "knocked out are born with a normal immune system yet die within 20 days, with massive T-cell expansion and tissue infiltration [28,29]. This T-cell proliferation and death can be prevented by the addition of CTLA4-lg to block CD28-mediated costimulation. This is in keeping with the model that CD28 is responsible for T-cell expansion but that CTLA4 is equally necessary to switch off the previously activated T cells.

C. Induction of Tolerance by Modulation of B7 Family–Mediated Costimulation

To determine the molecules critical for the prevention of anergy, fibroblasts were transfected with human MHC class II with or without B7-1 or B7-2. The functional ability of these artificial APCs was assessed by measuring proliferative responses of allogeneic T cells and results were compared with those induced by an EBV-transformed lymphoblastoid cell line (LBL) [9]. Transfectants expressing MHC class II did not induce proliferation and induced anergy and secondary rechallenge. These anergized cells are viable and proliferate on addition of exogenous IL-2. Transfectants coexpressing MHC class II and B7 could function effectively as artificial APCs to induce antigen-specific proliferation and IL-2 accumulation by either human T-cell clones [6,30] or unprimed alloreactive human T lymphocytes [9]. Under these circumstances, these cells proliferated normally on secondary rechallenge. Anergy was also induced when transfectants coexpressing MHC class II and B7 were used and B7/CD28 ligation was blocked with CTLA-4-lg. Similar results are obtained when the pathway is blocked by addition of anti-B7-1 and anti-B7-2 MAbs or anti-CD28 Fab. These experiments demonstrate that the presence of either B7-1 or B7-2 alone is sufficient to prevent the induction of anergy. Conversely, blockade of B7-1 and B7-2 on LBL is sufficient to induce anergy, suggesting that the other potentially costimulatory molecules present on the surface of the LBL and potentially other APCs are not sufficient to prevent the induction of anergy. Recent work has demonstrated that induction of anergy is not a passive process but rather the result of an active signaling pathway mediated by downstream mediators of the fyn pathway [31].

III. PREVENTION OF GVHD

A. Current Status of GVHD Prophylaxis

Since established GVHD has a high morbidity and mortality, considerable effort has been devoted to improving GVHD prophylaxis [32,33]. With increasing donor:host histoincompatibility, the incidence of GVHD, graft failure, and opportunistic infections increases markedly [34–41]. The mainstay of GVHD prophylaxis is in vivo immunosuppression using cyclosporine and methotrexate posttransplant; this is intended to prevent T-cell proliferation. Although aggressive immunosuppression has improved GVHD control significantly in matched family BMT, grade II–IV GVHD still occurs with a frequency of 10–35%, and is associated with significant toxicity [32,42–44]. Treatment related side-effects of such non-specific immunosuppression, including increased end-organ toxicity, susceptibility to infection and leukemic relapse, appear to have offset the advantages of improved GVHD control [41,43,45–48]. In the setting of alternative donor BMT (mismatched family or unrelated donors), immunosuppression has often been insufficient to control GVHD, yielding an extremely high incidence of grade III–IV acute and extensive chronic GVHD [39,49–53]. Further attempts have been made to eliminate or ameliorate GVHD by manipulation of the donor BM by T-cell depletion before infusion. T-cell depletion can be complete or partial, global or T cell subset–specific.

Whereas T-cell depletion has significantly decreased the incidence of severe acute and chronic GVHD, this has resulted in an increased incidence of graft failure and leukemic relapse. Follow-up studies of matched family BMT suggest that T-cell depletion may worsen long-term disease-free survival [47,54]. When alternative donors are used, T-cell depletion again appears equally or more efficacious in general than immunosuppression in decreasing the incidence of severe GVHD, but high rates of infection, B-cell lymphoproliferative disease, and graft failure are seen [36,38,39,49,55–59].

B. Strategies to Prevent or Ameliorate GVHD by Blockade of B7-Mediated Costimulation

Strategies to inhibit GVHD have previously employed either immunosuppression or T-cell depletion, as described above. An alternative strategy is blockade of the B7 pathway to induce anergy. Several in vivo murine transplantation studies have previously demonstrated that blockade of the B7:CD28 pathway can be used to induce tolerance. Treatment with human CTLA-4-Ig resulted in long-lasting tolerance to human xenoantigens in mice [7], suppressed antibody responses to sheep red blood cell in vivo [60], and prolonged survival of cardiac allografts in rats and mice [8]. Administration of donor-specific transfusions of peripheral blood mononuclear cells to the host animals before cardiac allografting prolonged cardiac allograft survival and suppressed responses to donor-specific but not to third-party skin grafts [61]. In a murine model of BMT, CTLA-4-Ig treatment reduced the incidence of lethal GVHD without effect on hematopoietic reconstitution [62]. These experiments are described in more detail in Chapter 3.

In fully mismatched human mixed-lymphocyte reactions (MLRs), blockade of either alloantigen recognition, adhesion, or complete blockade of both B7-1 and B7-2 inhibits maximal proliferation by greater than 90%. On secondary rechallenge, blockade of adhesion or alloantigen recognition during the primary response leads to equivalent levels of proliferation against both donor and third-party antigens. In contrast, complete blockade of B7 family–mediated costimulation during the primary MLR with either CTLA-4-Ig or the combination of anti-B7-1 and anti-B7-2 resulted in markedly decreased proliferation to donor but has no effect against third party. Maximal hyporesponsiveness required blockade of both B7-1 and B7-2 by the addition of either anti-B7-1 and anti-B72 MAbs or

CTLA-4-Ig and can be achieved within 36 to 48 h [63]. However, nonreactivity in a matched sibling MLR is a poor predictor of subsequent GVHD. In contrast, in HLA-identical sibling BMT recipients, a high frequency of alloreactive donor precursor helper T lymphocytes (pHTL) is associated with subsequent development of acute GVHD [64,65]. Complete blockade of B7 family–mediated costimulation markedly reduces the pHTL frequency against donor on rechallenge [63]. The addition of anti-B7-1 MAb has little effect, whereas anti-B7-2 had very modest effect. Even in fully HLA-disparate individuals blockade of B7 family–mediated costimulation by the addition of CTLA-4-Ig during the primary culture markedly decreases the PHTL frequency against donor but not third-party alloantigen. Ex vivo incubation of BM cells alone, in the presence of irradiated allogeneic stimulator cells alone, with the addition of CTLA-4-Ig had no effect on hematopoietic progenitor cells in either committed progenitor cells or long-term culture-initiating cell [63].

These results are highly encouraging, since they suggest that we shall be

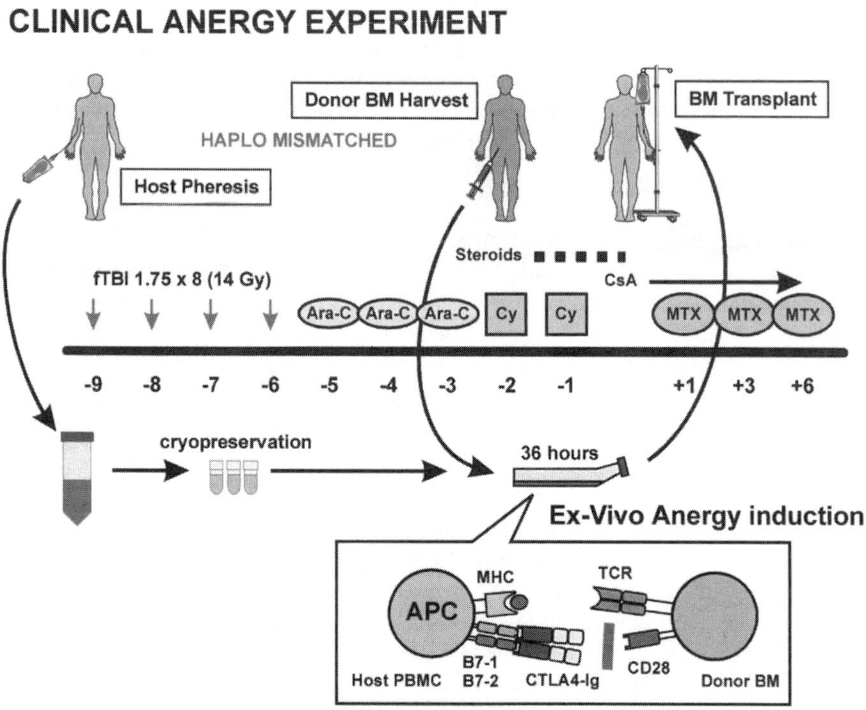

Figure 2 Clinical protocol for induction of alloantigen-specific anergy in haploidentical bone marrow transplantation.

able to reduce the pHTL frequency not only for matched sibling donors to levels below that predictive for GVHD but also for more disparate donor:recipient pairs. Based on these studies, we have commenced a clinical trial of ex vivo incubation of haploidentical donor and recipient cells in the presence of CTLA-4-lg to induce alloantigen hyporesponsiveness in addition to standard immunosuppression for the prevention of GVHD, as outlined in Figure 2. Initial studies are ongoing and have yielded preliminary data that such an approach is feasible and allows engraftment in haploidentical transplantation without significant GVHD. Following high-dose chemoradiotherapy, there is release of cytokines that have been implicated in the pathogenesis of GVHD [66]. Whether this will result in sufficient signaling to enable reversal of anergy may be determined by the results of these clinical trials. The aim is to determine whether this ex vivo manipulation of bone marrow will lead to reproducible decrease in the pHTL frequency and whether this will have any effect on subsequent engraftment. An important factor to consider will be whether the induction of host alloantigen–specific tolerance will also lead to loss of the GVL effect, as has been seen for T cell–depletion studies.

IV. IMMUNOLOGICAL STRATEGIES TO INCREASE TUMOR IMMUNITY

A. Tumor-Specific Immunological Strategies to Maximize GVL

Alternatively or in addition to reducing GVHD is the approach to enhance the GVL effect. In contrast to donor lymphocyte infusions (DLI), the goal of this approach would be to generate only tumor-specific T-cell responses without targeting alloantigen expressed on normal host cells. Theoretically, this could be achieved by two different strategies. First, tumor-specific T cells from the donor could be generated and adoptively transferred to the patient (passive immunotherapy). Alternatively, the patient could be vaccinated with tumor-specific antigens or whole-tumor-cell vaccines once donor T lymphocytes are detectable after HSCT (active immunotherapy). Although increasing numbers of tumor-specific peptide antigens have been described for many different tumors over the last 5 years [1–4], the usage of these peptide epitopes has several disadvantages in this particular setting. First, the binding of the peptide to the HLA molecule might differ from donor to host; therefore, the T cell–mediated immune response elicited might be strong on the donor's HLA background but weak on the host's background. This additional variable would make it even more difficult to find suitable peptides for a large group of patients. Moreover, even if peptides that elicit strong tumor-specific T-cell responses could be identified, it has already been shown in melanoma patients that the therapy with single peptides induces immunoselection of peptide-negative tumor cells and subsequent relapse with peptide tumor [67]. To circumvent the down side of the peptide approach, we and others have studied the use of whole tumor cells to elicit a T-cell response in vivo and ex vivo.

B. Tumor Cells as Antigen-Presenting Cells

The use of tumor cells to stimulate T cells in vivo or ex vivo, however, also has several disadvantages. For example, although many tumor-cell lines have been established over the last decades, it is still a difficult task for many primary tumors to be cultured and expanded in vitro to generate sufficient numbers of tumor cells for T-cell stimulation [68]. Moreover, the study of tumor-cell lines has elicited many molecular defects that might hamper their use as APCs for the stimulation of T cells.

C. Molecular Basis of Poor APC Function of Tumor Cells

Increasing numbers of tumor-specific antigens are being identified, especially in melanoma but also in breast, pancreatic, and renal cancer. It is not yet clear whether tumor-specific or associated antigens exist for all tumors, although this remains an extremely active area of research. However, even if tumor-specific antigens exist in almost every tumor patient, it will be important to identify tumor antigens that are not only specific for the tumor but that also lead to tumor regression when effectively targeted by the immune response [69,70]. Preliminary evidence for some of the melanoma-derived tumor antigens suggests that immune responses elicited against these antigens can result in eradication of disease [71–73].

Assuming that tumors present tumor regression antigens, the tumor cells can evolve additional mechanisms to escape an antitumor immune response. Recent research in many laboratories has revealed important mechanisms of tumor-cell escape from immune surveillance [74–82]. Potential mechanisms of tumor-cell escape are shown in Figure 3. Tumor cells may fail to express MHC class I and II molecules [74,79], or may fail to process and express tumor antigens in the context of MHC molecules [83]. They may lack expression of requisite costimulatory molecules [84–87] or secrete factors that inhibit the immune response [75]. It has been found that, in many solid tumors at presentation but especially during tumor progression the majority of the tumor cells lose expression of MHC molecules and therefore cannot be attacked by tumor-specific T cells [74]. Although this might lead to increased detection by natural killer (NK) cells due to the loss of MHC as NK cell–suppressor molecules, the impact on immunosurveillance is not well studied and even less understood. Lack of expres-

Tumor cell	T Cell Response					
	Antigen Recognition	Proliferation	Cytolysis	Ignorance	Anergy	Suppression
No MHC	−	−	−	+	−	−
No Antigen	−	−	−	+	−	−
No costimulation	+	+/−	−	−	+	−
TGFβ, IL-10	+/−	−	−	−	−	+

Figure 3 Potential defects in the capacity of tumor cells to function as competent antigen-presenting cells and consequent T-cell responses against tumor.

sion of antigens and/or lack of MHC will lead to the tumor cells being ignored by the immune system.

Even if the tumor cells express both tumor antigens and MHC on the surface, the lack of important accessory molecules, including adhesion and costimulatory molecules, could be responsible for the lack of a clinically efficient antitumor immune response [84–86].

Most or all solid tumors lack surface expression of B7 molecules, and this is also true for many hematological malignancies. Germinal center–derived B-cell lymphomas [86], plasma-cell leukemia [88], and some pre-B acute lymphoblastic leukemias (ALLs) [89] seem to be exceptions, since we have been able to demonstrate surface expression of B7-1 and/or B7-2 on these tumor cells. However, in most cases the expression of B7 was very weak, and these cells induced only weak proliferative responses of allogeneic T cells, suggesting that the level of B7 expression was insufficient [90]. Indeed, comparison with professional APCs, such as dendritic cells, clearly demonstrated that these malignant cells expressed insufficient levels of adhesion and costimulatory molecules [88].

Following the two-signal model of T-cell activation, lack of expression of B7 on tumor cells might induce antigen-specific T-cell anergy in vitro and potentially T-cell tolerance in vivo. Using an allogeneic in vitro system, we have been able to further substantiate the important role of B7 expression on tumor cells for the prevention of T-cell anergy. Follicular lymphoma cells expressing B7 at very low levels, only detectable by a highly sensitive immunohistochemistry method, prevented the induction of T-cell anergy [90]. In contrast, blockade using

CTLA4-Ig during priming of the allogeneic T cells lead to T-cell anergy. Similarly, B7-pre-B-ALL cells also induced T-cell anergy [89].

In addition to the lack of important surface molecules, tumor cells have been shown to express a variety of immune modulators, in particular inhibitory cytokines. More than 10 years ago, supernatants from glioblastoma cells were demonstrated to suppress T-cell proliferation, and the factor responsible for this phenomenon has been identified as transforming growth factor beta 1 (TGF-β_1) [91]. TGF-β has been demonstrated to be expressed in large quantities by a variety of tumor cells [92]. One of the potential mechanisms for the dysregulated expression of TGF-β by the tumor is down-regulation of the TGF-β receptors on the tumor cells, which does not allow a negative feedback mechanism controlling TGF-β production by the tumor cells [93–95]. Another example of the expression of an immunoinhibitory cytokine by tumor cells is the expression of IL-10 by many Non-Hodkin-Lymphoma (NHL) [96–98]. We and others have demonstrated that both cytokines can play an important role in the down-regulation of T cell–mediated immune responses [98–107].

Another mechanism of tumor-cell escape from immunosurveillance is the ectopic expression of FAS ligand on tumor cells, as demonstrated for colon cancer, melanoma, lung and colon carcinoma, multiple myeloma, glioblastoma, and lymphomas [108–120]. Since the expression of FAS ligand in the eye, placenta, and testis has been shown to be important to establish immune privilege [113,121–123], it is perhaps not surprising that such a mechanism has been adopted by many tumors. Taken together, it is important to understand the mechanisms that define tumor cells as poor APCs compared with professional APCs. Once these mechanisms have been identified, strategies can be developed to overcome these obstacles.

D. Strategies to Repair Defective APC Function of Tumor Cells

With increasing knowledge in basic immunology, molecular biology, and advanced biotechnology, the generation of tumor APCs has come into our reach and clinical experimentation using such biologically engineered cells has already begun. There are several different methodologies that could be applied, and these principals are summarized in Figure 4. Clearly, much recent clinical and preclinical research to enhance the APC function of tumor cells has focused on the transfer of genes into the tumor cells. Many different strategies have been proposed and are already in clinical trials. Retroviral gene transfer, lipofection, receptor-mediated gene transfer, adenoviral vectors, or adeno- or adeno-associated viral vectors as well as the gene gun have all been proposed for clinical experimentation. Many different genes for the transfer to tumor cells are under study, with an emphasis on cytokine genes including IL-2, IL-4, and GM-CSF [124,125].

Strategy	Example	T Cell Response					
		Antigen Recognition	Proliferation	Cytolysis	Ignorance	Anergy	Suppression
Gene transfer	Transfection of B7-1 and MHC	+	+	+	−	−	−
Physiological signal	CD40 activation	+	+	+	−	−	−
Tumor cell APC fusion		+	+	+	−	−	−
Downregulation of suppressors	TGFβ IL-10	+	+	+	−	−	−
Use of professional APC	Dendritic cells CD40-activated B cells	+	+	+	−	−	−

Figure 4 Strategies to repair defective antigen-presenting capacity of tumor cells. Successful repair of the defect will lead to productive immunity.

Cell-surface molecules such as MHC and B7 are also under investigation. All these trials are based on findings in mouse models that have yielded quite impressive results. Here we shall only summarize the extensive work in murine models, studying the role of B7 and GM-CSF expression on neoplastic cells, since this area has been recently extensively reviewed [124,126,127]. Vaccination with B7-transfected tumor cells has been shown in several models to induce protection on rechallenge with the transfected tumor and the wild-type tumor. Although the induction of systemic immunity could be demonstrated for specific antigen and immunogenic tumors, the manipulation of the B7:CD28 pathway in nonimmunogenic tumors appears relatively ineffective in eliciting tumor-specific reactions [85]. This result is not surprising, and these experiments underscore the fact that there is an absolute requirement for adequate signaling through the TCR as well as a costimulatory pathway for effective antigen-specific immunity.

Clinically more relevant is the outcome of vaccination in animals with established tumor. When tumor-bearing animals were vaccinated with B7-1–transfected tumor cells, protection was observed only in animals with low tumor load and if vaccination with tumor cells transfected with B7-1 was given early after tumor inoculation [126]. Dranoff and collegues demonstrated in their models that GM-CSF does seem to be superior to B7 [124,125]. This might be due to the lack of T-cell help, which could not be provided by the tumor cells expressing B7, since the tumor cells were negative for MHC class II. Baskar and colleagues have demonstrated the important role of MHC class II on the tumor cell [128].

Vaccination with B7-I+ sarcoma cells of mice with high tumor burden provided no protection, whereas vaccination with B7-1+ MHC class II+ sarcoma cells protected more than 50% of the mice. By depleting CD4+ or CD8+ T cells, it could be shown that both T-cell subsets were important for tumor regression. In context with data from others [129] this emphasizes on the important role of tumor-specific T-helper (Th) cells is a prerequisite for the induction of a sufficient antitumor immune response in the tumor-bearing host. Moreover, tumor cells function as efficient APCs only if they express MHC class I, II, and B7.

Although data from murine model systems led to great expectations and hope early on, the clinical implementation of gene therapy as a strategy for cancer immunotherapy has been far more frustrating, and the results have been depressing. This was due mainly to unexpected technical difficulties and insufficient transfection efficiency using primary human tumor cells. As is true for every new biotechnology, second and third generations of gene-transfer technology will probably solve these technical issues and allow this strategy to become more effective in the future.

Another approach to induce tumor cells to present antigen is the up-regulation or induction of the molecules necessary for antigen presentation. It was shown many years ago that IFN-γ up-regulates the expression of MHC class I and II molecules on endothelial cells and solid tumors derived from endothelial cells [130–135]. However, it has not been shown that costimulatory molecules can be induced on these tumor cells. Therefore, although specific effector T cells can detect peptides in the context of MHC class I and II molecules on these tumor cells after IFN-γ treatment, these tumor cells likely fail to induce a specific T-cell immune response, since they still lack the necessary costimulatory molecules. Induction of costimulatory molecules is a natural consequence of B-cell activation [14,136]. Studies using monoclonal antibodies to the CD40 molecule have identified this pathway of activation as one of the major pathways of activation of B cells [137]. Indeed we and others have recently shown that the interaction of CD40 ligand with CD40 on malignant B cells is the major pathway of inducing and or up-regulating MHC, adhesion and costimulatory molecules [86,90,138,139]. Moreover, the level of expression of these molecules is comparable with that of dendritic cells [99]. Using CD40-activated B-lymphoma cells, we have been able to generate autologous and allogenic T cells capable of killing the unstimulated primary lymphoma cells, suggesting that CD40-activated lymphoma cells are sufficient to induce T-cell activation and proliferation. However, once the T cells have been sufficiently activated, they are less dependent on the expression of accessory molecules on the target cells [138]. Studies using chronic lymphocytic leukemia (CLL) cells, plasma-cell leukemia cells, or pre-B ALL cells have confirmed that virtually all CD40 B-cell malignancies can be induced to become efficient APCs after CD40 activation. We have already been able to optimize this culture system for clinical use, and ongoing vaccination trials using CD40-activated follicular lymphoma cells will answer the question of whether such a therapy is safe, feasible, and ultimately efficacious [88]. Although other tumors, including endothelial tumors, express CD40, it has not been demonstrated and reported to date that cross linking CD40 on these tumor cells can induce costimulatory molecules. Further study will be necessary to determine if other CD40+ tumor cells can be induced to express costimulatory molecules and, if not, which signaling cascades are missing in these tumor cells. Clearly, this strategy cannot be applied to tumors unreactive to CD40 activation or to CD40 tumors. An alternative strategy has been proposed in murine model systems. Guo and colleagues proposed to fuse dendritic cells with tumor cells leading to a ''fusidoma'' probably expressing the tumor antigens derived from the tumor and the accessory molecules derived from the dendritic cells [140].

Although this study elegantly demonstrated feasibility in the mouse, studies in the human have not been reported to date, and our own attempts have also failed. It appears unlikely that the many technical difficulties of this approach will be resolved in the near future.

The strategies described above all attempt to improve APC function by inducing or adding a stimulatory signal. However, we should not forget that it might be important to suppress or block inhibitory factors or cell-surface molecules produced by the tumor cells. Clearly, our current knowledge about successful strategies in this area is very limited. Again, effects have been demonstrated in murine models, but these strategies have not yet entered the preclinical or clinical arena. For example, blockade of CTLA-4 using anti-CTLA-4 MAbs in the mouse could provide tumor outgrowth in a murine model. This suggests that blockade of the down-regulatory ligand for B7-1 and B7-2 can inhibit interactions between B7-1 and B7-2 and CD28 on the T cells, ultimately leading to enhanced T-cell activation, proliferation, and expansion [127]. Another example is blockade of TGF-β_1 production by antisense approaches to reduce or abrogate the production of inhibitory cytokine [141]. Again, although successful in murine model systems, it remains unclear how this would be translated into the clinic.

E. Induction of Tumor-Specific T-Cell Responses

As outlined earlier, tumor-specific T-cell responses can be induced either ex vivo or in vivo. Whereas the in vivo induction via vaccination is currently favored in the autologous setting, it is rather unlikely to be successful in the context of allogeneic HSCT. The probability of inducing GVHD using competent tumor-APCs is rather high. Therefore it will be more likely that ex vivo strategies using specific T cells will be applicable. Multiple clinical trials have demonstrated the efficacy of adoptively transferred matched allogeneic antigen-specific T cells for both treatment and prophylaxis of viral diseases after HSCT [142,143]. However, so far, the technology to induce tumor-specific T cells for clinical testing has not been established. Beginning with CD40+ B-cell malignancies [138,144], we have initiated preclinical experiments testing the hypothesis whether tumor-specific autologous or allogeneic T cells could be generated for adoptive T-cell immunotherapy. These initial studies have been performed with T-cell lines rather than T-cell clones [138,144]. First, in follicular lymphoma and subsequently in PCL, CLL, and pre-B ALL, we identified tumor-specific T cells by expanding T cells with CD40-activated tumor cells. The expansion of these short-term cultured T-cell lines varied widely between patients. Further, increase in expansion was induced by the addition of a cytokine such as IFN-γ or IL-7. Most of our preclinical studies have been performed with cryopreserved cells therefore expansion might be significantly higher when using fresh T cells. Moreover, it remains to be determined whether T cells from peripheral blood can be used as a source for the generation of tumor-specific T cells. Although cytotoxic T cells were generated from the peripheral blood of patients with pre-B ALL, we could easily generate tumor-specific T cells from peripheral blood in patients with plasma cell leukemia and follicular lymphoma. Further studies will be necessary to understand whether this observation is an intrinsic property of pre-B ALL. Clearly, for clinical practice, the use of peripheral blood would be of advantage. Another issue is the use of T-cell lines versus T-cell clones. For clinical practice, T-cell lines are easier to generate than T-cell clones. However, since these lines are polyclonal and nonspecific T cells are not excluded, they might have the disadvantage of inducing GVHD. Ongoing research focuses on these important questions.

V. FUTURE DIRECTIONS–INDUCTION OF GVL WITHOUT GVHD APPLYING GVHD REDUCED HSCT FOLLOWED BY TUMOR-SPECIFIC COMBINATION IMMUNOTHERAPY

To make allogeneic HSCT available for more patients with cancer, the ultimate goal is to decrease the side effects and increase the tumor-specific effects. We have outlined current and novel methodologies of decreasing GVHD and novel principles for inducing or increasing a specific GVL effect. How can we combine these efforts?

To increase the pool of allogeneic HSC donors, methodologies including those outlined here will be implemented at the time of HSCT. Patients will undergo high-dose chemotherapy followed by modified HSCT. Using surrogate endpoints such as PCR detection of tumor cells after HSCT, we will identify patients who did not achieve molecular remission. These patients can then be treated to increase tumor-specific immunity. Figure 5 depicts our current model. Strategies to increase immune responsiveness in vivo will be based upon knowl-

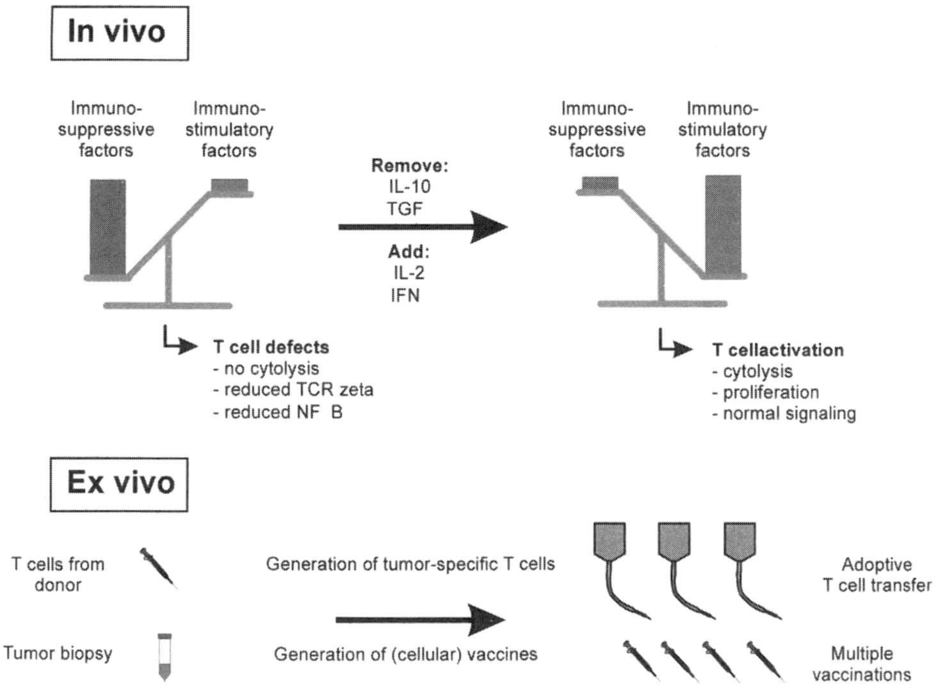

Figure 5 Model for in vivo and ex vivo immune manipulations to induce effective tumor immunity.

edge of the underlying molecular mechanism whereby immune recognition is defective for an individual tumor. These patients will be further treated with a combination immunotherapy using donor-derived tumor-specific T cells generated ex vivo for adoptive T-cell therapy followed by cytokine therapy and potentially boost immunizations using either tumor regression antigen-derived peptides or whole-tumor-cell vaccines.

REFERENCES

1. Van Pel A, Van der Bruggen P, Coulie PG, Brichard VG, Lethe B, Vail den Eynde B, Uyttenhove C, Renauld J-C, Boon T. Genes coding for tumor antigens recognized by cytolytic T lymphocytes. Immunol Rev 1995; 145:229.
2. Pardoll DM. Tumor antigens: a new look for the 1990s. Nature 1994; 369:357.

3. Boon T, Cerottini JC, Eynde B, Braggen P, Pel AV. Tumor antigens recognized by T lymphocytes. Annu Rev Immunol 1994; 12:337.
4. Pardoll DM. Cancer vaccines. Immunol Today 1993; 14:310.
5. Harding FA, McArthur JG, Gross JA, Raulet DH, Allison JP. CD28-mediated signaling co-stimulates murine T cells and prevents induction of anergy in T-cell clones. Nature 1992; 356:607.
6. Gimmi CD, Freeman GJ, Gribben JG, Gray G, Nadler LM. Human T-cell clonal anergy is induced by antigen presentation in the absence of B7 costimulation. Proc Natl Acad Sci USA 1993; 90:65–86.
7. Lenschow DJ, Zeng Y, Thistlethwaite JR, Montag A, Brady W, Gibson G, Linsley PS, Bluestone JA. Long-term survival of xenogeneic pancreatic islet grafts induced by CTLA41g (see comments). Science 1992; 257:789.
8. Turka LA, Linsley PS, Lin H, Brady W, Leiden JM, Wei RQ, Gibson ML, Zheng XG, Myrdal S, Gordon D, Bailey T, Bolling SF, Thompson CB. T-cell activation by the CD28 ligand B7 is required for cardiac allograft rejection in vivo. Proc Natl Acad Sci USA 1992; 89:11102.
9. Boussiotis VA, Freeman GJ, Gray GS, Gribben JG, Nadler LM. B7 but not intercellular adhesion molecule- I costimulation prevents the induction of human alloantigen-specific tolerance. J Exp Med 1993; 178:1753.
10. Linsley PS, Clark EA, Ledbetter JA. T-cell antigen CD28 mediates adhesion with B cells by interacting with activation antigen B7/BB-1. Proc Natl Acad Sci USA 1990; 87:5031.
11. Linsley PS, Brady W, Grosmaire L, Aruffo A, Damle NK, Ledbetter JA. Binding of the B cell activation antigen B7 to CD28 costimulates T cell proliferation, and interleukin 2 mRNA accumulation. J Exp Med 1991; 173:721.
12. Gimmi CD, Freeman GJ, Gribben JG, Sugita K, Freedman AS, Morimoto C, Nedler LM. B-cell surface antigen B7 provides a costimulatory signal that induces T cells to proliferate and secrete interleukin 2. Proc Natl Acad Sci USA 1991; 88:6575.
13. Freeman GJ, Gribben JG, Boussiotis VA, Ng JW, Restivo VAJ, Lombard LA, Gray GS, Nadler LM. Cloning of B7-2: a CTLA-4 counter-receptor that costimulates human T cell proliferation (see comments). Science 1993; 262:909.
14. June CH, Bluestone JA, Nadler LM, Thompson CB. The B7 and CD28 receptor families. Immunol Today 1994; 15:321.
15. Gross JA, St. John T, Allison JP. The murine homologue of the T lymphocyte antigen CD28: molecular cloning and cell surface expression. J Immunol 1990; 144:320.
16. Cerdan C, Martin Y, Courcoul M, Brailly H, Mawas C, Birg F, Olive D. Prolonged IL-2 receptor alpha/CD25 expression after T cell activation via the adhesion molecules CD2 and CD28: demonstration of combined transcriptional and post-transcriptional regulation. J Immunol 1992; 149:2255.
17. Freeman GJ, Boussiotis VA, Anumanthan A, Bernstein GM, Ke X-Y, Rennert PD, Gray GS, Gribben JG, Nadler LM. B7-1 and B7-2 do not deliver identical costimulatory signals since B7-2 but not B7-1 preferentially costimulates the initial production of IL-4. Immunity 1995; 2:523.
18. Fraser JD, Weiss A. Regulation of T-cell lymphokine gene transcription by the accessory molecule CD28. Mol Cell Biol 1992; 12:43–57.

19. de Boer M, Kasran A, Kwekkeboom J, Walter H, Vandenberghe P, Ceuppens JL. Ligation of B7 with CD28/CTLA-4 on T cells results in CD40 ligand expression, interleukin-4 secretion and efficient help for antibody production by B cells. Eur J Immunol 1993; 23:3120.
20. Lindsten T, Lee KP, Harris ES, Petryniak B, Craighead N, Reynolds PJ, Lombard DB, Freeman GJ, Nadler LM, Gray GS, Thompson CB, June CH. Characterization of CTLA-4 structure and expression on human T cells. J Immunol 1993; 151: 3489.
21. Thompson CB, Lindsten T, Ledbetter JA, Kunkel SL, Young HA, Emerson SG, Leiden JM, June CH. CD28 activation pathway regulates the production of multiple T-cell-derived lymphokines/cytokines. Proc Natl Acad Sci USA 1989; 86:1333.
22. Boise LH, Minn AJ, Noel PJ, June CH, Accavitti MA, Lindsten T, Thompson CB. 28 Costimulation can promote T cell survival by enhancing the expression of Bcl-XL. Immunity 1995; 3:87.
23. Brunet JF, Denizot F, Luciani MF, Roux-Dosseto M, Suzan M, Mattei MG, Golstein P. A new member of the immunoglobulin superfamily—CTLA-4. Nature 1987; 328:267.
24. Harper K, Balzano C, Rouvier E, Mattei MG, Luciani MF, Golstein P. CTLA-4 and CD28 activated lymphocyte molecules are closely related in both mouse and human as to sequence, message expression, gene structure, and chromosomal location. J Immunol 1991; 147:1037.
25. Freeman GJ, Lombard DB, Gimmi CD, Brod SA, Lee K, Laning JC, Hafler DA, Dorf ME, Gray G, Reiser H, June CH, Thompson CB, Nadler LM. CTLA-4 and CD28 mRNA are coexpressed in most T cells after activation: expression of CTLA-4 and CD28 mRNA does not correlate with the pattern of lymphokine production. J Immunol 1992; 149:3795.
26. Linsley PS, Greene JL, Tan P, Bradshaw J, Ledbetter JA, Anasetti C, Damle NK. Coexpression and functional cooperation of CTLA-4 and CD28 on activated T lymphocytes. J Exp Med 1992; 176:1595.
27. Gribben JG, Freeman GJ, Boussiotis VA, Rennert P, Jellis CL, Greenfield E, Barber M, Restivo VAJ, Ke X-Y, Gray GS, Nadler LM. CTLA4 mediates antigen-specific apoptosis of human T cells. Proc Natl Acad Sci USA 1995; 92:811.
28. Tivol EA, Boriello F, Schweitzer AN, Lynch WP, Bluestone JA, Sharpe AH. Loss of CTLA-4 leads to massive lymphoproliferation and fatal multi-organ tissue destruction, revealing a critical negative regulatory role for CTLA-4. Immunity 1995; 3:541.
29. Waterhouse P, Penninger JM, Timms E, Wakeharn A, Shahinian A, Lee KP, Thompson CB, Griesser H, Mak TW. Lymphoproliferative disorders with early lethality in mice deficient in CTLA-4. Science 1995; 270:985.
30. Boussiotis VA, Freeman GJ, Griffin JD, Gray GS, Gribben JG, Nadler LM. CD2 is involved in maintenance and reversal of human alloantigen specific clonal anergy. J Exp Med 1994; 180:1665.
31. Boussiotis VA, Barber DL, Lee BJ, Gribben JG, Freeman GJ, Nadler LM. Differential association of protein tyrosine kinases with the T cell receptor is linked to the induction of anergy and its prevention by B7 family-mediated costimulation. J Exp Med 1996; 184:365.

32. Martin PJ, Schoch G, Fisher L, Byers V, Appelbaum FR, McDonald GB, Storb R, Hansen JA. A retrospective analysis of therapy for acute graft-versus-host disease: secondary treatment. Blood 1991; 77:1821.
33. Vogelsang GB, Hess AD, Santos GW. Acute graft-versus-host disease: clinical characteristics in the cyclosporine era. Medicine 1988; 67:163.
34. Anasetti C, Amos D, Beatty PG, Appelbaum FR, Bensinger W, Buckner CD, Clift R, Doney K, Martin PJ, Mickelson E, Nisperos B, O'Quigley J, Ramberg R, Sanders JE, Stewart P, Storb R, Sullivan KM, Witherspoon RP, Thomas ED, Hansen JA. Effect of HLA compatibility on engraftment of bone marrow transplants in patients with leukemia or lymphoma. N Engl J Med 1989; 320:197.
35. Anasetti C, Beatty PG, Storb R, Martin PJ, Mori M, Sanders JE, Thomas ED, Hansen JA. Effect of HLA incompatibility on graft-versus-host disease, relapse and survival after marrow transplantation for patients with leukemia and lymphoma. Hum Immunol 1990; 29:79.
36. Pirsch JD, Maki DO. Infectious complications in adults with bone marrow transplantation and T-cell depletion of donor marrow: increased susceptibility to fungal infections. Ann Intern Med 1986; 104:619.
37. Nademanee A, Schmidt GM, Parker P, Dagis AC, Stein A, Snyder DS, O'Donnell M, Smith EP, Stepan DE, Molina A, Wong KK, Margolin K, Somlo G, Littrell B, Woo D, Sniecinski I, Niland JC, Forman SJ. The outcome of matched unrelated donor bone marrow transplantation in patients with hematologic malignancies using molecular typing for donor selection and graft-versus-host disease prophylaxis regimen of cyclosporine, methotrexate, and prednisone. Blood 1995; 86:1228.
38. Marks DI, Cullis JO, Ward KN, Lacey S, Syzdlo R, Hughes TP, Schwarer AP, Lutz E, Barrett AJ, Hows JM, Batchelor JR, Goldman JM. Allogeneic bone marrow transplantation for chronic myeloid leukemia using sibling and volunteer unrelated donors. Ann Intern Med 1993; 119:207.
39. Kernan NA, Bartsch G, Ash RC, Beatty PG, Champlin R, Filipovich A, Gajewski J, Hansen JA, Henslee-Downey J, McCullough J, McGlave P, Perkins HA, Phillips GL, Sanders J, Stroncek D, Thomas ED, Blume KG. Analysis of 462 transplantation from unrelated donors facilitated by the national marrow donor program. N Engl J Med 1993; 328:593.
40. Beatty PG, Clift RA, Mickelson EM, Nisperos BB, Flournoy N, Martin PJ, Sanders JE, Stewart P, Buckner CD, Storb R, Thomas ED, Hansen JA. Marrow transplantation from related donors other than HLA-identical siblings. N Engl J Med 1985; 313:765.
41. O'Reilly RJ. T-cell depletion and allogeneic bone marrow transplantation. Semin Hematol 1992; 29(2 suppl 1):20.
42. Storb R, Deeg HJ, Pepe M, Doney K, Appelbaum F, Beatty P, Bensinger W, Buckner CD, Clift R, Hansen J, et al. Graft-versus-host disease prevention by methotrexate combined with cyclosporin compared to methotrexate alone in patients given marrow grafts for severe aplastic anaemia: long-term follow-up of a controlled trial (see comments). Br J Haematol 1989; 72:567.
43. Storb R, Deeg HJ, Pepe M, Appelbaum F, Anasetti C, Beatty P, Bensinger W, Berenson R, Buckner CD, Clift R, Doney K, Longton G, Hansen J, Hill R, Loughran T, Jr., Martin P, Singer J, Sanders J, Stewart P, Sullivan K, Witherspoon R,

Thomas ED. Methotrexate and cyclosporine versus cyclosporine alone for prophylaxis of graft-versus-host disease in patients given HLA-identical marrow grafts for leukemia: long-term follow-up of a controlled trial. Blood 1989; 73:1729.

44. Chao NJ, Schmidt GM, Niland JC, Amylon MD, Dagis AC, Long GD, Nademanee AP, Negrin RS, O'Donnell MR, Parker PM, Smith EP, Snyder DS, Stein AS, Wong RM, Blume KG, Forman SJ. Cyclosporine, methotrexate and prednisone compared with cyclosporine and prednisone for prophylaxis of acute graft-versus-host disease. N Engl J Med 1993; 329:1225.
45. Storb R, Deeg HJ, Whitehead J, Appelbaum F, Beatty P, Bensinger W, Buckner D, Clift R, Doney K, Farewell V, Hansen J, Hill R, Lum L, Martin P, McGuffin R, Sanders J, Stewart P, Sullivan K, Witherspoon R, Yee G, Thomas ED. Methotrexate and cyclosporine compared with cyclosporine alone for prophylaxis of acute graft-versus-host disease after marrow transplantation for leukemia. N Engl J Med 1986; 314:729.
46. Storb R, Sanders JE, Pepe M, Anasetti C, Appelbaum FR, Buckner CD, Deeg HJ, Doney K, Hansen J, Martin P, Stewart P, Sullivan KM, Thomas ED, Witherspoon RP. Graft-versus-host disease prophylaxis with methotrexate/cyclosporine in children with severe aplastic anemia treated with cyclophosphamide and HLA-identical marrow grafts (letter). Blood 1991; 78:1144.
47. Blaise D, Gravis G, Marinichi D. Long-term follow-up of T-cell depletion for bone marrow transplantation. Lancet 1993; 341:51.
48. Soiffer RJ, Murray C, Mauch P, Anderson KC, Freedman AS, Rabinowe SN, Takvorian T, Robertson MJ, Spector N, Gonin R, Miller KB, Rudders RA, Freeman A, Blake K, Coral F, Nadler LM, Ritz J. Prevention of graft-versus-host disease by selective depletion of CD6-positive T lymphocytes from donor bone marrow. J Clin Oncol 1992; 10:1191.
49. McGlave P, Bartsch G, Anasetti C, Ash R, Beatty P, Gajewski J, Kernan NA. Unrelated donor marrow transplantation therapy for chronic myelogenous leukemia: initial experience of the national marrow donor program. Blood 1993; 81:543.
50. McGlave PB, Beatty P, Ash R, Hows JM. Therapy for chronic myelogenous leukemia with unrelated donor bone marrow transplantation: results in 102 cases [published erratum appears in Blood 1990; 76:654]. Blood 1990; 75:1728.
51. Beatty PG. Results of allogeneic bone marrow transplantation with unrelated or mismatched donors. Semin Oncol 1992; 19(3 suppl 7):13.
52. Beatty PG, Hansen JA, Longton GM, Thomas ED, Sanders JE, Martin PJ, Bearman SI, Anasetti C, Petersdorf EW, Mickelson EM, Pepe MS, Appelbaum FR, Buckner CD, Clift RA, Petersen FB, Stewart PS, Storb RF, Sullivan KM, Tesler MC, Witherspoon RP. Marrow transplantation from HLA-matched unrelated donors for treatment of hematologic malignancies. Transplantation 1991; 51:443.
53. Petersdorf EW, Longton GM, Anasetti C, Martin PJ, Mickelson EM, Smith AG, Hansen JA. The significance of HLA-DRBI matching on clinical outcome after HLA. A, B, DR identical unrelated donor marrow transplantation. Blood 1995; 86:1606.
54. Marmont AM, Horowitz MM, Gale RP, Sobocinski K, Ash RC, Van Bekkum DW, Champlin RE, Dicke KA, Goldman JM, Good RA, Herzig RH, Hong R, Masaoka T, Rimm AA, Ringden O, Speck B, Weiner RS, Bortin M. T-cell depletion of HLA-identical transplants in leukemia. Blood 1991; 78:2120.

55. Hows JM, Yin JL, Marsh J, Swirsky D, Jones L, Apperley JF, James DCO, Smithers S, Batchelor JR, Goldman JM, Gordon-Smith EC. Histocompatible unrelated volunteer donors compared with HLA nonidentical family donors in marrow transplantation for aplastic anemia and leukemia. Blood 1986; 68:1322.
56. Hows JM. Unrelated donor bone marrow transplantation for severe aplastic anaemia and Fanconi's anaemia. Bone Marrow Transplant 1989; 4:126.
57. Antin J, Bierer N, Smith B, Ferrara J, Guinan EC, Selff C, Golon DE, Macklis RM, Tarbell NJ, Lynch E, Reichert TA, Blythman H, Bouloux C, Rappeport JM, Burakoff SJ, Weinstein HJ. Selective depletion of bone marrow T lymphocytes with anti-CD5 monoclonal antibodies: effective prophylaxis for graft-versus-host disease in patients with hematologic malignancies. Blood 1991; 76:1464.
58. Ash RC, Casper JT, Chitambar CR, Hansen R, Bunin N, Truitt RL, Lawton C, Murray K, Hunter J, Baxter-Lowe LA, Gottschall JL, Oldham K, Anderson T, Camitta B, Menitove J. Successful allogeneic transplantation of T-cell-depleted bone marrow from closely HLA-matched unrelated donors. N Engl J Med 1990; 322: 485.
59. Casper J, Camitta B, Truitt R, Baxter-Lowe LA, Bunin N, Lawton C, Murray K, Hunter J, Pietryga D, Garbrecht F, Taylor CK, Drobyski W, Horowitz M, Flomenberg N, Ash R. Unrelated bone marrow donor transplants for children with leukemia or myelodysplasia. Blood 1995; 85:2354.
60. Linsley PS, Wallace PM, Johnson J, Gibson MG, Greene JL, Ledbetter JA, Singh C, Tepper MA. Immunosuppression in vivo by a soluble form of the CTLA4 T cell activation molecule. Science 1992; 257:792.
61. Lin H, Bolling SF, Linsley PS, Wei RQ, Gordon D, Thompson CB, Turka LA. Long-term acceptance of major histocompatibility complex mismatched cardiac allografts induced by CTLA4-lg plus donor-specific transfusion. J Exp Med 1993; 178:1801.
62. Blazar BR, Taylor PA, Linsley PS, Vallera DA. In vivo block of CD28/CTLA4: By/BBI interaction with CTLA4-lg reduces lethal murine graft-versus-host disease across the major histocompatibility complex barrier in mice. Blood 1994; 83: 3815.
63. Gribben JG, Guinan EC, Boussiotis VA, Ke XY, Linsley L, Sieff C, Gray G, Freeman GJ, Nadler LM. Complete blockade of B7 mediated costimulation is necessary to induce human alloantigen specific anergy: a method to ameliorate graft versus host disease and extend the donor pool. Blood 1996; 87:4887.
64. Theobald M, Nierle T, Bunjes D, Arnold R, Heimpel H. Host-specific interleukin 2–secreting donor T-cell precursors as predictors of acute graft-versus-host-disease in bone marrow transplantation between HLA-identical siblings. N Engl J Med 1992; 327:1613.
65. Schwarer AP, Jiang YZ, Brookes PA, Barrett AJ, Batchelor JR, Goldman JM, Lechler RI. Frequency of anti-recipient alloreactive helper T-cell precursors in donor blood and graft-versus-host disease after HLA-identical sibling bone-marrow transplantation. Lancet 1993; 341:203.
66. Ferrara JLM, Deeg HJ. Mechanisms of disease: graft-versus-host disease. N Engl J Med 1991; 324:667.
67. Jager E, Ringhoffer M, Altmannsberger M, Arand M, Karbach J, Jager D, Oesch

F, Knuth A. Immunoselection in vivo: independent loss of MHC class land melanocyte differentiation antigen expression in metastatic melanoma. Int J Cancer 1997; 71:142.

68. Lahn M, Kohler G, Schmoor C, Dengler W, Veelken H, Brennscheidt U, Mackensen A, Kulmburg P, Hentrich I, Jesuiter H, Rosenthal FM, Fiebig HH, Sommerkamp H, Farthmann EH, Hasse J, Mertelsmann R, Lindemann. Processing of tumor tissues for vaccination with autologous tumor cells. Eur Surg Res 1997; 29: 292.
69. Kawakami Y, Eliyahu S, Jennings C, Sakaguchi K, Kang X, Southwood S, Robbins PF, Sette A, Appella E, Rosenberg SA. Recognition of multiple epitopes in the human melanoma antigen gp100 by tumor-infiltrating T lymphocytes associated with in vivo tumor regression. J Immunol 1995; 154:3961.
70. Kawakami Y, Eliyahu S, Delgado CH, Robbins PF, Sakaguchi K, Appella E, Yannelli JR, Adema GJ, Miki T, Rosenberg SA. Identification of a human melanoma antigen recognized by tumor-infiltrating lymphocytes associated with in vivo tumor rejection. Proc Natl Acad Sci USA 1994; 91:6458.
71. Carcelain G, Rouas-Freiss N, Zorn E, Chung-Scott V, Viel S, Faure F, Bosq J, Hercend T. In situ T-cell responses in a primary regressive melanoma and subsequent metastases: a comparative analysis. Int J Cancer 1997; 72:241.
72. Marchand M, Weynants P, Rankin E, Arienti F, Belli F, Parmiani G, Cascinelli N, Bourlond A, Vanwijck R, Humblet Y, et al. Tumor regression responses in melanoma patients treated with a peptide encoded by gene MAGE-3 (letter). Int J Cancer 1995; 63:883.
73. Mackensen A, Carcelain G, Viel S, Raynal MC, Michalaki H, Triebel F, Bosq J, Hercend T. Direct evidence to support the immunosurveillance concept in a human regressive melanoma. J Clin Invest 1994; 93:1397.
74. Ferrone S, Marincola FM. Loss of HLA class I antigens by melanoma cells: molecular mechanisms, functional significance and clinical relevance. Immunol Today 1995; 16:487.
75. Chouaib S, Asselin-Paturel C, Mami-Chouaib F, Caignard A, Blay JY. The host-tumor immune conflict: from immunosuppression to resistance and destruction. Immunol Today 1997; 18:493.
76. Zier K, Gansbacher B, Salvadori S. Preventing abnormalities in signal transduction of T cells in cancer: the promise of cytokine gene therapy (see comments). Immunol Today 1996; 17:39.
77. Mizoguchl H, JJ OS, Longo DL, Loeffler CM, McVicar DW, Ochoa AC. Alterations in signal transduction molecules in T lymphocytes from tumor-bearing mice (see comments). Science 1992; 258:1795.
78. Ochoa AC, Longo DL. Alteration of signal transduction in T cells from cancer patients. Important Adv Oncol 1995:43.
79. Garrido F, Cabrera T, Concha A, Glew S, Ruiz-Cabello F, Stern PL. Natural history of HLA expression during tumor development. Immunol Today 1993; 14:491.
80. Clayberger C, Wright A, Medeiros Li, Koller TD, Link MP, Smith SD, Warnke RA, Krensky AM. Absence of cell surface LFA-1 as a mechanism of escape from immunosurveillance. Lancet 1987; 2:533.
81. Vasmel WL, Sijts EJ, Leupers CJ, Matthews EA, Melief CJ. Primary virus-induced

lymphomas evade T cell immunity by failure to express viral antigens. J Exp Med 1989; 169:1233.
82. Billaud M, Rousset F, Calender A, Cordier M, Aubry JP, Laisse V, Lenoir GM. Low expression of lymphocyte function-associated antigen (LFA)-I and LFA-3 adhesion molecules is a common trait in Burkitt's lymphoma associated with and not associated with Epstein-Barr virus. Blood 1990; 75:1827.
83. Wiertz EJ, Mukherjee S, Ploegh HL. Viruses use stealth technology to escape from the host immune system. Mol Med Today 1997; 3:116.
84. Chen L, Linsley PS, Hellstrom KE. Costimulation of T cells for tumor immunity. Immunol Today 1993; 14:483.
85. Chen L, McGowan P, Ashe S, Johnston J, Li Y, Hellstrom I, Hellstrom KE. Tumor immunogenicity determines the effect of B7 costimulation on T cell–mediated tumor immunity. J Exp Med 1994; 179:523.
86. Schultze JL, Cardoso AA, Freeman GJ, Seamon MJ, Daley J, Pinkus GS, Gribben JG, Nadler LM. Follicular lymphomas can be induced to present alloantigen efficiently: a conceptual model to improve their tumor immunogenicity. Proc Natl Acad Sci USA 1995; 92:8200.
87. Johnston JV, Malacko AR, Mizuno MT, McGowan P, Hellstrom I, Hellstrom KE, Marquardt H, Chen L. B7-CD28 costimulation unveils the hierarchy of tumor epitopes recognized by major histocompatibility complex class I-restricted CD8+ cytolytic T lymphocytes. J Exp Med 1996; 183:791.
88. Schultze JL. Unpublished results, 1999.
89. Cardoso AA, Schultze JL, Boussiotis VA, Freeman GJ, Seamon MJ, Laszlo S, Billet A, Sallan SE, Gribben JG, Nadler LM. Pre-B acute lymphoblastic leukemia cells may induce T-cell anergy to alloantigen. Blood 1996; 88:41.
90. Dorfman DM, Schultze JL, Shahsafaei A, Michalak S, Gribben JG, Freeman GJ, Pinkus GS, Nadler LM. In vivo expression of B7-1 and B7-2 on follicular lymphoma is not sufficient to induce significant T cell proliferation but is sufficient to prevent T cell anergy in vitro. Blood 1997; 90:4297.
91. Schwyzer M, Fontana A. Partial purification and biochemical characterization of a T cell suppressor factor produced by human glioblastoma cells. J Immunol 1985; 134:1003.
92. Kingsley DM. The TGF-beta superfamily: new members, new receptors, and new genetic tests of function in different organisms. (review). Genes Dev 1994; 8:133.
93. Kopper L, Ladanyi A, Mlhalik R, Nagy P. Loss of transforming growth factor beta I regulatory activity in human non-Hodgkin lymphomas. Anticancer Res 1994; 14:119.
94. Markowitz S, Wang J, Myeroff L, Parsons R, Sun L, Lutterbaugh J, Fan RS, Zborowska E, Kinzler KW, Vogelstein B, Brattain M, Willson JKV. Inactivation of the type II TGF–beta receptor in colon cancer cells with microsatellite instability (see comments). Science 1995; 268:1336.
95. Kadin ME, Cavaille-Coll MW, Gertz R, Massague J, Cheifetz S, George D. Loss of receptors for transforming growth factor beta in human T-cell malignancies. Proc Natl Acad Sci USA 1994; 91:6002.
96. Masood R, Zhang Y, Bond MW, Scadden DT, Moudgil T, Law RE, Kaplan MH, Jung B, Espina BM, Lunardi-Iskandar Y, Levine AM, Gill PS. Interleukin-10 is

an autocrine growth factor for acquired immunodeficiency syndrome–related B-cell lymphoma. Blood 1995; 85:3423.

97. Blay JY, Burdin N, Rousset F, Lenoir G, Biron P, Philip T, Banchereau J, MC. Serum interleukin-10 in non-Hodgkin's lymphoma: a prognostic factor. Blood 1993; 82:2169.

98. Voorzanger N, Toultou R, Garcia E, Delecluse HJ, Rousset F, Joab 1, Favrot MC, Blay JY. Interleukin (IL)-10 and IL-6 are produced in vivo by non-Hodgkin's lymphoma cells and act as cooperative growth factors. Cancer Res 1996; 56:5499.

99. Schultze JL, Michalak S, Seamon MJ, Gribben JG, Nadler LM. CD40 activated follicular lymphoma cells are resistant to and can overcome generalized T cell unresponsiveness induced by IL-IO and TGFB 1. Blood 1996; 86(suppl):2534.

100. Kehrl JH, Wakefield LM, Roberts AB, Jakowlew S, Alvarez-Mon M, Derynck R, Sporn MB, Fauci AS. Production of transforming growth factor beta by human T lymphocytes and its potential role in the regulation of T cell growth. J Exp Med 1986; 163:1037.

101. Bodmer S, Strommer K, Frei K, Siepl C, de Tribolet N, Heid I, Fontana A. Immunosuppression and transforming growth factor-beta in glioblastoma: preferential production of transforming growth factor-beta 2. J Immunol 1989; 143:3222.

102. de Waal Malefyt R, Haanen J, Spits H, Roncarolo MG, te Velde AF, Johnson C, Kastelein K, Yssel H R, de Vries JE. Interleukin 10 (IL-10) and viral IL-10 strongly reduce antigen-specific human T cell proliferation by diminishing the antigen-presenting capacity of monocytes via downregulation of class II major histocompatibility complex expression. J Exp Med 1991; 174:915.

103. Ralph P, Nakoinz I, Sampson-Johannes A, Fong S, Lowe D, Min HY, Lin L. IL-10, T lymphocyte inhibitor of human blood cell production of IL-1 and tumor necrosis factor. J Immunol 1992; 148:808.

104. Wang L, Goillot E, Tepper RI. IL-10 inhibits alloreactive cytotoxic T lymphocyte generation in vivo. Cellular Immunology 1994; 159:152.

105. Powrie F, Menon S, Coffrnan RL. Interleukin-4 and interleukin-10 synergize to inhibit cell-mediated immunity in vivo. Eur J Immunol 1993; 23:2223.

106. Peguet-Navarro J, Moulon C, Caux C, Dalbiez-Gauthier C, Banchereau J, Schmitt D. Interleukin-10 inhibits the primary allogenic T cell response to human epidermal Langerhans cells. Eur J Immunol 1994; 24:884.

107. de Waal Malefyt R, Yssel H, de Vries JE. Direct effects of IL-10 on subsets of human CD4+ T cell clones and resting T cells: specific inhibition of, IL-2 production and proliferation. J Immunol 1993; 150:4754.

108. O'Connell J, O'Sullivan GC, Collins JK, Shanahan F. The Fas counterattack: Fas-mediated T cell killing by colon cancer cells expressing Fas ligand. J Exp Med 1996; 184:1075.

109. Hahne M, Rimoldi D, Schroter M, Romero P, Schreier M, French LE, Schneider P, Bornand T, Fontana A, Lienard D, Cerottini J, Tschopp J. Melanoma cell expression of Fas(Apo-1/CD95) ligand: implications for tumor immune escape (see comments). Science 1996; 274:1363.

110. Williams N. Tumor cells fight back to beat immune system (news; comment). Science 1996; 274:1302.

111. Strand S, Hofmann WJ, Hug H, Muller M, Otto G, Strand D, Mariani SM, Stremmel

W, Krammer PH, Galle PR. Lymphocyte apoptosis induced by CD95 (APO-1/Fas) ligand-expressing tumor cells-a mechanism of immune evasion? (see comments). Nature Med 1996; 2:1361.

112. Niehans GA, Brunner T, Frizelle SP, Liston JC, Salerno CT, Knapp DJ, Green DR, Kratzke RA. Human lung carcinomas express Fas ligand. Cancer Res 1997; 57:1007.

113. Saas P, Walker PR, Hahne M, Quiquerez AL, Schnuriger V, Perrin G, French L, Van Meir EG, de Tribolet N, Tschopp J, Dietrich PY. Fas ligand expression by astrocytoma in vivo: maintaining immune privilege in the brain? J Clin Invest 1997; 99:1173.

114. Walker PR, Saas P, Dietrich PY. Role of Fas ligand (CD95L) in immune escape: the tumor cell strikes back. J Immunol 1997; 158:4521.

115. Shiraki K, Tsuji N, Shioda T, Isselbacher KJ, Takahashi H. Expression of Fas ligand in liver metastases of human colonic adenocarcinomas. Proc Natl Acad Sci USA 1997; 94:6420.

116. Villunger A, Egle A, Marschitz I, Kos M, Bock G, Ludwig H, Geley S, Kofler R, Greil R. Constitutive expression of Fas (Apo-1/CD95) ligand on multiple myeloma cells: a potential mechanism of tumor-induced suppression of immune surveillance. Blood 1997; 90:12.

117. Bamberger AM, Schulte HM, Thuneke I, Erdmann I, Bamberger CM, Asa SL. Expression of the apoptosis-inducing Fas ligand (FasL) in human first and third trimester placenta and choriocarcinoma cells. J Clin Endocrinol Metab 1997; 82: 3173.

118. Gratas C, Tohma Y, Van Meir EG, Klein M, Tenan M, Ishii N, Tachibana O, Kleihues P, Ohgaki H. Fas ligand expression in glioblastoma cell lines and primary astrocytic brain tumors. Brain Pathol 1997; 7:863.

119. Zeytun A, Hassuneh M, Nagarkatti M, Nagarkatti PS. Fas-Fas ligand-based interactions between tumor cells and tumor-specific cytotoxic T lymphocytes. a lethal two-way street. Blood 1997; 90:1952.

120. Xerri L, Devilard E, Hassoun J, Haddad P, Birg F. Malignant and reactive cells from human lymphomas frequently express Fas ligand but display a different sensitivity to Fas-mediated apoptosis. Leukemia 1997; 11:1868.

121. Griffith TS, Brunner T, Fletcher SM, Green DR, Ferguson TA. Fas ligand–induced apoptosis as a mechanism of immune privilege (see comments). Science 1995; 270: 1189.

122. Stuart PM, Griffith TS, Usui N, Pepose J, Yu X, Ferguson TA. CD95 Ligand (FasL)-induced apoptosis is necessary for corneal allograft survival. J Clin Invest 1997; 99:396.

123. Guller S. Role of Fas ligand in conferring immune privilege to non-lymphoid cells. Ann NY Acad Sci 1997; 828:268.

124. Dranoff G, Mulligan RC. Gene transfer as cancer therapy. Adv Immunol 1995; 58: 417.

125. Dranoff G, Jaffee E, Lazenby A, Golumbek P, Levitsky H, Brose K, Jachson V, Hamada H, Pardoll D, Mulligan RC. Vaccination with irradiated tumor cells engineered to secrete murine granulocyte-macrophage colony-stimulating factor stimulates potent, specific, and long-lasting anti-tumor immunity. Proc Natl Acad Sci USA 1993; 90:3539.

126. Hellstrom KE, Hellstrom I, Chen L. Can co-stimulated tumor immunity be therapeutically efficacious? Immunol Rev 1995; 145:123.
127. Allison JP, Hurwitz AA, Leach DR. Manipulation of costimulatory signals to enhance antitumor T-cell responses. Curr Opin Immunol 1995; 7:682.
128. Baskar S, Glimcher L, Nabavi N, Jones RT, Ostrand-Rosenberg S. Major histocompatibility complex class II+B7−1+ tumor cells are potent vaccines for stimulating tumor rejection in tumor-bearing mice. J Exp Med 1995; 181:619.
129. Topalian SL. MHC class II restricted tumor antigens and the role of CD4+ T cells in cancer immunotherapy. Curr Opin Immunol 1994; 6:741.
130. Funa K, Gazdar AF, Mattson K, Niiranen A, Koivuniemi A, Oberg K, Wilander E, Doyle A, Linnoila RI. Interferon-mediated in vivo induction of beta 2-microglobulin on small-cell lung cancers and mid-gut carcinoids. Clin Immunol Immunopathol 1986; 41:159.
131. Leeuwenberg JF, Van Damme J, Meager T, Jeunhomme TM, Buurman WA. Effects of tumor necrosis factor on the interferon-gamma-induced major histocompatibility complex class II antigen expression by human endothelial cells. Eur J Immunol 1988; 18:1469.
132. Renkonen R, Ristimaki A, Hayry P. Interferon-gamma protects human endothelial cells from lymphokine-activated killer cell-mediated lysis. Eur J Immunol 1988; 18:1839.
133. Klar D, Hammerling GJ. Induction of assembly of MHC class I heavy chains with beta 2 microglobulin by interferon-gamma. Embo J 1989; 8:475.
134. Sugimoto T, Horii Y, Hino T, Kemshead JT, Kuroda H, Sawada T, Morioka H, Imanishi J, Inoko H. Differential susceptibility of HLA class II antigens induced by gamma-interferon in human neuroblastoma cell lines. Cancer Res 1989; 49:1824.
135. Guadagni F, Schlom J, Johnston WW, Szpak CA, Goldstein D, Smalley R, Simpson JF, Borden EC, Pestka S, Greiner JW. Selective interferon-induced enhancement of tumor-associated antigens on a spectrum of freshly isolated human adenocarcinoma cells. J Natl Cancer Inst 1989; 81:502.
136. Nabavi N, Freeman GJ, Gault A, Godfrey D, Nadler LM, Glimcher LH. Signalling through the MHC class II cytoplasmic domain is required for antigen presentation and induces B7 expression. Nature 1992; 360:266.
137. Ranheim EA, Kipps TJ. Activated T cells induce expression of B7/BB1 on normal or leukemic B cells through a CD40-dependent signal. J Exp Med 1993; 177:925.
138. Schultze JL, Seamon MJ, Michalak S, Gribben JG, Nadler LM. Autologous tumor infiltrating T cells cytotoxic for follicular lymphoma cells can be expanded in vitro. Blood 1997; 89:3806.
139. Schultze JL, Michalak S, Seamon MJ, Dranoff G, Jung K, Daley J, Delgado JC, Gribben JG, Nadler LM. CD40 activated human B cells: an alternative source of highly efficient antigen presenting cells to generate autologous antigen-specific T cells for adoptive immunotherapy. J Clin Invest 1997; 100:2757.
140. Guo Y, Wu M, Chen H, Wang X, Liu G, Li G, Ma J, Sy MS. Effective tumor Vaccine generated by fusion of hepatoma cells with activated b cells. Science 1994; 263:518.
141. Fitzpatrick DR, Bielefeldt-Ohmann H, Himbeck RP, Jamicki AG, Marzo AL,

Robinson BW. Transforming growth factor-beta: antisense RNA-mediated inhibition affects anchorage-independent growth, tumorigenicity and tumor-infiltrating T-cells in malignant mesothelioma. Growth Factors 1994; 11:29.

142. Riddell SR, Gilbert MJ, Greenberg PD. CD8+ cytotoxic T cell therapy of cytomegalovirus and HIV infection. Curr Opin Immunol 1993; 5:484.

143. Riddell SR, Greenberg PD. Principles for adoptive T cell therapy of human viral diseases. Annu Rev Immunol 1995; 13:545.

144. Cardoso AA, Seamon MJ, Afonso HM, Ghia P, Boussiotis VA, Freeman GJ, Gribben JG, Sallan SE, Nadler LM. Ex vivo generation of human anti-pre-B leukemia-specific autologous cytolytic T cells. Blood 1997; 90:549.

17

Genetic Modulation of Effector Cells to Enhance GVL Effects

Helen E. Heslop and Koichi Moriwaki
Baylor College of Medicine
Houston, Texas

I. INTRODUCTION

Over the past few years, adoptive transfer studies, described in detail in other chapters of this book, have shown that donor T cells can be effective in the therapy of relapsed malignancy or viral infection in recipients of allogeneic hematopoietic stem-cell transplants [1,2]. Although administration of donor T cells has produced clinical benefit, it has been complicated by the frequent development of graft-versus-host disease (GVHD) due to alloreactive T cells present in the infused product. Gene transfer offers the possibility of improving such strategies by several means; infused T cells may be marked to monitor therapy, allogeneic T cells may be eradicated in the event of GVHD or other adverse events, or the function of infused T cells may be augmented by providing novel recognition properties or cytokine secretion. In this chapter we review current methodologies for gene transfer to immune system effector cells and then discuss strategies in preclinical and clinical use for using gene transfer to modulate T-cell function.

II. METHODS OF GENE DELIVERY TO IMMUNE EFFECTORS

A requirement for gene transfer to immune system effectors is an efficient delivery system to transfer the gene of interest to the immune system cells. An ideal vector for gene delivery would be selectively targeted to T cells, have a high efficiency of transduction, and result in long-term expression of the transferred gene. None of the currently available vectors meet these requirements, and limitations of current gene-transfer techniques represent a major constraint on approaches for genetic modulation of T cells. Most current clinical protocols use replication-defective viral vectors, while a few utilize physical methods of gene delivery [3]. The most widely used delivery systems in clinical studies have been retroviruses [4,5]. Adenoviruses [6], adeno-associated virus [7], and liposomes [8] have also been used, while other delivery systems are under clinical evaluation. Table 1 summarizes features of the most widely used vectors.

A. Retrovirus Vectors

Figure 1 shows the structure of a retrovirus vector [9]. The wild-type retrovirus consists of two long terminal repeats (LTRs), responsible for transcriptional control, polyadenylation, replication and integration, and three structural genes: *gag*, which encodes structural proteins and confers high packaging efficiency; *pol*, which codes for replicative polymerases and integrase; and *env*, which codes for envelope proteins. In a clinical vector, the structural and replicative genes (*gag*, *pol*, and *env*) of a murine retrovirus are replaced by one or more genes of interest, driven either by the retroviral promoter in the 5′ LTR or by an internal promoter (Figure 1). The retroviral constructs are made in cell lines in which the missing retrovirus genes are present in *trans* and thus reproduce and package a vector that is not replication-competent. After replication, defective viral vectors infect a target cell, the virus is uncoated in the cytosol, and RNA is transcribed via reverse transcriptase into DNA, which integrates into the host genome. The host range of MoMuLV viruses is determined by the gp70 envelope protein interacting

Table 1 Vector Delivery Systems

Property	Retrovirus	Adenovirus	AAV	Herpesvirus
Genome	RNA	ds DNA	ss DNA	ds DNA
Integration	Yes (in dividing cells)	No	Yes (in dividing and nondividing cells)	No
Insert size	6–8 kb	8–35 kb	4.5 kb	10–100 kb
Packaging system	Stable	No	Developmental	Complex
Potential problems	Insertional mutagenesis, productive retroviral infection	Immunogenicity	Insertional mutagenesis	Cytotoxic

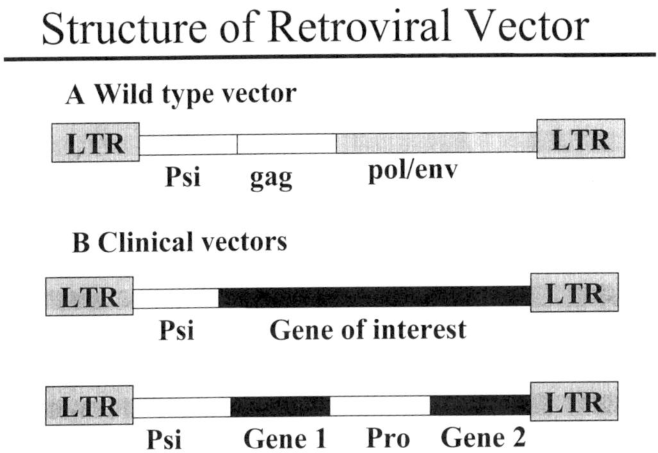

Figure 1 Structure of retroviral vectors. Diagrammatic wild-type retroviral vector (A) consisting of 5′ and 3′ LTRs which contain promoter, enhancer, and polyadenylation sequences as well as inverted repeats, a packaging signal (Ψ), and three structural genes—*gag*, *pol*, and *env*—which are required in trans for replication and packaging. B. Examples of clinical vectors. The transgene may be a single gene regulated by the LTR or the retroviral vector may contain two genes, one of which is driven by an external promoter (pro) and the other regulated by the LTR.

with their cellular receptors, which are transmembrane polypeptides normally involved in ion transport [10–12]. Poor transduction efficiencies of human lymphocytes and the limited number of amphotropic receptors on the cell surface have prompted studies to improve specific viral targeting [13]. One approach is to modify the viral envelope to include ligand-binding proteins such as erythropoietin [14]. An alternate strategy is to change the viral envelope to the gibbon ape leukemia virus envelope (GaLV) [15,16] or vesicular stomatitis virus G glycoprotein (VSV-g) [12], which helps stabilize the vector, allowing physical methods of concentration to be used, and which may also broaden the target-cell range. Both these approaches have increased transduction efficiencies into T cells [12,16]. Colocalization of retrovirus and target cells by culturing cells on stromal support components [17], by centrifugation [18], or by flow through transduction [19] may also increase transduction efficiency. Finally, a delivery system that produces transient high expression may be used to express the retroviral receptor on the surface of nonpermissive cells, thereby increasing retroviral entry [20].

Because the genetic information that retroviral vectors convey is integrated into the host-cell DNA, the transferred gene persists for the entire life span of the transduced cell and is also present in that cell's progeny. Hence, these vectors are ideal for transferring genes into a rapidly dividing cell population, such as lymphocytes. However, retroviral vectors have several disadvantages. Expression of the transferred gene requires integration, which occurs only in dividing cells, so lymphocytes must be activated for efficient transduction. Further, because the integration events themselves occur at largely random sites in the host cell's DNA, regulatory genes could conceivably be damaged, contributing to later oncogenesis [21]. Finally, retrovirus vectors are not well suited for use in vivo [22], since they are generally unstable in primate complement.

B. Adenovirus Vectors

Most adenovirus vectors are based on AD5 with deletions in E1 and E3 regions [6]. Adenoviruses infect a wide range of cell types and, unlike retrovirus vectors, can transfer genes into nondividing cells. The vectors are reasonably stable in vivo but are generally nonintegrating, so that the gene products are expressed from episomal DNA [23]. The episome is often lost after cell division and can be inactivated or lost even in a nondividing cell [24]. Thus, adenovirus vectors are unsuited for any application that requires long-term expression, and their role in transferring genes to T cells would be limited to situations where short-term expression is adequate. Another limitation is that most adenovirus vectors are immunogenic [6]. Immune responses are generated against the vector proteins themselves and often prevent readministration of the vector. Recently second-generation vectors, where more viral proteins are deleted, have been developed in an effort to overcome this limitation [25]. In the meantime, however, adenoviral vectors could be potentially used for transient expression of ecotropic viral receptors on nonpermissive human hematopoietic cells.

C. Adeno-Associated Virus Vector

Adeno-associated virus (AAV) [26] is a "dependovirus," which can replicate only when an AAV infected cell is coinfected with adenovirus or herpesvirus. The 4.7-kb genome is bordered by inverted terminal repeat (ITR) sequences of 145 nt. Two sets of structural genes, rep and cap, provide replicative and capsid proteins respectively. In addition, Rep is required for site-specific integration of the virus into human chromosome 19, with consequent establishment of a latent state [7]. Thus, AAV, like retroviruses, should be present for the entire life span of the host cell and in its progeny. It was initially thought that integration of AAV was relatively site-specific, which reduces the risk of insertional mutagenesis. Moreover, it has been claimed that integration occurs in nondividing cells, so that, in contrast to retroviruses, AAV should be permanently expressed even in resting or postmitotic cells. These expectations have not yet been met. The rep gene products that contribute to site-specific integration are toxic to virus producer cells and are usually deleted from vectors. Rep-deficient vectors have a reduced ability to integrate and site specificity is lost [26]. It has also proved difficult to scale up current vector production systems to develop high-titer producer cell lines, free of contaminating helper adenoviruses. Recent studies show that this problem may be soluble [27].

D. Liposomes and Other Physical Methods

Clinical experience with the available physical methods of gene transfer has primarily involved cationic liposome/DNA complexes [8,28–30], which fuse with the cell membrane and enter the endosomal uptake pathway. DNA released from these endosomes may then pass through the nuclear membrane and be expressed. The main advantage of liposomes is that they are nontoxic and can be given repeatedly. In some cell types, high levels of gene transfer have been obtained [8]. Liposomes are unstable in vivo and cannot effectively be given systemically, but liposomal transfer by local injection of human melanoma cells in situ has resulted in expression of a new gene (HLA-B7) [8]. However, the DNA transferred by liposomes is nonintegrating, and despite the incorporation of a variety of ligands into the liposome-DNA complex [30], the ability to target these vectors is still quite limited.

E. Other Vectors

Other vectors, including herpesviruses [31,32] and lentiviruses [33], have been proposed as high-efficiency transducers of normal and malignant hematopoietic cells and will likely enter clinical trials within the next few years. Several other viral vector systems are currently in the early stages of development. These include the spumavirus human foamy virus [34,35], other parvoviruses, and the poxviruses. However, in most cases efficient packaging systems have not been developed. Lentiviruses in particular appear promising, as they can transduce nondividing cells. Recent second-generation vectors have increased safety by deleting the virulence genes most associated with HIV pathogenesis, and the attenuated vector maintains its ability to transduce resting cells [36]. However, while these viruses may become future substitutes for currently available vector systems, a longer-term solution may be to develop new synthetic vectors [37]. Possibilities include the generation of hybrid viral vectors, which may combine, for example, the in vivo stability of adenoviruses and the integrating capacity of retroviruses. At present, however, protocols for gene transfer to immune effector cells will require the investigators to choose their agent on the basis of the most important feature required. In general the requirement for long-term expression will require a retroviral vector or perhaps, in the future, a lentiviral vector. For applications where transient expression is adequate, adenovirus- or herpes-based vectors may be used.

III. GENE TRANSFER TO T CELLS

There are some particular considerations with gene transfer to T cells (see Figure 2). In early studies the level of gene transfer to T cells was low [38,39]. Recent improvements in methodologies for transduction incorporating centrifugation and the use of a GaLV or VSV-G envelope have resulted in increases in levels of transduction obtained in vitro and in primate studies [12,15,16], and these results should hopefully translate to human clinical trials. Colocalization of virus and target cell on fibronectin fragments produces similar effects. Use of a construct containing a selectable marker, such as CD24 [40] or NGFR [41], is an alternate approach that allows sorting of transduced cells ex vivo to ensure high level transduction of an infused population.

A second problem is that transferred genes may not be well expressed in T cells. This may reflect heterogeneity in terms of viral insertion and expression and may be potentially overcome by the use of clones [42]. However, it may also reflect the propensity of T cells to down-regulate various types of message such as cytokines, so that the solution to this problem may require more basic research in gene regulation.

IV. CLINICAL STUDIES

Table 2 lists the current clinical immunotherapy studies in which gene transfer is used to modify therapy [3]. These studies fall into two categories; gene-marking studies and therapeutic studies, where gene transfer provides a suicide mechanism or aims to enhance immune recognition and function.

A. Gene-Marking Studies Using T Cells

Transfer of a marker gene has allowed monitoring of adoptive transfer approaches to determine survival of infused T cells. In addition, the fate of T cells can be tracked to learn if they can home to sites of disease and if they mediated adverse effects such as GVHD. In most studies, the marker gene used has been the neomycin phosphotransferase (*neo*) gene, which provides phenotypic resistance to neomycin and its analogues. The gene can also be detected genotypically in transduced cells by PCR.

1. Gene Transfer to TIL Cells

The rationale for the first clinical gene-transfer study approved by regulatory authorities in the United States was to learn if tumor-infiltrating lymphocytes (TILs) had tumor-specific homing properties [38]. To address this question, TIL

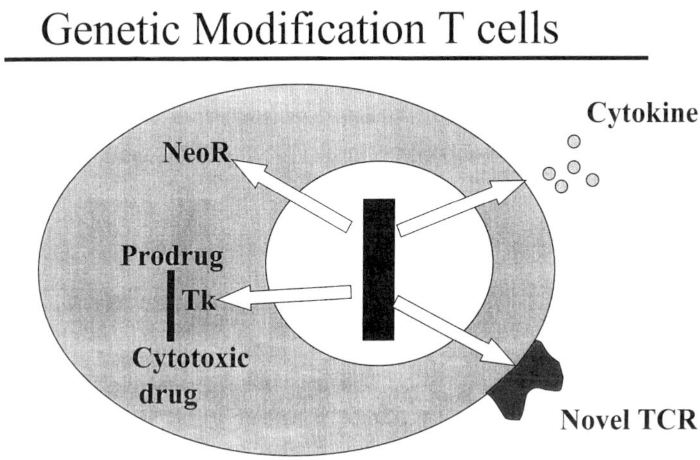

Figure 2 Gene transfer to T cells. Illustration of how transfection of a T cell with a marker gene, a suicide gene, a cytokine gene, or a novel recognition molecule may modify function or allow the infused T cell to be tracked.

cells were marked with *neo* to track their fate and persistence [38]. Analysis of peripheral blood and tumor deposits for presence of the marker gene suggested that TILs could persist for up to 2 months [38]. Studies in one patient showed presence of the marker gene in biopsy tissue from a tumor deposit [43]. In a French study, marked TILs were detected for up to 260 days and TILs were also detected in 4 of 8 tumor biopsies after therapy [44]. Recently, a double-marking study compared the survival and tracking of peripheral blood lymphocytes (PBLs) and TILs by marking with distinguishable retroviral vectors [45]. Both marked PBLs and TILs could be detected in peripheral blood for 4 months and no selective homing of TIL cells to tumor sites compared with unmanipulated PBLs was seen [45]. None of these studies, therefore, provide any evidence to support the theory that TIL cells are capable of selective homing.

2. Gene Transfer to Track Adoptive Transferred Cytotoxic T Lymphocytes

Gene marking has also been used in an adoptive transfer study to determine if donor-derived EBV-specific cytotoxic T lymphocytes are effective prophylaxis for EBV lymphomas that arise after BMT. The pathogenesis of EBV lymphoproliferation is outgrowth of EBV-infected B cells that express a number of EBV-encoded antigens and are therefore highly immunogenic. Normally, outgrowth

Table 2 Immunotherapy Trials Using Genetic Modification of T Lymphocytes

Target Cell	Vector	Purpose	Investigator
TIL	neo	Track fate and trafficking pattern	Rosenberg [38]
TIL	TNF	Augment function TILs	Rosenberg [68]
TIL	neo	Track fate and trafficking pattern	Lotze [74]
TIL and PBM	neo	Track fate and trafficking pattern	Economou [45]
TIL	neo	Trafficking pattern ovarian TIL	Freedman [3]
HIV specific CTL	Tk/hygromycin	Track fate and function Destroy if adverse effects	Riddell [67]
CTL	neo	Track syngeneic T cells in HIV affected patients with uninfected twins	Walker [75]
Allogeneic EBV-specific CTL	neo	Track fate and determine if cause GVHD	Heslop/Rooney [39,50,51]
Autologous EBV-specific CTL	neo	Track fate and persistence	Heslop/Rooney [53]
Tyrosinase-specific CTL	neo	Track fate and persistence of tyrosinase specific CTL in patients with melanoma	Greenberg/Yee [3]
Allogeneic PBL	Tk	Destroy if adverse effect	Tiberghien [66]
Allogeneic PBL	Tk	Destroy if adverse effect	Link [3]
Allogeneic PBL	Tk/NGFR/neo	Select prior to infusion Destroy if adverse effect	Bordignon [55]
Donor PBL	Tk	Suicide if produce GVHD	Munshi/Barlogie [65]
T cells	CC94-zeta	Colorectal carcinomas expressing the tumor associated antigen TAG-72	Venook [3]
Anti-CD3 stimulated PBL	Chimeric T cell receptor reactive with folate-binding protein	Enhance effector function in patients with ovarian cancer	Hwu [3]

is prevented by EBV-specific CTLs [46] and can occur only in severely immunosuppressed individuals, such as patients receiving T cell–depleted allogeneic bone marrow from HLA-mismatched family members or HLA-matched unrelated donors [47,48]. Because the frequency of EBV-specific CTL precursors (CTLp) in seropositive individuals is high, donor-derived peripheral blood leukocytes are effective therapy for this complication [2,49]. However, the frequency of alloreactive CTLp is also high, resulting in a significant risk of severe GVHD. In addition, treatment of established disease can lead to toxicity from inflammatory responses to virus-infected cells [2,48].

In a recent protocol at St. Jude Children's Research Hospital, patients at high risk of developing EBV lymphoproliferation after receiving T cell–depleted BMT from HLA-mismatched family members or unrelated donors were eligible to receive donor-derived, EBV-specific CTLs as prophylaxis for EBV-associated lymphoma, from day 45 post-BMT [50]. To allow tracking of infused cells and to determine if they produced adverse effects, CTLs were marked with the *neo* gene. Over fifty patients have received CTL lines on the prophylaxis component of this study, and no immediate adverse effects from infusion have been seen. In particular, there was no induction of GVHD. The marker gene was detected by PCR for up to 16 weeks in unmanipulated peripheral blood mononuclear cells and for up to 37 months in EBV-specific CTL lines regenerated from patients following treatment with gene-marked CTLs [39,51]. There is also evidence for efficacy, in that six of the patients receiving prophylactic CTL developed greatly elevated levels of EBV DNA prior to administration of CTLs, a result strongly predictive of the onset of lymphoma [52]. In all six, levels returned to baseline following infusion. Moreover in two patients who received CTLs therapeutically rather than prophylactically, there was a dramatic therapeutic response to CTL infusion. In one of these patients, the marking component of the study allowed us to show, by in situ hybridization and semiquantitative PCR, that the infused cells had selectively accumulated at disease sites. However while prophylactic CTLs did not produce any adverse effects, the patient who received therapeutic CTLs for bulky established disease developed initial tumor swelling and respiratory obstruction prior to response. This patient illustrates that even when alloreactivity is absent, it is possible to get morbidity from tissue inflammation during therapy to bulky disease.

In follow-up studies, the effects of autologous EBV-specific CTLs are being evaluated in patients with EBV genome-positive Hodgkin's disease [53]. Five patients with multiply relapsed disease have received gene-marked CTLs. The CTLs persisted for more than 13 weeks postinfusion and retained their potent anti-viral effects in vivo, thereby enhancing the patient's immune response to EBV. Moreover, in one patient who had a malignant pleural effusion, the marker gene was detected in the pleural fluid at a 10-fold higher level than in peripheral blood, indicating that the infused CTLs can traffic to sites of active disease [53].

B. Gene Transfer to Confer Drug Sensitivity (Suicide-Gene Strategy)

Infusing donor-derived T cells following allogeneic BMT can lead to GVHD initiated by alloreactive T cells. Even if CTL clones are used, cross reaction with histocompatibility polymorphisms may cause GVHD in an allogeneic setting. In addition, as discussed in the previous section, therapy of established disease with T cells can result in tissue damage from inflammatory reactions. One solution to this problem is the transduction of T cells with a ''suicide gene,'' so that cell death may be induced if adverse effects occur [54,55]. Suicide genes encode enzymes that convert prodrugs to active metabolites. The most commonly used encodes the herpes simplex thymidine kinase (Tk) gene. Unlike mammalian Tk, viral Tk can phosphorylate nucleotide analogues such as ganciclovir, rendering dividing host cells sensitive to the cytotoxic effects produced by incorporation of these molecules. Many other prodrug systems have been described over the past few decades, including cytosine deaminase [56–58], which converts 5-fluorocytosine to 5-fluorouracil. However, application of these and other agents [59,60] will require improved methods of targeting their expression to the desired cells [61], and most studies using T cells as the target have focused on the Tk system.

If transfer of a suicide gene is to be successful and to result in destruction of infused cells if they produce adverse effects, it is necessary that all infused cells contain the suicide gene and that expression is maintained in vivo. To accomplish this, suicide-gene constructs generally include a selectable marker such as *neo* [54] or a cell-surface marker such a truncated nerve growth factor receptor that allows selection of transduced cells [55]. Another potential problem is that not only must all cells be transduced but expression must be maintained long term in vivo, an aim that proved difficult in studies where TIL cells are transduced with cytokines [62]. Finally, even if the infused cells that initiate GVHD are all destroyed, the recruited immune effectors such as NK cells, endogenous T cells, and monocytes may still mediate tissue damage.

The suicide gene approach has been evaluated in several preclinical models. Two murine models provided proof of concept [63,64] by administering spleen cells from mice transgenic for the HSV Tk gene. Recipient mice who received ganciclovir did not develop GVHD while control mice did. While these studies show the feasibility of controlling GVHD, ganciclovir was administered before GVHD developed; whereas in clinical studies, administration is delayed until signs of GVHD develop. In human preclinical studies, Munshi and colleagues showed 90% killing of T cells transduced with a Tk-*neo* construct and selected in G418 [65].

Suicide genes are currently being evaluated in several clinical trials of adoptive immunotherapy posttransplant [66]. Bonini and colleagues have reported the results of the first eight patients in their study of donor T cells to treat leukemia relapse or EBV lymphoma following BMT [55]. In this protocol, they transfect lymphocytes, after a brief 24- to 48-h primary stimulation with antigen, with a construct containing a suicide gene and a truncated version of the low-molecular-weight nerve growth factor gene to serve as a selectable marker. Of the 8 patients, 3 of those treated developed GVHD; in 2, administration of ganciclovir resulted in complete remission of GVHD. In the third patient, there was a reduction in circulating cells expressing the transgene, but it proved impossible to eliminate all transduced cells [55].

One limitation of suicide-gene therapy that became apparent in clinical studies was the potential immunogenicity of the Tk gene. Riddell and colleagues have administered autologous *gag*-specific CTLs transduced with a construct encoding Tk and the hygromycin resistance gene to HIV-infected patients [67]. In this study, 5 of 6 patients developed CTL responses specific for the transgene, which destroyed the infused cells [67]. One patient in the Italian study also developed CTLs specific for the HSV-Tk-neo fusion protein [55], so this approach may be limited by the immunogeneicity of the transgene.

C. Gene Transfer to Enhance Effector Function

Gene transfer might also provide a means of enhancing the function of infused T cells. Several approaches are being evaluated, including transfer of cytokine genes to augment cytotoxic function, promotion of helper function of CD8 clones, and enhancement of T-cell recognition by introduction of novel receptors.

1. Transfer of Cytokine Genes

The antitumor activity of T cells may also be enhanced by increasing the levels of cytotoxic cytokines that they produce at local tumor sites. Eleven patients at the NIH have received TIL cells transduced with TNF [62,68]. However the lack of TIL homing and the tendency of T cells to down-regulate their own TNF production has hampered this study: the amount of TNF produced by transduced TIL cells was around 2 logs lower than that produced by tumor cells transduced with the same vector [62].

2. Promotion of Helper Independence

An alternate approach developed by Greenberg and colleagues is to modify CD8 clones in order to confer helper independence, so that exogenous IL-2 or CD4 help is not required [69]. The strategy they employed was to introduce a chimeric receptor composed of the cytoplasmic domain of IL-2 and the extracellular domain of granulocyte-macrophage colony-stimulating factor (GM-CSF). When GM-CSF is produced by this CD8 clone in response to antigenic stimulus, signaling through the chimeric receptor will result in provision of help [69]. Minamoto and colleagues used a similar strategy to avoid the T-cell requirement for IL-2 and introduced a chimeric receptor encoding the extracellular portion of the erythropoietin receptor and the intracellular portion of the IL-2 receptor subunits β and γ [70]. T-cell lines transduced with such a construct proliferated in response to erythropoietin, and the authors hypothesized that erythropoietin, which is less toxic than IL-2, could be administered in vivo to promote proliferation and antitumor activity of infused T cells.

3. Gene Transfer to Confer Novel Recognition Properties

The function of T cells may also be modified by transducing them with appropriate antigen-specific T-cell receptors to confer novel tumor-recognition properties [45,71,72]. Many tumors express surface antigens that may be recognized by specific antibodies. In the "T-body" [71] or "universal receptor" [73] approach, T cells are transduced with a construct encoding a chimeric gene that contains an antibody-derived single-chain variable region linked with the T-cell receptor constant region or a T-cell signaling molecule such as ZAP-70 [71]. The transduced CTLs then possesses the antibody-determined specificity and will recognize the tumor cell via the chimeric receptor and trigger effector function. Moreover, these modified lymphocytes would recognize a tumor-specific antigen in an MHC-unrestricted fashion. This approach has been evaluated in several preclinical models. T cells expressing chimeric receptors with anti-neu/HER2 specificity are able to lyse tumor lines expressing HER-2 [72]. When a construct encoding the extracellular domain of CD4 linked to the ζ chain of the TCR was transduced into murine hemopoietic stem cells, which were transplanted into SCID mice, high-level expression was seen in myeloid and NK cells. In addition, recipient mice were protected from an otherwise lethal dose of leukemia-expressing HIV envelopes [73]. Two clinical studies to evaluate this approach have been initiated [3] (Table 2). In one study, patients with colon cancer expressing the tumor-associated antigen TAG 72 receive autologous CC94-zeta chain–modified T cells, while the other patients with ovarian cancer receive a chimeric TCR reactive with folate-binding protein. If CTLs targeted to proteins specifically expressed on leukemic cells could be generated, their administration post-BMT may produce GVL without GVHD.

V. FUTURE DIRECTIONS

Gene transfer is already being used to monitor and modify many immunotherapy strategies. It seems likely that the use of gene transfer will increase as more tumor-defined antigens that may be targets for specific immune responses are defined. The major challenges are to develop improved gene delivery systems and to define the basic mechanisms to regulate gene expression in T cells, so that expression of transgenes may be more precisely controlled.

REFERENCES

1. Kolb H, Schattenberg A, Goldman JM, Hertenstein B, Jacobsen N, Arcese W, Ljungman P, Ferrant A, Verdonck L, Niederwieser D, van Rhee F, Mittermueller J, de Witte T, Holler E, Ansari H. Graft-versus-leukemia effect of donor lymphocyte infusions in marrow grafted patients. Blood 1995; 86:2041–2050.
2. Papadopoulos EB, Ladanyi M, Emanuel D, MacKinnon S, Boulad F, Carabasi MH, Castro-Malaspina H, Childs BH, Gillio AP, Small TN, Young JW, Kernan NA, O'Reilly RJ. Infusions of donor leukocytes to treat Epstein-Barr virus–associated lymphoproliferative disorders after allogeneic bone marrow transplantation. N Engl J Med 1994; 330:1185–1191.
3. Rosenberg SA, Blaese RM, Brenner MK, Deisseroth AB, Ledley FD, Lotze MT, Wilson JM, Nabel GJ, Cornetta K, Economou JS, Freeman SM, Riddell SR, Oldfield EH, Gansbacher B, Dunbar C, Walker RE, Schuening FG, Roth JA, Crystal RG, Welsh MJ, Culver K, Heslop HE, Simons J, Wilmott RW, Tiberghien P, et al. Human gene marker/therapy clinical protocols. Hum Gene Ther 1997; 8:2301–2338.
4. Miller AD. Retroviral vectors. Curr Top Microbiol Immunol 1992; 158:1–24.
5. Crystal RG. Transfer of genes to humans: early lessons and obstacles to success. Science 1995; 270:404–410.
6. Wilson JM. Adenoviruses as gene delivery vehicles. N Engl J Med 1996; 334:1185–1187.
7. Muzyczka N. Adeno-associated virus (AAV) vectors: will they work? J Clin Invest 1994; 94:1351.
8. Nabel GJ, Nabel EG, Yang ZY, Fox BA, Plautz GE, Gao X, Huang L, Shu S, Gordon D, Chang AE. Direct gene transfer with DNA-liposome complexes in melanoma: expression, biologic activity, and lack of toxicity in humans. Proc Natl Acad Sci USA 1993; 90:11307–13111.
9. Bender MA, Palmer TD, Gelinas RE, Miller AD. Evidence that the packaging signal of Moloney murine leukemia virus extends into the gag region. J Virol 1987; 61: 1639–1646.
10. Weiss RA, Tailor CS. Retrovirus receptors. Cell 1995; 82:532–533.
11. Miller DG, Edwards RH, Miller AD. Cloning of the cellular receptor for amphotropic murine retroviruses reveals homology to that for gibbon ape leukemia virus. Proc Natl Acad Sci USA 1994; 91:78–82.
12. Miller AD. Cell-surface receptors for retroviruses and implications for gene transfer. Proc Natl Acad Sci USA 1996; 93:11407–11413.
13. Cosset F, Russell SJ. Targeting retrovirus entry. Gene Ther 1996; 3:946–956.
14. Kasahara N, Dozy AM, Kan YW. Tissue-specific targeting of retroviral vectors through ligand-receptor interactions. Science 1994; 266:1373–1376.
15. Bunnell BA, Muul LM, Donahue RE, Blaese RM, Morgan RA. High-efficiency ret-

roviral-mediated gene transfer into human and nonhuman peripheral blood lymphocytes. Proc Natl Acad Sci USA 1995; 92:7739–7743.
16. Bunnell BA, Metzger M, Byrne E, Morgan RA, Donahue RE. Efficient in vivo marking of primary CD4+ T lymphocytes in nonhuman primates using a gibbon ape leukemia virus-derived retroviral vector. Blood 1997; 89:1987–1995.
17. Hanenberg H, Xiao XL, Dilloo D, Hashino K, Kato I, Williams DA. Co-localization of retrovirus and target cells on specific fibronectin adhesion domains for increased genetic transduction of mammalian cells. Nature Med 1996; 2:876–882.
18. Bahnson AB, Dunigan JT, Baysal BE, Mohney T, Atchison RW, Nimgaonkar MT, Ball ED, Barranger JA. Centrifugal enhancement of retroviral mediated gene transfer. J Virol Meth 1995; 54:131–143.
19. Palsson B, Andreadis S. The physico-chemical factors that govern retrovirus-mediated gene transfer. Exp Hematol 1997; 25:94–102.
20. Bertran J, Miller JL, Yang Y, Fenimore-Justman A, Rueda F, Vanin EF, Nienhuis AW. Recombinant adeno-associated virus-mediated high-efficiency, transient expression of the murine cationic amino acid transporter (ecotropic retroviral receptor) permits stable transduction of human HeLa cells by ecotropic retroviral receptors. J Virol 1996; 70:6759–6766.
21. Donahue RE, Kessler SW, Bodine D, McDonagh K, Dunbar C, Goodman S, Agricola B, Byrne E, Raffeld M, Moen R, Bacher J, Zsebo KM, Nienhuis AW. Helper virus induced T cell lymphoma in nonhuman primates after retroviral mediated gene transfer. J Exp Med 1992; 176:1125–1135.
22. Cornetta K, Morgan RA, Anderson WF. Safety issues related to retrovirus-mediated gene transfer in humans. Hum Gene Ther 1991; 2:5–14.
23. Engelhardt JF, Yang Y, Stratford-Perricaudet LD, Allen ED, Kozarsky K, Perricaudet M, Yankaskas JR, Wilson JM. Direct gene transfer of human CFTR into human bronchial epithelia of xenografts with E1-deleted adenoviruses. Nature Genet 1993; 4:27–34.
24. Smith TA, Mehaffey MG, Kayda DB, Saunders JM, Yei S, Trapnell BC, McClelland A, Kaleko M. Adenovirus mediated expression of therapeutic plasma levels in human factor IX in mice. Nature Genet 1993; 5:397–402.
25. Wang Q, Finer MH. Second-generation adenovirus vectors. Nature Med 1996; 2: 714–716.
26. Muzyczka N. Use of adeno-associated virus as a general transduction vector for mammalian cells. Curr Top Microbiol Immunol 1992; 158:97–129.
27. Ferrari FK, Xiao X, McCarty D, Samulski RJ. New developments in the generation of Ad-free, high titer rAAV gene therapy vectors. Nature Med 1997; 3:1295–1297.
28. Nabel EG, Simari R, Yang Z, San H, Nabel GJ. In vivo gene transfer: a biological tool. Ann NY Acad Sci 1997; 811:289–292.
29. Gao X, Huang L. A novel cationic liposome reagent for efficient transfection of mammalian cells. Biochem Biophys Res Commun 1991; 179:280–285.
30. Trubetskoy VS, Torchilin VP, Kennel SJ, Huang L. Cationic liposomes enhance targeted delivery and expression of exogenous DNA mediated by N-terminal modified poly-L-lysine-antibody conjugate in mouse lung endothelial cells. Biochem Biophys Acta 1992; 1131:311–313.

dent tumor immunity after transplantation of universal receptor-modified bone marrow into SCID mice. J Exp Med 1996; 184:2261–2269.
74. Cai Q, Rubin JT, Lotze MT. Genetically marking human cells: results of the first clinical gene transfer studies. Cancer Gene Ther 1995; 2:125–136.
75. Walker R, Blaese RM, Carter CS, Chang L, Klein H, Lane HC, Leitman SF, Mullen CA, Larson M. A study of the safety and survival of the adoptive transfer of genetically marked syngeneic lymphocytes in HIV infected identical twins. Hum Gene Ther 1993; 4:659–680.

31. Glorioso JC, Goins WF, Schmidt MC, Ologino T, Krisky DM, Marconi PC, Cavalcoli JD, Ramakrishnan R, Poliani PL, Fink DJ. Engineering herpes simplex virus vectors for human gene therapy. Adv Pharmacol 1997; 10:103–136.
32. Glorioso JC, DeLuca NA, Fink DJ. Development and application of herpes simplex virus vectors for human gene therapy. Annu Rev Microbiol 1995; 49:675–710.
33. Naldini L, Blomer U, Gallay P, Ory D, Mulligan R, Gage FH, Verma IM, Trono D. In vivo gene delivery and stable transduction of nondividing cells by a lentiviral vector. Science 1996; 272:263–267.
34. Russell DW, Miller AD. Foamy virus vectors. J Virol 1996; 70:217–222.
35. Nestler U, Heinkelein M, Lucke M, Meixensberger J, Scheurlen W, Kretschmer A, Rethwilm A. Foamy virus vectors for suicide gene therapy. Gene Ther 1997; 4: 1270–1277.
36. Zufferey R, Nagy D, Mandel RJ, Naldini L, Trono D. Multiply attenuated lentiviral vector achieves efficient gene delivery in vivo. Nat Biotechnol 1997; 15:871–875.
37. Schofield JP, Caskey CT. Non-viral approaches to gene therapy. Br Med Bull 1995; 51:56–71.
38. Rosenberg SA, Aebersold P, Cornetta K, Kasid A, Morgan RA, Moen R, Karson EM, Lotze MT, Yang JC, Topalian SL, Merino MJ, Culver J, Miller D, Blaese RM, Anderson WF. Gene transfer into humans—immunotherapy of patients with advanced melanoma, using tumor-infiltrating lymphocytes modified by retroviral gene transduction. N Engl J Med 1990; 323:570–578.
39. Rooney CM, Smith CA, Ng C, Loftin SK, Li C, Krance RA, Brenner MK, Heslop HE. Use of gene-modified virus-specific T lymphocytes to control Epstein-Barr virus–related lymphoproliferation. Lancet 1995; 345:9–13.
40. Pawliuk R, Kay R, Lansdorp P, Humphries RK. Selection of retrovirally transduced hematopoietic progenitor cells using CD24 as a marker of gene transfer. Blood 1994; 84:2868–2877.
41. Mavilio F, Ferrari G, Rossini S, Nobili N, Bonini C, Casorati G, Traversari C, Bordignon C. Peripheral blood lymphocytes as target cells of retroviral vector-mediated gene transfer. Blood 1994; 83:1988–1997.
42. Gallot G, Hallet M, Gaschet J, Moreau J, Vivien R, Bonneville M, Milpied N, Vie H. Human HLA-specific T-cell clones with stable expression of a suicide gene: a possible tool to drive and control a graft-versus host-graft-versus-leukemia reaction? Blood 1996; 88:1098–1103.
43. Aebersold P, Kasid A, Rosenberg SA. Selection of gene-marked tumor infiltrating lymphocytes from post-treatment biopsies: a case study. Hum Gene Ther 1990; 1: 373–384.
44. Merrouche Y, Negrier S, Bain C, Combaret V, Mercatello A, Coronel B, Moskovtchenko J, Tolstoshev P, Moen R, Philip T, Favrot MC. Clinical application of retroviral gene transfer in oncology: results of a French study with tumor-infiltrating lymphocytes transduced with the gene of resistance to neomycin. J Clin Oncol 1995; 13:410–418.
45. Economou JS, Belldegrun AS, Glaspy J, Toloza EM, Figlin R, Hobbs J, Meldon N, Kaboo R, Tso C, Miller A, Lau R, McBride W, Moen RC. In vivo trafficking of

adoptively transferred interleukin-2 expanded tumor-infiltrating lymphocytes and peripheral blood lymphocytes: results of a double gene marking trial. J Clin Invest 1996; 97:515–521.

46. Rickinson AB, Moss DJ. Human cytotoxic T lymphocyte responses to Epstein-Barr virus infection. Annu Rev Immunol 1997; 15:405–431.

47. O'Reilly RJ, Small TN, Papadopoulos E, Lucas K, Lacerda J, Koulova L. Biology and adoptive cell therapy of Epstein-Barr virus-associated lymphoproliferative disorders in recipients of marrow allografts. Immunol Rev 1997; 157:195–216.

48. Heslop HE, Rooney CM. Adoptive immunotherapy of EBV lymphoproliferative diseases. Immunol Rev 1997; 157:217–222.

49. Heslop HE, Brenner MK, Rooney CM. Donor T cells to treat EBV-associated lymphoma. N Engl J Med 1994; 331:679–680.

50. Heslop HE, Brenner MK, Rooney CM, Krance RA, Roberts WM, Rochester R, Smith CA, Turner V, Sixbey J, Moen R, Boyett JM. Administration of neomycin-resistance-gene-marked EBV-specific cytotoxic T lymphocytes to recipients of mismatched-related or phenotypically similar unrelated donor marrow grafts. Hum Gene Ther 1994; 5:381–387.

51. Heslop HE, Ng CYC, Li C, Smith CA, Loftin SK, Krance RA, Brenner MK, Rooney CM. Long-term restoration of immunity against Epstein-Barr virus infection by adoptive transfer of gene-modified virus-specific T lymphocytes. Nature Med 1996; 2:551–555.

52. Rooney CM, Loftin SK, Holladay MS, Brenner MK, Krance RA, Heslop HE. Early identification of Epstein-Barr virus-associated post-transplant lymphoproliferative disease. Br J Haematol 1995; 89:98–103.

53. Roskrow MA, Suzuki N, Gan Y, Sixbey JW, Ng CYC, Kimbrough S, Hudson MM, Brenner MK, Heslop HE, Rooney CM. EBV-specific cytotoxic T lymphocytes for the treatment of patients with EBV positive relapsed Hodgkin's disease. Blood 1998; 91:2925–2934.

54. Tiberghien P, Reynolds CW, Keller J, Spence S, Deschaseaux M, Certoux J, Contassot E, Murphy WJ, Lyons R, Chiang Y, Herve P, Longo DL, Ruscetti FW. Ganciclovir treatment of herpes simplex thymidine kinase-transduced primary T lymphocytes: an approach for specific in vivo donor T-cell depletion after bone marrow transplantation? Blood 1994; 84:1333–1341.

55. Bonini C, Ferrari G, Verzeletti S, Servida P, Zappone E, Ruggieri L, Ponzoni M, Rossini S, Malvilio F, Traversari C, Bordignon C. HSV-TK gene transfer into donor lymphocytes for control of allogeneic graft versus leukemia. Science 1997; 276: 1719–1724.

56. Wei K, Huber BE. Cytosine deaminase gene as a positive selection marker. J Biol Chem 1996; 271:3812–3816.

57. Huber BE, Austin EA, Richards CA, Davis ST, Good SS. Metabolism of 5-fluorocytosine to 5-fluorouracil in human colorectal tumor cells transduced with the cytosine deaminase gene: significant antitumor effects when only a small percentage of tumor cells express cytosine deaminase. Proc Natl Acad Sci USA 1994; 91:8302–8306.

58. Mullen CA, Coale MM, Lowe R, Blaese RM. Tumors expressing the cytosine deaminase suicide gene can be eliminated in vivo with 5-fluorocytosine and induce protective immunity to wild type tumor. Cancer Res 1994; 54:1503–1506.

59. Mroz PJ, Moolten FL. Retrovirally transduced *Escherichia coli gpt* genes combine selectability with chemosensitivity capable of mediating tumor eradication. Hum Gene Ther 1993; 4:589–595.

60. Sorscher EJ, Peng S, Bebok Z, Allan PW, Bennett LL, Parker WB. Tumor cell bystander killing in colonic carcinoma utilizing the *Escherichia coli* DeoD gene to generate toxic purines. Gene Ther 1994; 1:233–238.

61. Huber BE, Richards CA, Austin EA. Virus-directed enzyme/prodrug thera
(VDEPT): selectively engineering drug sensitivity into tumors. Ann NY Acad
1994; 716:104–114.

62. Hwu P, Rosenberg SA. The use of gene-modified tumor infiltrating lympho
for cancer therapy. Ann NY Acad Sci 1994; 716:188–197.

63. Cohen JL, Boyer O, Salomen B, Onclercq R, Charlotte F, Bruel S, Boiss
Klatzmann D. Prevention of graft-versus-host disease in mice using a suic
expressed in T lymphocytes. Blood 1997; 89:4636–4645.

64. Lake-Bullock MHV, Bryson JS, Jennings CD, Kaplan AM. Inhibition of
sus-host disease: use of a T cell–controlled suicide gene. J Immunol
5079–5082.

65. Munshi N, Govindarajan R, Drake R, Ding LM, Iyer R, Saylors R,
Marcus S, Chiang Y, Ennist D, Kwak L, Reynolds C, Tricot G, Barlo
dine kinase (TK) gene–transduced human lymphocytes can be hig
main fully functional, and are killed efficiently with ganciclovir.
1334–1340.

66. Tiberghien P, Cahn J, Brion A, Deconinck E, Racadot E, Herve P,
B, Gluckman E, Bordigoni P, Jacob W, Chiang Y, Marcus S,
D. Use of donor T-lymphocytes expressing herpes-simplex thyn
geneic bone marrow transplantation: a phase I–II study. Hum
615–624.

67. Riddell SR, Elliot M, Lewinsohn DA, Gilbert MJ, Wilson
SD, Overell RW, Reynolds TC, Corey L, Greenberg PD.
of gene-modified HIV-specific cytotoxic T lymphocytes
Nature Med 1996; 2:216–223.

68. Ettinghausen SE, Rosenberg SA. Immunotherapy and
Surg 1995; 28:223–254.

69. Nelson BH, Lord JD, Greenberg PD. Cytoplasmic do
ceptor beta and gamma chains mediate the signal f
1994; 369:333–336.

70. Minamoto S, Treisman J, Hankins WD, Sugamu
erythropoietin responsiveness of interleukin-2 dep
transduced with genes encoding chimeric eryt
Blood 1995; 86:2281–2287.

71. Eshhar Z. Tumor-specific T-bodies: towards
Immunother 1997; 45:131–136.

72. Hwu P, Yang JC, Cowherd R, Treisman J,
vivo antitumor activity of T cells redirected
genes. Cancer Res 1995; 55:3369–3373.

73. Hege KM, Cooke KS, Finer MH, Zsebo K

18

Leukemia-Reactive T Cells in Adoptive Immunotherapy for Relapsed Leukemia After Allogeneic Transplantation

J.H. Frederick Falkenburg and Roelof Willemze
Leiden University Medical Center
Leiden, The Netherlands

I. INTRODUCTION

In allogenic stem-cell transplantation (SCT), the observation that graft-versus-host disease (GVHD) after the transplantation is associated with a decreased risk of relapse of the malignant disease for which the patient is treated has led to the conclusion that alloreactive T cells may be capable of suppressing the outgrowth of leukemic cells in vivo [1–7]. The graft-versus-leukemia (GVL) effect of donor T cells has been further supported by the successful treatment of relapsed leukemia after allogenic SCT with donor lymphocyte infusions (DLIs) [8–15]. Although it has been tempting to postulate that alloreactive T cells are the mediators of the GVL effect, formal proof has not been provided in humans. T cells probably play a crucial role in the induction of GVL, but other effector cells, including natural killer (NK) cells or cytokines produced by effector cell populations, may be essential for the full clinical effect resulting in eradication of the malignant cells [16–19]. Support for a role of NK cells in the antileukemic effect has come from the observation that after allogeneic SCT, an association was found between NK activity and a decreased incidence of relapse [16,17].

II. DONOR LYMPHOCYTE INFUSIONS FOR TREATMENT OF RELAPSED LEUKEMIA

In relapsed chronic myeloid leukemia (CML), after allogeneic SCT, DLIs infusions have been shown to be a very potent antileukemic therapy (see Chapter 9). Successful DLIs have also been reported for acute myeloid leukemia (AML), multiple myeloma (MM), and some cases of acute lymphoblastic leukemia (ALL) as well as myelodysplastic syndrome (MDS), although the success rate has been lower. However, this treatment is frequently associated with GVHD. This may lead to the suggestion that the same T cells that mediate GVHD are also responsible for the GVL effect. Although this assumption is probably in part true, since most alloreactive T cells in HLA-identical donor/recipient combinations are capable of suppressing the leukemic cells [20–22], it can only be concluded from the clinical observations that both GVHD-inducing T cells and antileukemic T cells are present within the same T-cell transfusate. Previously, we have shown that the frequency of leukemia-reactive T cells in normal individuals may be as low as 1–10 per million T cells [23]. Similarly, in HLA-identical combinations, the frequency of alloreactive T cells directed against normal blood cells from the recipient is also approximately 1–10 per 10^6 T cells. Therefore, these T cells may be identical, may overlap, but may also be different T cells. If the degree of mismatch between donor and recipient increases, the frequency of alloreactive T cells increases, which may lead to a more negative balance between GVHD and GVL effects. In closely matched donor/recipient pairs, however, it may be possible to demonstrate the presence of donor T cells that are capable of more specific recognition of the leukemic cells, leading to complete remissions without GVHD following DLI [14,24].

III. DONOR-DERIVED LEUKEMIA-REACTIVE T CELLS

The existence of donor-derived T cells showing relative specificity for the leukemic cells has been demonstrated in a number of cases. Leukemia-reactive T cells recognizing AML cells but not PHA blasts and EBV-transformed B cells from the same individual have been reported, as well as T cells recognizing acute lymphoblastic leukemic (ALL) cells and EBV cells from the same individual, but not non-transformed B cells, T cells, monocytes, or fibroblasts [25–31]. In addition, minor histocompatibility antigen (mHAg)–specific T-cell responses have been described showing that hematopoiesis-specific polymorphic antigens can be recognized by alloreactive T cells, which led to the eradication of all recipient hematopoietic cells including the leukemic cells [32–35]. The same T cells do not react with other nonhematopoietic tissues from the recipient and are also not capable of reacting with donor hematopoiesis in the patient, indicating that such T cells may lead to an antileukemic effect without GVHD. From these observations, it has been suggested that donor-derived T cells can be found that show relative specificity for the leukemic cells and may therefore be capable of exhibiting an antileukemic effect with a decreased risk of GVHD following infusion as a treatment of relapsed leukemia following allogenic SCT [7].

IV. LEUKEMIA-REACTIVE T CELLS AS MEDIATORS OF ANTILEUKEMIC EFFECT IN VIVO

To establish which T cells may be mediators of the GVL effect following DLI, we have recently demonstrated that T cells capable of suppressing the CML precursor cells circulate at increased frequencies during clinical response following DLI for relapsed CML after allogeneic SCT [7,24]. This was demonstrated by a newly developed assay measuring the frequency of progenitor-cell inhibitory lymphocyte precursors (PCILp) reactive with the CML progenitor cells. In this assay, similar to a classical cytotoxic T lymphocyte precursor (CTLp) frequency analysis, limiting dilution experiments are performed [36]. Graded numbers of responder cells are stimulated with irradiated leukemic cells from the patient and expanded in the presence of CML cells and interleukin-2 (IL-2). After approximately 21 days, when proliferation of the T cells can be observed, the T cells are irradiated, and cocultured with CML cells from the patient in the presence of multiple hematopoietic growth factors. The proliferation of these CML precursor cells can be measured using ^{3}H-thymidine incorporation assays. The growth of CML precursor cells in the presence of T cells can be compared with the proliferation of CML cells in the absence of effector cells. Using this assay, a frequency of PCILp can be calculated using Poisson statistics [36]. With this assay, we demonstrated that up to a 100-fold increase in a frequency of PCILp reactive with the leukemic cells could be observed in patients responding to DLI both in the presence and in the absence of GVHD. A correlation between CTLp frequencies recognizing leukemic cells in a ^{51}Cr release assay was less significantly correlated with the clinical response. From these studies it may be concluded that T cells recognizing the leukemic precursor cells are responsible for the antileukemic effect in vivo.

V. INFUSION OF LEUKEMIA-REACTIVE T CELLS CAN MEDIATE AN ANTILEUKEMIC EFFECT

Based on the observations that the antileukemic effect following DLI was associated with an increased frequency of PCILp against CML precursor cells, we generated cytotoxic T-cell lines that recognized the leukemic cells from patients, and not the PHA blasts of donor or recipient [27]. We studied a patient who relapsed following allogeneic SCT and failed to respond to DLI despite developing GVHD. We tested whether donor T-cell lines generated against the leukemia had an antileukemic effect. At intervals of 5 weeks, three CTL lines fulfilling these criteria were infused with a total number of 3.7×10^9 T cells. Shortly after the third infusion, aplasia developed, with complete eradication of the leukemic cells followed by conversion to normal donor hematopoiesis and disappearance of the t(9;22)-positive cells as measured by cytogenetic analysis and reverse transcriptase PCR using bcr/abl–specific primers. No acute GVHD was observed. Since this patient already suffered from chronic GVHD, no conclusions can be drawn on a possible effect on chronic GVHD [37]. These observations showed that leukemia-reactive T cells can be expanded in vitro, infused in vivo without major toxicity or acute GVHD, and can exhibit a potent antileukemic effect.

VI. TREATMENT OF RELAPSED LEUKEMIA AFTER ALLOGENEIC SCT WITH T CELLS WITH DEFINED SPECIFICITY

Although the successful treatment of a patient with refractory leukemia following allogeneic SCT with leukemia-reactive CTL lines shows the feasibility of adoptive immunotherapy using such in vitro expanded T cells, treatment with T cells directed against more defined antigens is desirable, since no good prediction can be made whether or not such T cells will exhibit GVHD and cross-reactivity with other tissues can be only partially examined. Therefore, attempts are being made to generate T-cell responses against mHAg specific for hematopoietic tissues or antigens that are even more specific for the leukemic cells. These target antigens may include polymorphic proteins derived from the normal counterpart of the malignant cells. For example, T-cell responses against polymorphic antigens derived from the proteinase 3 protein as described by Molldrem et al. can behave as a leukemia-specific antigen after allogeneic SCT with full donor chimerism [38,39]. Although T-cell responses against such proteins are not completely leukemia-specific, in the context of allogeneic SCT, CTLs against such antigens may fulfil the criteria of being completely leukemia-specific since only residual patient-derived myeloid cells will be eliminated. Hematopoiesis in these patients is preferentially and frequently exclusively of donor origin. Therefore, absence of significant side effects can be expected after treatment with cytotoxic T cells specific for such proteins expressed in the context of MHC molecules. If specific T-cell responses can be generated against synthetic peptides identical to the polymorphic site of the protein, the presence of large numbers of malignant cells from the recipient would no longer be required to generate leukemia-specific T cells for adoptive immunotherapy. Even in this situation, however, it is still possible that CTLs against mHAg specific for hematological cells induce GVHD by an indirect effect. If large numbers of leukemic or normal hematological cells are present in the GVHD target organs, the ''cytokine storm'' induced by the mHAg-specific CTLs may also induce GVHD (see Chapter 14).

VII. LEUKEMIA-SPECIFIC T CELLS

Many leukemic cell populations exhibit a leukemia-specific protein. This protein is encoded by a fusion of genes resulting from a translocation leading to fusion peptides consisting of two truncated parts of a normal protein [40]. For instance, the t(9;22) translocation in CML leads to the production of the bcr/abl protein by the malignant cells. The t(9;22) translocation is expressed in all malignant CML cells and appears to be necessary for the malignant phenotype of the cell. The fusion part of the protein contains unique sequences not expressed by normal cells. T-cell responses directed against the fusion region expressed in MHC molecules may lead to a specific eradication of the leukemic cells [41–46]. Such a T-cell response would have the major advantage that immunotherapy can be used in the autologous situation without the necessity to perform an allogenic SCT (Table 1). Therefore, several investigators have looked into the possibility of generating T-cell responses against peptides identical to the fusion region of bcr/abl. Although both T cells could be isolated recognizing bcr/abl in the context of HLA class I or class II antigens, only limited evidence is available that such T cells do also recognize bcr/abl in the context of MHC in primary leukemic cells. Presumably, bcr/abl proteins are not endogenously processed or appropriately expressed in most MHC molecules, alternatively the presence of bcr/abl protein in the cell is so low in patients who developed CML that insufficient bcr/abl is expressed in the context of MHC on the cell membrane.

Recently, epidemiological studies have indicated that expression of certain

Table 1 Possible Beneficial Target Antigens Presented in MHC Molecules on Leukemic Cells in the Context of Allogeneic or Autologous T-Cell Responses

Antigen	Allogeneic	Autologous
Recipient-specific mHAg	(+)	−
Hematopoiesis-specific mHAg	+	−
Cell lineage–specific mHAg not expressed on stem cells	+	+
Overexpressed cell differentation–associated antigen	(+)	(+)
Translocation-specific antigen	+	+
Virus-specific antigen	(+)	(+)

polymorphic MHCs that are capable of binding bcr/abl specific proteins may protect against developing CML, suggesting that in healthy individuals an autologous leukemia-specific T cell may have occurred [47].

Since CML is a stem-cell disease, attempts have been made to modify the leukemic cells to become more appropriate antigen-presenting cells. It has been demonstrated that culturing CML precursor cells in the presence of cytokines capable of inducing differentiation into dendritic cells (DC) can lead to the formation of cells with a DC phenotype derived from CML precursor cells exhibiting the t(9;22) translocation and expressing bcr/abl [45,46,48]. It has been reported by Choudhury et al. that autologous T-cell responses can be generated against CML cells, suggesting that CML-reactive autologous T-cell responses may be capable of suppressing the leukemic cells, although no specificity for bcr/abl has been demonstrated. While T-cell responses against fusion parts of leukemia-specific proteins may be the most sophisticated approach for the immunotherapy of hematological malignancies, at the present time the only clinical evidence for successful immunotherapy mediated by T cells has been demonstrated in the context of allogeneic SCT.

REFERENCES

1. Weiden PL, Flournoy N, Thomas ED, Prentice R, Fefer A, Buckner CD, Storb R. Antileukemic effect of graft-versus-host disease in human recipients of allogeneic-marrow grafts. N Engl J Med 1979; 300:1068–1073.
2. Goldman JM, Gale RP, Horowitz MM, Biggs JC, Champlin RE, Gluckman E, Hoffmann RG, Jacobsen SJ, Marmont AM, McGlave PB, Messner HA, Rimm AA, Rozman C, Speck B, Tura S, Weiner RS, Bortin MM. Bone marrow transplantation for chronic myelogenous leukemia in chronic phase: increased risk for relapse associated with T-cell depletion. Ann Intern Med 1988; 108:806–814.
3. Barrett AJ, Horowitz MM, Gale RP, Biggs JC, Camitta BM, Dicke KA, Gluckman E, Good RA, Herzig RH, Lee MB, Marmont AM, Masoaka T, Ramsay NKC, Rimm AA, Speck B, Zwaan FE, Bortin MM. Marrow transplantation for acute lymphoblastic leukemia: factors affecting relapse and survival. Blood 1989; 74:862–871.
4. Horowitz MM, Gale RP, Sondel PM, Goldman JM, Kersey J, Kolb HJ, Rimm AA, Ringden O, Rozman C, Speck B, Truitt RL, Zwaan FE, Bortin MM. Graft-versus-leukemia reactions after bone marrow transplantation. Blood 1990; 75:555–562.
5. Jones RJ, Ambinder RF, Piantodosi S, Santos GW. Evidence of a graft-versus-lymphoma effect associated with allogeneic bone marrow transplantation. Blood 1991; 77:649–653.
6. Antin JH. Graft-versus-leukemia: no longer an epiphenomenon. Blood 1993; 82: 2273–2277.
7. Falkenburg JHF, Smit WM, Willemze R. Cytotoxic T-lymphocyte (CTL) responses against acute or chronic myeloid leukemia. Immunol Rev 1997; 157:223–230.
8. Kolb HJ, Mittermüller J, Clemm Ch, Holler E, Ledderiose G, Brehm G, Heim M,

Wilmanns W. Donor leukocyte transfusions for treatment of recurrent chronic myelogenous leukemia in marrow transplant patients. Blood 1990; 76:2462–2465.

9. Cullis JO, Jiang YZ, Schwarer AP, Hughes TP, Barrett AJ, Goldman JM. Donor Leukocyte infusions for chronic myeloid leukemia in relapse after allogeneic bone marrow transplantation. Blood 1992; 79:1379–1380.
10. Bär BMAM, Schattenberg A, Mensink EJBM, Geurts van Kessel A, Smetsers TFCM, Knops GHJN, Linders EHP, de Witte T. Donor leukocyte infusions for chronic myeloid leukemia relapsed after allogeneic bone marrow transplantation. J Clin Oncol 1993; 11:513–519.
11. Porter DL, Roth MS, McGarigle C, Ferrara JLM, Antin JH. Induction of graft-versus-host disease as immunotherapy for relapsed chronic myeloid leukemia. N Engl J Med 1994; 330:100–106.
12. van Rhee F, Lin F, Cullis JO, Spencer A, Cross NCP, Chase A, Garicochea B, Bungey J, Barrett J, Goldman JM. Relapse of chronic myeloid leukemia after allogeneic bone marrow transplant: the case of giving donor leukocyte transfusions before the onset of hematologic relapse. Blood 1994; 83:3377–3383.
13. Kolb HJ, Schattenberg A, Goldman JM, Hertenstein B, Jacobsen N, Arcese W, Ljungman P, Ferrant A, Verdonck L, Niederwieser D, van Rhee F, Mittermueller J, de Witte T, Holler E, Ansari H. Graft-versus-leukemia effect of donor lymphocyte transfusions in marrow grafted patients. Blood 1995; 86:2041–2050.
14. Mackinnon S, Papadopoulos EB, Carabasi MH, Reich L, Collins NH, Boulad F, Castro-Malaspina H, Childs BH, Gillio AP, Kernan NA, Small TN, Young JW, O'Reilly RJ. Adoptive immunotherapy evaluating escalating doses of donor leukocytes for relapse of chronic myeloid leukemia after bone marrow transplantation: separation of graft-versus-leukemia from graft-versus-host disease. Blood 1995; 86: 1261–1268.
15. Collins RH, Shpilberg O, Drobyski WR, Porter DL, Giralt S, Champlin R, Goodman SA, Wolff SN, Hu W, Verfaille C, List A, Dalton W, Ognoskie N, Chetrit A, Antin JH, Nemunaitis J. Donor leukocyte infusions in 140 patients with relapsed malignancy after allogeneic bone marrow transplantation. J Clin Oncol 1997; 15:433–444.
16. Hauch M, Gazzola MV, Small T, Bordignon C, Barnett L, Cunningham I, Castro-Malaspinia H, O'Reilly RJ, Keever CA. Antileukemia potential of interleukin-2 activated natural killer cells after bone marrow transplantation for chronic myelogenous leukemia. Blood 1990; 75:2250–2262.
17. Mackinnon S, Hows JM, Goldman JM. Induction of in-vitro graft-versus-leukemia activity following bone marrow transplantation for chronic myeloid leukemia. Blood 1990; 76:2037–2045.
18. Maraninchi D, Blaise D, Viens P, Brandely M, Olive D, Lopez M, Sainty D, Marit G, Stoppa AM, Reiffers J, Gratecos N, Bertau-Perez P, Mannoni P, Mawas C, Hercend T, Sebahoun G, Carcassonne Y. High-dose recombinant interleukin-2 and acute myeloid leukemias in relapse. Blood 1991; 78:2181–2187.
19. Soiffer RJ, Murray C, Cochran K, Cameron C, Wang E, Schow PW, Daley JF, Ritz J. Clinical and immunologic effects of prolonged infusion of low-dose recombinant interleukin-2 after autologous and T-cell-depleted allogeneic bone marrow transplantation. Blood 1992; 79:517–526.
20. Falkenburg JHF, Goselink HM, Van der Harst D, Van Luxemburg-Heijs SA, Kooy-

Winkelaar YM, Faber LM, De Kroon J, Brand A, Fibbe WE, Willemze R, Goulmy E. Growth inhibition of clonogenic leukemic precursor cells by minor histocompatibility antigen-specific cytotoxic T lymphocytes. J Exp Med 1991; 174:27–33.
21. van der Harst D, Goulmy E, Falkenburg JHF, Kooij-Winkelaar YMC, Van Luxemburg-Heijs SAP, Goselink HM, Brand A. Recognition of minor histocompatibility antigens on lymphocytic and myeloid leukemic cells by cytotoxic T cell clones. Blood 1994; 83:1060–1066.
22. Faber LM, van Luxemburg-Heijs SAP, Veenhof WFJ, Willemze R, Falkenburg JHF. Generation of CD4+ cytotoxic T lymphocyte clones from a patient with severe graft-versus-host disease after allogeneic bone marrow transplantation: implications for graft-versus-leukemia reactivity. Blood 1995; 86:2821–2828.
23. Smit WM, Rijnbeek M, van Bergen CAM, Willemze R, Falkenburg JHF. Generation of leukemia reactive cytotoxic T lymphocytes from HLA-identical donors of patients with chronic myeloid leukemia using modifications of a limiting dilution assay. Bone Marrow Transplant 1998; 21:553–560.
24. Smit WM, van Bergen CAM, Fibbe WE, Willemze R, Falkenburg JHF. The antileukemic effect of donor leukocyte transfusions (DLT) for relapsed chronic myeloid leukemia (CML) is mediated by cytotoxic T lymphocytes (CTL). Blood 1997; 90: 548a.
25. Faber LM, van Luxemburg-Heijs SAP, Willemze R, Falkenburg JHF. Generation of leukemia-reactive cytotoxic T lymphocyte clones from the HLA-identical donor of a patient with leukemia. J Exp Med 1992; 176:1283–1289.
26. van Lochem E, de Gast B, Goulmy E. In vitro separation of host specific graft-versus-host and graft-versus-leukemia cytotoxic T cell activities. Bone Marrow Transplant 1992; 10:181–183.
27. Falkenburg JHF, Faber LM, van den Elshout M, van Luxemburg-Heys SAP, Hooftman-den Otter A, Smit WM, Voogt PJ, Willemze R. Generation of donor-derived antileukemic cytotoxic T lymphocyte responses for treatment of relapsed leukemia after allogeneic HLA-identical bone marrow transplantation. J Immunother 1993; 14:305–309.
28. Faber LM, Van der Hoeven J, Goulmy E, Hooftman-den Otter AL, Van Luxemburg-Heijs SAP, Willemze R, Falkenburg JHF. Recognition of clonogenic leukemic cells, remission bone marrow and HLA-identical donor bone marrow by $CD8^+$ or $CD4^+$ minor histocompatibility antigen specific cytotoxic T lymphocytes. J Clin Invest 1995; 96:877–883.
29. Oettel KR, Wesly OH, Albertini MR, Hank JA, Iliopolis O, Sosman JA, Voelkerding K, Wu SQ, Clark SS, Sondel PM. Allogeneic T-cell clones able to selectively destroy Philadelphia chromosome-bearing (Ph^{1+}) cells from the same patient. Blood 1994; 83:3390–3402.
30. Mutis T, Schrama E, van Luxemburg-Heijs SAP, Falkenburg JHF, Melief CJM, Goulmy E. HLA class II restricted T-cell reactivity to a developmentally regulated antigen shared by leukemic cells and $CD34^+$ early progenitor cells. Blood 1997; 90: 1083–1090.
31. Dolstra H, Fredrix H, Preijers F, Goulmy E, Figdor CG, de Witte TM, van de Weel-van Kemenade E. Recognition of a B-cell-leukemia-associated minor histocompatibility antigen by CTL. J Immunol 1997; 158:560–565.

32. de Bueger M, Bakker A, van Rood JJ, van der Woude F, Goulmy E. Tissue distribution of human minor histocompatibility antigens: ubiquitous versus restricted tissue distribution indicates heterogeneity among human cytotoxic T-lymphocyte defined non-MHC antigens. J Immunol 1992; 149:1788–1794.
33. den Haan JMM, Sherman NE, Blokland E, Huczko E, Koning F, Drijfhout JW, Skipper J, Shabanowitz, Hunt DF, Engelhard VH, Goulmy E. Identification of a graft versus host disease-associated human minor histocompatibility antigen. Science 1995; 268:1476–1480.
34. den Haan JMM, Meadows LM, Wang W, Pool J, Blokland E, Bishop TL, Reinhardus C, Shabanowitz J, Offringa R, Hunt DF, Engelhard VH, Goulmy E. The minor histocompatibility antigen HA-1: diallelic gene with a single amino acid polymorphism. Science 1998; 279(5353):1054–1057.
35. Niederwieser D, Grassegger A, Auböck J, Herold M, Nachbaur D, Rosmayer A, Gächter A, Nussbaumer W, Gaggl S, Riter M, Huber Ch. Correlation of minor histocompatibility antigen-specific cytotoxic T lymphocytes with graft-versus-host-disease status and analyses of tissue distribution of their target antigens. Blood 1993; 81:2200–2208.
36. Strijbosch LWG, Buurman WA, Does RJMM, Zinken PH, Groenewegen G. Limiting dilution assays: experimental design and statistical analysis. J Immunol Methods 1987; 97:133–140.
37. Falkenburg JHF, Wafelman AR, van Bergen CAM, Bongaerts R, Lurvink EGA, Posthuma EFM, Smit WM, Joosten P, Landegent JE, Kluin-Nelemans JC, Fibbe WE, Willemze R. Clinical transplantation-recurrence, secondary neoplasia and late events. Blood 1997; 90:589a.
38. Molldrem J, Dermime S, Parker K, Jiang YZ, Mavroudis D, Hensel N, Fukushima P, Barrett AJ. Targeted T-cell therapy for human leukemia: cytotoxic T lymphocytes specific for a peptide derived from proteinase 3 preferentially lyse human myeloid leukemia cells. Blood 1996; 88:2450–2457.
39. Clave E, Molldrem J, Hensel N, Raptis A, Barrett AJ. Donor-recipient polymorphism of the proteinase 3 gene in bone marrow transplantation. Blood 1997; 90:534a.
40. Rowley JD. Recurring chromosome abnormalities in leukemia and lymphoma. Semin Hematol 1990; 27:122–136.
41. Chen W, Peace DJ, Rovira DK, You SG, Cheever MA. T-cell immunity to the joining region of $p210^{bcr\text{-}abl}$ protein. Proc Natl Acad Sci USA 1992; 89:1468–1472.
42. Bocchia M, Wentworth PA, Southwood S, Sidney J, McGraw K, Scheinberg DA, Sette A. Specific binding of leukemia oncogene fusion peptides to HLA class I molecules. Blood 1995; 85:2680–2684.
43. Bocchia M, Korontsvit T, Xu Q, Mackinnon S, Yang SY, Sette A, Scheinberg DA. Specific human cellular immunity to bcr-abl oncogene-derived peptides. Blood 1996; 87:3587–3592.
44. ten Bosch GJA, Joosten AM, Kessler JH, Melief CJM, Leeksma OC. Recognition of BCR-ABL positive leukemic blasts by human $CD4^+$ T cells elicited by primary in vitro immunization with a BCR-ABL breakpoint peptide. Blood 1996; 9:3522–3527.
45. Choudhury A, Gajewski JL, Liang JC, Popat U, Claxton DF, Kliche KO, Andreeff M, Champlin RE. Use of leukemic dendritic cells for the generation of antileukemic

cellulary cytotoxicity against Philadelphia chromosome-positive chronic myelogenous leukemia. Blood 1997; 89:1133–1142.

46. Eibl B, Ebner S, Duba C, Böck G, Romani N, Erdel M, Gächter A, Niederwieser D, Schuler G. Dendritic cells generated from blood precursors of chronic myelogenous leukemia patients carry the Philadelphia translocation and can induce a CML-specific primary cytotoxic T cell response. Genes, Chromosomes Cancer 1997; 20:215–223.
47. Posthuma EFM, Falkenburg JHF, Apperley JF, Jeannet M, Schipper RE, Schreuder GMT, D'Amaro J, van Biezen JH, Hermans J, Willemze R, Niederwieser D. HLA-A3 and HLA-B8 may protect against acquiring chronic myeloid leukemia. Blood 1997; 90:250a.
48. Smit WM, Rijnbeek M, Van Bergen CAM, De Paus RA, Vervenne HAW, Van de Keur M, Willemze R, Falkenburg JHF. Generation of dendritic cells expressing bcr/abl from CD34-positive chronic myeloid leukemia precursor cells. Human Immunol 199; 53:216–223.

19

The BCR-ABL Oncoprotein and Immunological Targeting

Vaccination for Tumor Prevention and Therapy

George J.A. ten Bosch, Onno C. Leeksma, and Cornelis J.M. Melief
Leiden University Medical Center
Leiden, The Netherlands

I. INTRODUCTION

During the last decade, efforts to define the molecular nature of tumor-associated antigens and our increased understanding of the antitumor immune response have helped us find ways to manipulate T cell–mediated antitumor responses. Current efforts are directed at applying this knowledge in the development of new modalities of cancer treatment. Despite the expression of malignancy-related antigens, tumors develop in patients without obvious immunodeficiencies, indicating that, even if the immune system responds to specific alterations in these tumors, this response is often inadequate. Very intriguing in this regard is the demonstration by sensitive RT-PCR of the leukemia-associated gene translocations t(8;21), t(14; 18) [1], and t(9;22) [2] in apparently healthy individuals. Assuming a predisposition in these people for malignancies associated with these gene translocations, intervention immunotherapy might also play a role in primary disease prevention of malignancies arising from these initially benign conditions. The potential of the immune system to control cancer is perhaps best illustrated by the effects of donor T cells in chronic myeloid leukemia (CML) patients relapsing after allogeneic bone marrow transplantation [3,4]. This clinical success provides impetus to develop bcr/abl oncoprotein-related, tumor antigen–directed immunotherapy for patients with CML.

II. ANTIGEN RECOGNITION AND TUMOR-ASSOCIATED EPITOPES

Major histocompatibility complex (MHC) molecules on the cell surface present peptides derived from endogenous or exogenous proteins to the immune system. CD8-positive cytotoxic T lymphocytes (CTL) recognize peptides, derived from processed cellular proteins, by means of their T-cell receptor (TCR) in the context of MHC class I molecules (membrane glycoprotein heavy chains associated with the light chain β2 microglobulin) [5–7]. The generation of these peptides from cytoplasmic or nuclear proteins is facilitated by cellular proteolytic machineries, of which the proteasome [8] is currently best known. After protein ubiquitination [9], proteasomal digestion results in peptides that may be translocated to the endoplasmic reticulum (ER) by two transporters associated with antigen processing (TAP) [10]. In the ER, MHC molecule assembly is stabilized by MHC class I–peptide complex formation [11]. The resulting MHC class I–peptide complex is then transported through the Golgi apparatus to the cell surface. Most MHC class I binding peptides have a length of 8 to 11 amino acids (aa) [12,13] and usually contain two conserved anchor residues (binding motif) required for binding to a specific MHC class I allele [13–15]. CD4-positive T lymphocytes can be activated by interaction of their TCR with MHC class II molecules [16]. These heterodimer α and β-chain membrane glycoproteins are complexed with antigenic peptides, which are variable in size but generally longer than class I–presented peptides. MHC class II–bound peptides show less stringent MHC allele-restricted aa sequence motifs [7,17,18]. The MHC class II heterodimer molecule assembles in the ER with the invariant chain (Ii) [19]. Ii is thought to prevent binding of peptide to class II molecules within the ER, and it functions as a targeting signal directing the class II molecules to the endocytic route. MHC class II–peptide complex assembly takes place in the endocytic MHC class II compartment (MIIC) [20]. The degradation of Ii by cathepsin B [21] and subsequent removal by HLA-DM of class II–associated invariant chain peptide (CLIP) from the MHC class II molecule allows class II–peptide complex formation [22] and precedes transport of the complex to the cell surface.

The identification of tumor-associated antigens and tumor-specific peptide epitopes (i.e., antigenic determinants) is a key issue in the development of anticancer vaccines. Tumor immunology research focuses on proteins exclusively synthesized by tumor cells or proteins overexpressed in tumor cells. Well-characterized antigens related to the process of neoplastic transformation or stabilization of malignant behavior are by definition attractive targets for immunotherapy.

Recent years have witnessed a rapidly increasing knowledge of T cell–defined tumor antigens [23]. Human malignancy–associated T-cell epitopes—recognized as such by use of tumor-specific CTL combined with tumor cell cDNA library expressing antigen presenting cells (APCs) [24] or by isolation and subsequent sequencing of peptides extracted from MHC molecules on the tumor cell surface as well as by peptide-binding studies [25,26]—are mainly derived from cellular proteins that are encoded by mutated or translocated (onco)-genes (for instance p53, BCR-ABL, pml-RAR), ectopically expressed malignancy-related but nonmutated genes (MAGE, BAGE, and GAGE, which are not expressed in normal tissues except in testis, and PRAME), shared expression of lineage-specific genes (tyrosinase, Melan A/MART-1, CEA, gp100, PSA), or from virus-encoded oncoproteins (HPV-E6, HPV-E7).

Sequencing of peptides eluted from different HLA alleles as well as peptide-binding studies have revealed motifs in peptides showing HLA allele specificity. This knowledge, combined with insights in intracellular protein cleavage preferences, allows a limited degree of epitope prediction within given oncoproteins. Recently an effort was made to map HLA class I binding motifs in the fusion regions of 44 fusion proteins involved in human cancers [27]. However, from a given protein, at this time no properly processed MHC class I or class II epitopes can be predicted with a high degree of probability [28].

Various clinical observations and the identification of tumor antigens and antigenic peptides have firmly established the existence of tumor-associated T-cell targets. Evidence that T cells can potentiate antitumor responses came from animal tumor models, in which adoptive transfer of tumor-specific T cells resulted in eradication of established tumors [29]. Also, CTLs have been reported to exert antitumor activity in human beings. For example, ex vivo expanded autologous tumor-infiltrating lymphocytes displayed therapeutic activity in patients with malignant melanoma [30]. In cervical carcinoma, an increased prevalence of HPV-associated proliferative diseases in immunosuppressed patients indicates that progression of HPV infection is affected by the cellular arm of the immune response [31].

III. THE BCR-ABL ONCOPROTEIN AS IMMUNOLOGICAL TARGET

In CML, the translocation t(9;22)(q34;q11) results in a BCR-ABL fusion gene [32], which in general encodes chimeric 210 kDa ($p210^{BCR\text{-}ABL}$) [33] and often also relatively low amounts of 190 kDa BCR-ABL ($p190^{BCR\text{-}ABL}$) oncoproteins [34,35]. The $p190^{BCR\text{-}ABL}$ oncoprotein is primarily associated with acute lymphoblastic leukemia [36]. Strong indications have accumulated that the $p190^{BCR\text{-}ABL}$ and $p210^{BCR\text{-}ABL}$ fusion products are involved in the process of leukemogenesis [37–

40]. Depending on the location of the BCR-ABL fusion site and mRNA splicing pattern [41], the BCR-ABL fusion gene in CML leads to the expression of mainly two, sometimes simultaneously expressed [33], p210$^{BCR-ABL}$ oncoproteins known as b2a2 and b3a2, but alternative BCR-ABL proteins can occur [42]. Peptides corresponding to the fusion regions in the nonphysiological CML (and ALL) BCR-ABL hybrid proteins can therefore be considered tumor-specific T-cell targets.

Fusion region sequences of the BCR-ABL b3a2 oncoprotein have initially been found to induce BCR-ABL peptide specific T cells upon in vivo immunization in mice [43]. A few years later, for the first time, HLA class II (DR2/DRB1*1501)–restricted human T cells were generated in our laboratory by primary in vitro immunization with BCR-ABL peptides in human volunteers [44]. Since then several other BCR-ABL peptide-specific human T-cell lines and clones not only directed to the b3a2 but to the b2a2 fusion as well were obtained by us. One of these BCR-ABL b3a2 peptide-specific T-cell lines showed an HLA-DR4 restriction and was induced to proliferate by HLA DR4 and BCR-ABL b3a2 mRNA positive blasts from a CML patient in blast crisis [45]. No responses were observed with DR4 positive p210 BCR-ABL–negative cells or with p210 b3a2–positive leukemic cells with absent or insufficient expression of DR4. These data provided a first suggestion of processing of endogenous BCR-ABL protein by CML cells into MHC-peptide ligands. Peptides corresponding to the b3a2 fusion sequence were shown to bind to HLA A3 [46,47], A11, B8 [46], and A68 (our unpublished observation) HLA DRB1*0402, DRB1*0301 and DR11 [48]. HLA A3 and A11 restricted cytotoxic T cells have been obtained [47,49] as well as HLA DR1 [50], DR2(DRB1*1501) [44], DR4(DRB1*0401) [45], DR11 [49], and DR3(DR17) [48] restricted helper T cells. Although a 23mer b2a2 peptide appeared to bind with intermediate affinity to HLA DR3 [48], no HLA-DR restricted T-cell responses to the b2a2 breakpoint sequence have been described. Recently we have been able to elicit human HLA-DR2 restricted cytotoxic T-cell clones via primary in vitro BCR-ABL peptide immunization. These clones showed lysis of partially HLA-matched APC-pulsed with BCR-ABL b2a2 breakpoint representing peptide [64].

IV. PROTECTIVE IMMUNE RESPONSES INDUCED BY PEPTIDE-BASED VACCINES

The first animal tumor model in which peptide-based immunotherapy led to complete tumor protection involved an HPV16 E7-encoded CTL epitope (aa 49-57) presented by the murine H-2D^b molecule [51,52]. Vaccination with this peptide (in incomplete Freund's adjuvant) protected mice from a subsequent challenge with a lethal dose of HPV16-transformed syngeneic tumor cells. CTL induced by this immunization protocol were capable of lysing peptide-pulsed target cells as well as tumor cells in vitro. In this model, the expression of the endogenously processed antigenic peptide on the tumor cells appeared to be sufficient for immune recognition but not for efficient induction of a CTL response against this peptide. This demonstrates that selective stimulation of a T-cell specificity of choice by immunogenic peptide vaccination can provide extra capacity exceeding that of the failing immune system and possibly also of immunization with entire antigens [53]. Besides preventive induction of antitumor immunity, peptide vaccination can also result in eradication of small established tumors. This phenomenon has been reported for a cellular tumor antigen consisting of a mutated connexin 37 gap-junction protein [54]. Alternatively, dendritic APC pulsed with antigenic peptides provide antigen in combination with costimulatory molecules, and this strategy has been shown effective in the induction of specific T-cell responses. Treatment of HPV16-containing tumors was also achieved by vaccination with bone marrow-derived dendritic cells pulsed with acid-eluted peptides from these tumors [55].

Apart from vaccination with tumor-derived CTL epitopes, CD4 positive T-helper cell epitopes may be needed to induce antitumor immunity. It was observed from experiments with murine skin allografts that CD4-positive cells have a crucial role in providing efficient help for in vivo CTL generation [56], and vaccination with a synthetic peptide encoding a CD4-positive T-helper epitope present in the envelope gp70 protein induces protective immunity against murine leukemia virus–induced lymphoma [57]. In vivo depletion of CD4-positive T cells completely abrogated the protective effect, strongly indicating the importance of T-helper cells in the immune control of these lymphomas. In CML, CD4-positive lymphocytes are claimed to be important effector cells involved in cytotoxicity following allogeneic bone marrow transplantation (BMT): CD8-positive T cell–depleted donor marrow cells did not impair graft-versus-leukemia effects observed after allogeneic BMT for CML [58] and donor lymphocyte infusions, depleted of CD8-positive T cells (in order to reduce the risk of graft-versus host disease) still induced remissions in patients with relapsed CML after allogeneic BMT [59].

Vaccination with peptides may consistently achieve protective and therapeutic T-cell immunity. However, in the design of epitope-based vaccines, the inclusion of tumor specific T-helper epitopes appears essential. A trial coordinated by the Memorial Sloan-Kettering Cancer Center in New York is currently under way using a BCR-ABL breakpoint–based peptide vaccine in CML patients. Other clinical trials based on vaccination with peptides, with protein loaded dendritic cells (DC) or other antigen delivery systems, such as viral vectors, are in progress. All aim at somehow augmenting the autologous immune response. The feasibility of specific antiviral and antitumor (adoptive) immunotherapy after

BMT has been demonstrated [60] and refinements of present-day donor lymphocyte infusion therapies in post-BMT relapses in disorders like CML are within reach.

A BCR-ABL breakpoint peptide vaccination approach or adoptive transfer of breakpoint peptide-specific T cells would become very attractive if peptide elution from HLA class I or class II molecules isolated from CML or t(9;22) positive ALL tumor cells reveals BCR-ABL oncoprotein-derived epitopes. But even if such peptides were isolated and identified as tumor-specific, the best vaccination strategies with tumor-specific synthetic peptides are not known. Although, in murine models, vaccination with peptides has been shown to induce protective and even therapeutic T-cell immunity, in other cases vaccination with peptide down-regulated T cell–mediated responses [61] and even enhanced tumor growth in conjunction with in vitro T-cell unresponsiveness to the respective epitopes has been reported [62]. The mechanisms behind these phenomena are unclear, but there are indications that the context in which peptides are presented to the immune system determines the protective outcome of immunization. To bypass unfavorable consequences in the use of isolated peptide, autologous (patient-derived) DCs have been peptide pulsed before vaccination [63]. These efficient antigen-processing DCs can also be preincubated with the complete target protein to initiate or activate class I and class II–restricted T-cell responses. When only autologous tumor cells are the source of tumor antigens, autologous DCs pulsed with unfractionated MHC acid–eluted peptides from tumor cells may induce protection and remission [55]. This option, or, in the case of CML, BCR-ABL–positive DC originating from the malignant stem cell, would become important if strategies with BCR-ABL fusion protein alone prove ineffective.

REFERENCES

1. Limpens J, Stad R, Vos C, de Vlaam C, De Jong D, van Ommen GJ, Schuuring E, Kluin PM. Lymphoma associated translocation t(14;18) in blood B cells of normal individuals. Blood 1995; 85:2528–2536.
2. Biernaux C, Loos M, Sels A, Huez G, Strykmans P. Detection of bcr-abl gene expression at a very low level in blood cells of some healthy individuals. Blood 1995; 86:3118–3122.
3. Horowitz MM, Gale RP, Sondel PM, Goldman JM, Kersey J, Kolb HJ, Rimm AA, Ringden O, Rozman C, Speck B, Truitt RL, Zwaan FE, Bortin MM. Graft-versus-leukemia reactions after bone marrow transplantation. Blood 1990; 75:555–562.
4. Kolb HJ, Schattenberg A, Goldman JM, Hertenstein B, Jacobsen N, Arcese W, Ljungman P, Ferrant A, Verdonck L, Niederwieser D, van Rhee F, Mittermuller J, de Witte T, Holler E, Ansari H. Graft-versus-leukemia effect of donor lymphocyte transfusions in marrow grafted patients. European Group for Blood and Marrow Transplantation Working Party Chronic Leukemia. Blood 1995; 86:2041–2050.

5. Townsend A, Bodmer H. Antigen recognition by class I-restricted T lymphocytes. Annu Rev Immunol 1989; 7:601–624.
6. Bjorkman PJ, Parham P. Structure, function, and diversity of class I major histocompatibility complex molecules. Annu Rev Biochem 1990; 59:253–288.
7. Neefjes JJ, Momburg F. Cell biology of antigen presentation. Curr Opin Immunol 1993; 5:27–34.
8. Rock KL, Gramm C, Rothstein L, Clark K, Stein R, Dick L, Hwang D, Goldberg AL. Inhibitors of the proteasome block the degradation of most cell proteins and the generation of peptides presented on MHC class I molecules. Cell 1994; 78:761–771.
9. Seufert W, Futcher B, Jeutsch S. Role of a ubiquitin-conjugating enzyme in degradation of S- and M-phase cyclins. Nature 1995; 373:78–81.
10. Kelly A, Powis SH, Kerr LA, Mockridge I, Elliott T, Nastin J, Uchauska-Ziegler B, Ziegler A, Trowsdale J, Townsend A. Assembly and function of the two ABC transporter proteins encoded in human major histocompatibility complex. Nature 1992; 355:641–644.
11. Ortmann B, Androlewicz MJ, Creswell P. MHC class I/β-microglobulin complexes associate with TAP transporters before peptide binding. Nature 1994; 368:864–867.
12. Elliott T, Cerundolo V, Elvin J, Townsend A. Peptide-induced conformational change of the class I heavy chain. Nature 1991; 351:402–406.
13. Falk K, Rötzschke O, Stevanovic S, Jung G, Rammensee HG. Allele-specific motifs revealed by sequencing of self-peptides eluted from MHC molecules. Nature 1991; 351:290–296.
14. Schumacher TNM, De Bruijn M, Vernie LN, Kast WM, Melief CJM, Neefjes JJ, Ploegh HL. Peptide selection by MHC class I molecules. Nature 1991; 350:703–706.
15. Rammensee HG, Friede H, Stevanovic S. MHC ligands and peptide motifs: first listing. Imunogenetics 1995; 41:178–228.
16. Brown JH, Jardetsky TS, Gorga JC, Stern LJ, Urban RG, Strominger JL, Wiley DC. Three-dimensional structure of the human class II histocompatibility antigen HLA-DR1. Nature 1993; 364:33–39.
17. Rudensky AY, Preston-Hulburt P, Hong S-C, Barlow A, Janeway CA: Sequence analysis of peptides bound to MHC class II molecules. Nature 1991; 360:622–627.
18. Chicz RM, Urban RG, Gorga JC, Vignali DAA, Lane WS, Strominger JL. Specificity and promiscuity among naturally processed peptides bound to HLA-DR alleles. J Exp Med 1993; 178:27–47.
19. Ghosh P, Amaya M, Mellins E, Wiley DC. The structure of an intermediate in class II MHC maturation: CLIP bound to HLA-DR3. Nature 1996; 378:457–462.
20. Peters PJ, Neefjes JJ, Oorschot V, Ploegh HL, Geuze HJ. Segregation of MHC class II molecules from MHC class I molecules in the Golgi complex for transport to lysosomal compartments. Nature 1991; 349:669–675.
21. Roche PA, Cresswell P. Proteolysis of the class II-associated invariant chain generates a peptide binding site in intracellular HLA-DR molecules. Proc Natl Acad Sci USA 1991; 88:3150–3154.

22. Sloan VS, Cameron P, Porter G, Gammon M, Amaya M, Mellins E, Zaller DM. Mediation by HLA-DM of dissociation of peptides from HLA-DR. Nature 1995; 375:802–806.
23. Van den Eynde BJ, Van der Bruggen P. T cell defined tumor antigens. Curr Opin Immunol 1997; 9:684–693.
24. Boon Th, Cerottini JC, Van den Eynde BJ, Van der Bruggen P, Van Pel A. Tumor antigens recognized by T lymphocytes. Annu Rev Immunol 1994; 12:337–365.
25. Cox AL, Skipper J, Chen Y, Henderson RA, Darrow TL, Shabanowitz J, Engelhard VH, Hunt DF, Slingluff CL. Identification of a peptide recognized by five melanoma-specific human cytotoxic T cell lines. Science 1994; 264:716–719.
26. Rammensee HG, Friede H, Stevanovic S. MHC ligands and peptide motifs: first listing. Immunogenetics 1995; 41:178–228.
27. Gambacorti Passerini C, Bertazzoli C, Dermime S, Scardino A, Schendel D, Parmiani G. Mapping HLA class I binding motifs in forty four fusion proteins involved in human cancers. Clin Cancer Res 1997; 3:675–683.
28. Van der Burg SH, Visseren MJW, Brandt RMP, Kast WM, Melief CJM. Immunogenicity of peptides bound to MHC class I molecules depends on the MHC peptide complex stability. J Immunol 1996; 156:3308–3314.
29. Melief CJM. Tumor eradication by adoptive transfer of cytotoxic T lymphocytes. Adv Cancer Res 1992; 58:143–175.
30. Rosenberg SA, Yanelli JR, Yang JC, Topalian SL, Schwartzentruber DJ, Weber JHS, Parkinson DR, Seipp CA, Einhorn JH, White DE. Treatment of patients with metastatic melanoma with autologous tumor-infiltrating lymphocytes and interleukin 2. J Natl Cancer Inst 1994; 15:1159–1166.
31. Benton C, Shahidullah H, Hunter JAA. Papilloma Virus Report 1992; 3:23–26.
32. Shtivelman E, Lifshitz B, Gale RP, Canaani E. Fused transcript of abl and bcr genes in chronic myelogenous leukemia. Nature 1985; 315:550–554.
33. Lee MS, LeMaistre A, Kantarjian HM, Talpaz M, Freireich EJ, Trujillo JM, Stass SA. Detection of two alternative bcr/abl mRNA junctions and minimal residual disease in Philadelphia chromosome positive chronic myelogenous leukemia by polymerase chain reaction. Blood 1989; 73:2165–2170.
34. Saglio G, Pane F, Gottardi E, Frigeri F, Buonaiuto MR, Guerrasio A, De Micheli D, Parziale A, Fornaci MN, Martinelli G, Salvatore F. Consistent amounts of acute leukemia-associated p190BCR/ABL transcripts are expressed by chronic myelogenous leukemia patients at diagnosis. Blood 1996; 87:1075–1080.
35. Rhee F van, Hochhaus A, Lin F, Melo JV, Goldman JM, Cross NC. P190 BCR-ABL mRNA is expressed at low levels in p210 chronic myeloid and acute lymphoblastic leukemias. Blood 1996; 87:5213–5217.
36. Priest JR, Robison LL, McKenna RW, Lindquist LL, Warkentin PI, LeBien TW, Woods WG, Kersey JH, Coccia PF, Nesbit ME. Philadelphia chromosome positive childhood acute lymphoblastic leukemia. Blood 1980; 56:15–23.
37. Daley GQ, Etten RA van, Baltimore D. Induction of chronic myelogenous leukemia in mice by the p210$^{bcr/abl}$ gene of the Philadelphia chromosome. Science 1990; 247: 824–830.
38. Voncken JW, Morris C, Pattengale P, Dennert G, Kikly C, Groffen J, Heister-

kamp N. Clonal development and karyotype evolution during leukemogenesis of BCR/ABL transgenic mice. Blood 1992; 79:1029–1036.

39. Honda H, Fujii T, Takatoku M, Mano H, Witte ON, Yazaki Y, Hirai H. Expression of p210bcr/abl by metallothionein promotor induced T-cell leukemia in transgenic mice. Blood 1995; 85:2853–2861.
40. Voncken JW, Kaartinen V, Pattengale PK, Germeraad WT, Groffen J, Heisterkamp N. BCR/ABL p210 and p190 cause distinct leukemia in transgenic mice. Blood 1995; 86:4603–4611.
41. Shtivelman E, Lifshitz B, Gale RP, Roe BA, Canaani E. Alternative splicing of RNAs transcribed from the human abl gene and from the BCR-ABL fused gene. Cell 1986; 47:277–284.
42. Melo JV. The diversity of BCR-ABL fusion proteins and their relationship to leukemia phenotype. Blood 1996; 88:2375–2384.
43. Chen W, Peace DJ, Rovira DK, You SG, Cheever MA. T cell immunity to the joining region of p210 BCR-ABL protein. Proc Natl Acad Sci USA 1992; 89:1468–1472.
44. Ten Bosch GJA, Toornvliet AC, Friede T, Melief CJM, Leeksma OC. Recognition of peptides corresponding to the joining region of p210 BCR-ABL protein by human T cells. Leukemia 1995; 9:1344–1348.
45. Ten Bosch GJA, Joosten AM, Kessler JH, Melief CJM, Leeksma OC. Recognition of BCR-ABL positive leukemic blasts by human CD4+ T cells elicited by primary in vitro immunization with a BCR-ABL breakpoint peptide. Blood 1996; 88:3522–3527.
46. Bocchia M, Wentworth PA, Southwood S, Sidney J, McGraw K, Scheinberg DA, Sette A. Specific binding of leukemia oncogene fusion protein peptides to HLA class I molecules. Blood 1995; 85:2680–2684.
47. Greco G, Fruci D, Accapezzato D, Barnaba V, Nisini R, Alimenta G, Montefusco E, Vigneti E, Butler R, Tanigaki N, Tosi R. Two bcr-abl junction peptides bind HLA-A3 molecules and allow specific induction of human cytotoxic T lymphocytes. Leukemia 1996; 10:693–699.
48. Pawelec G, Heiber M, Halder T, Bruserud Ø, Merl A, da Silva P, Kalbacher H. BCR/ABL leukemia oncogene fusion peptides selectively bind to certain HLA DR alleles and can be recognized by T cells found at low frequency in the repertoire of normal donors. Blood 1996; 88:2118–2124.
49. Bocchia M, Korontsvit T, Xu Q, Mackinnon S, Yang SY, Sette A, Scheinberg DA. Specific human cellular immunity to bcr-abl oncogene-derived peptides. Blood 1996; 87:3587–3592.
50. Mannering SI, McKenzie JL, Fearnley DB, Hart DNJ. HLA-DR1 restricted bcr-abl(b3a2)-specific CD4+ T lymphocytes respond to dendritic cells pulsed with b3a2 peptide and antigen-presenting cells exposed to b3a2 containing cell lysates. Blood 1997; 90:290–297.
51. Feltkamp MCW, Smits HL, Vierboom MPM, Minnaar RP, De Jongh BM, Drijfhout JW, Ter Schegget J, Melief CJM, Kast WM. Vaccination with cytotoxic T lymphocyte epitope-containing peptide protects against a tumor induced by human papillomavirus type 16-transformed cells. Eur J Immunol 1993; 23:2242–2249.

52. Feltkamp MCW, Vreugdenhil GR, Vierboom MPM, Ras E, Van der Burg SH, Ter Schegget J, Melief CJM, Kast WM. Cytotoxic T lymphocytes raised against a subdominant epitope offered as a synthetic peptide eradicate human papillomavirus type 16-induced tumors. Eur J Immunol 1995; 25:2638–2642.
53. Melief CJM, Kast WM. Prospects for T cell immunotherapy of tumours by vaccination with immunodominant and subdominant peptides. In: DJ Chadwick and J Marsh, eds. Vaccines Against Virally Induced Cancers. Chichester: Wiley, 1994; pp. 97–112.
54. Mandelboim O, Vadai E, Fridkin M, Katz-Hillel A, Feldman M, Berke G, Eisenbach L. Regression of established murine carcinoma metastases following vaccination with tumour-associated antigen peptides. Nature Med 1995; 1:1179–1183.
55. Zitvogel L, Mayordomo JI, Tjandrawan T, DeLeo AB, Clarke MR, Lotze MT, Storkus WJ. Therapy of murine tumors with tumor peptide-pulsed dendritic cells: dependence on T cells, B7 costimulation, and T helper cell 1-associated cytokines. J Exp Med 1996; 183:87–97.
56. Lee RS, Grusby MJ, Glimcher LH, Winn HJ, Auchincloss H. Indirect recognition by helper cells can induce donor specific cytotoxic T lymphocytes in vivo. J Exp Med 1994; 179:865–872.
57. Ossendorp F, Mengedé E, Camps M, Filius R, Melief CJM. Specific T helper cell requirement for optimal induction of cytotoxic T lymphocytes against Major Histocompatibility Complex class II negative tumors. J Exp Med 1998; 187:693–700.
58. Nimer SD, Giorgio J, Gajewski JL, Ku N, Schiller GJ, Lee K, Territo M, Ho W, Feig S, Selch M, Isacescu V, Reichert TA, Champlin RE. Selective depletion of CD8+ cells for prevention of graft-versus-host disease after bone marrow transplantation: a randomised controlled trial. Transplantation 1994; 57:82–87.
59. Giralt S, Hester J, Huh Y, Hirsch-Ginsberg C, Rondon G, Seong D, Lee M, Gajewski J, Van Besien K, Khouri I, Mehra R, Przepiorka D, Körbling M, Talpaz M, Kantarjian H, Fischer H, Deisseroth A, Champlin R. CD8-depleted donor lymphocyte infusion as treatment for relapsed chronic myelogenous leukemia after allogeneic bone marrow transplantation. Blood 1995; 86:4337–4343.
60. Kolb HJ, Holler E. Adoptive immunotherapy with donor lymphocyte transfusions. Curr Opin in Oncol 1997; 9:139–145.
61. Aichele P, Brduscha-Riem K, Zinkernagel RM, Hengartner H, Pircher H. T cell priming versus T cell tolerance induced by synthetic peptides. J Exp Med 1995; 182:261–266.
62. Toes REM, Offringa R, Blom HJJ, Melief CJM, Kast WM. Peptide vaccination can lead to enhanced tumor growth through specific T-cell tolerance induction. Proc Natl Acad Sci USA 1996; 93:7855–7860.
63. Toes REM, Van der Voort EIH, Schoenberger SP, Drijfhout JW, Van Bloois L, Storm G, Kast WM, Offringa R, Melief CJM. Enhancement of tumor outgrowth through CTL-tolerization after peptide vaccination is avoided by peptide presentation on dendritic cells. J Immunol 1998; 160:4449–4456.
64. ten Bosch G, Kessler J, Joosten A, et al. A BCR-ABL oncoprotein p210 b2a2 fusion region sequence is recognized by HLA-DR2a restricted cytotoxic T-lymphocytes and presented by HLA-DR matched cells transfected with an Ii^{b2a2} construct. Blood 1999; 94:1038–1045.

Index

About the Editors

JOHN BARRETT is Chief, Bone Marrow Transplant Unit, Hematology Branch, National Heart, Lung, and Blood Institute, National Institutes of Health, Bethesda, Maryland. The author or coauthor of over 135 professional papers, more than 50 book chapters and reviews, and the coauthor or coeditor of three books, Dr. Barrett is an active member of the International Bone Marrow Transplantation Registry and chairs its GVL chapter. He is a Fellow of the Royal College of Pathologists and the Royal College of Physicians, and a member of the British Society for Haematology, the Royal Society of Medicine, and the American Society of Hematology. He received the M.B. (1968), B.A. (1968), and M.D. (1977) degrees from the University of London, England.

YIN-ZHENG JIANG is a Medical Resident in the Department of Medicine, Bridgeport Hospital, Yale-New Haven Health System, Connecticut and formerly a Scientist with the National Institutes of Health, Bethesda, Maryland. The author or coauthor of more than 70 abstracts and peer-reviewed articles, Dr. Jiang is a member of the American College of Physicians, and a past member of the American Society of Hematology and the International Society for Experimental Hematology. He received the M.D. degree (1986) from Huabei Medical College, Tangshan, China, and the Ph.D. degree (1992) from the Royal Postgraduate Medical School, University of London, England.